CHF Clinic Book

Congestive Cardiac Failure

FUNDAMENTAL AND CLINICAL CARDIOLOGY

1. *Drug Treatment of Hyperlipidemia*, edited by Basil M. Rifkind
2. *Cardiotonic Drugs: A Clinical Review. Second Edition, Revised and Expanded*, edited by Carl V. Leier
3. *Complications of Coronary Angioplasty*, edited by Alexander J. R. Black, H. Vernon Anderson, and Stephen G. Ellis
4. *Unstable Angina*, edited by John D. Rutherford
5. *Beta-Blockers and Cardiac Arrhythmias*, edited by Prakash C. Deedwania
6. *Exercise and the Heart in Health and Disease*, edited by Roy J. Shephard and Henry S. Miller, Jr.
7. *Cardiopulmonary Physiology in Critical Care*, edited by Steven M. Scharf
8. *Atherosclerotic Cardiovascular Disease, Hemostasis, and Endothelial Function*, edited by Robert Boyer Francis, Jr.
9. *Coronary Heart Disease Prevention*, edited by Frank G. Yanowitz
10. *Thrombolysis and Adjunctive Therapy for Acute Myocardial Infarction*, edited by Eric R. Bates
11. *Stunned Myocardium: Properties, Mechanisms, and Clinical Manifestations*, edited by Robert A. Kloner and Karin Przyklenk
12. *Prevention of Venous Thromboembolism*, edited by Samuel Z. Goldhaber
13. *Silent Myocardial Ischemia and Infarction: Third Edition*, Peter F. Cohn
14. *Congestive Cardiac Failure: Pathophysiology and Treatment*, edited by David B. Barnett, Hubert Pouleur, and Gary S. Francis

Additional Volumes in Preparation

Heart Failure: Basic Science and Clinical Aspects, edited by Judith K. Gwathmey, G. Maurice Briggs, and Paul D. Allen

Cardiovascular Disease in the Elderly Patient, edited by Donald Tresch and Wilbert Aronow

The Heart as a Source of Systemic Embolization, edited by Michael Ezekowitz

Congestive Cardiac Failure

Pathophysiology and Treatment

edited by

David B. Barnett
University of Leicester and Leicester Royal Infirmary
Leicester, United Kingdom

Hubert Pouleur
University of Louvain
Brussels, Belgium

Gary S. Francis
University of Minnesota Hospital and Clinic
Minneapolis, Minnesota

Marcel Dekker, Inc. **New York • Basel • Hong Kong**

Library of Congress Cataloging-in-Publication Data

Congestive cardiac failure: pathophysiology and treatment / edited by David B. Barnett, Hubert Pouleur, Gary S. Francis.
p. cm. -- (Fundamental and clinical cardiology; 14)
Includes bibliographical references and index.
ISBN 0-8247-8821-4
1. Congestive heart failure. I. Barnett, David, B. II. Pouleur, Hubert. III. Francis, Gary S. IV. Series: Fundamental and clinical cardiology; v. 14.
[DNLM: 1. Heart Failure, Congestive--drug therapy. 2. Heart Failure, Congestive--physiopathology. 3. Heart Surgery. W1 FU538TD v. 14 1993 / WG 370 C7485 1993]
RC685.C53C62 1993
616.1'29--dc20
DNLM/DLC
for Library of Congress 93-7106
CIP

Great care has been taken to maintain the accuracy of the information contained in this volume. However, neither Marcel Dekker, Inc., nor the editors can be held responsible for errors or for any consequences arising from the use of the information contained herein.

The publisher offers discounts on this book when ordered in bulk quantities. For more information, write to Special Sales/Professional Marketing at the address below.

This book is printed on acid-free paper.

MARCEL DEKKER, INC.
270 Madison Avenue, New York, New York 10016

Current printing (last digit):
10 9 8 7 6 5 4 3 2 1

PRINTED IN THE UNITED STATES OF AMERICA

Series Introduction

Marcel Dekker, Inc., has focused on the development of various series of beautifully produced books in different branches of medicine. These series have facilitated the integration of rapidly advancing information for both the clinical specialist and the researcher.

My goal as editor of the Fundamental and Clinical Cardiology series is to assemble the talents of world-renowned authorities to discuss virtually every area of cardiovascular medicine. In the current monograph, *Congestive Cardiac Failure: Pathophysiology and Treatment*, Drs. Barnett, Pouleur, and Francis have edited a much needed and timely book. Future contributions to this series will include books on molecular biology, interventional cardiology, and clinical management of such problems as coronary artery disease and ventricular arrhythmias.

Samuel Z. Goldhaber

Preface

The status of cardiovascular disease and, in particular, heart disease as the major consumer of health care resources in the western world cannot be challenged. The total economic burden, if one includes the effects of morbidity/disability and loss of productivity on the general community, is immense. It is not surprising, therefore, that considerable financial and human resources are given over to the treatment of and research into cardiovascular disease. New approaches to therapy are regularly heralded as major breakthroughs by the pharmaceutical industry, although enthusiasm must be tempered until more information is gathered during clinical usage.

Our principal aim should be to abolish heart disease by attacking the root causes. In epidemiological terms and from the point of view of preventive medicine, we are gradually moving in this direction, albeit very slowly. In the meantime, however, it is necessary to treat the consequences of the disease process and reduce morbidity/mortality for the patient as far as we can.

Heart failure can be seen as the final common pathway for a wide variety of different causes of heart disease. Some of these are potentially amenable to "cure" as their root cause is identifiable and either directly treatable or preventable—for example, hypertensive heart disease and rheumatic valve disease. For the most part, however, the underlying cause of heart failure in a particular patient can only be ameliorated, at best, and therefore we are left to treat the consequences of the disease process rather than the disease itself.

In the past decade, the management of heart failure per se has dramatically changed and we have now entered a most exciting stage of this development. Thus the therapeutic objectives of reduction in morbidity, that is, symptom control and improvement in quality of life have become achievable for all but the most severely ill patients. This is principally the result of the application of improved understanding of the pathophysiology of heart failure to new drug development. The objective of reduction in mortality has been more difficult because, as far as heart disease is concerned, once established it is likely to be *the* cause of death unless some other misfortune occurs. Therefore, the objective should be to delay the inevitable, namely, to increase longevity. Recently, we have seen evidence that this objective is also achievable and that delay in heart failure progression is possible regardless of our ability to treat directly the underlying pathology.

The time is right, therefore, to bring together in one volume a statement of our present understanding of pathophysiological mechanisms in heart failure and the progress in therapeutic intervention that has been achieved. The authors of the various chapters are all heavily involved in research and clinical care of heart failure patients in the United Kingdom, Europe, and the United States. Final revisions of the chapters were possible up to the last minute and this has allowed the inclusion of results from all the relevant major trials published during 1992. Hopefully, this has resulted in a balanced and very current review of the subject for clinicians and researchers in this field.

All of us who deal with heart failure are aware that, although we have come a long way, we are not yet at the end of the road for future development of care for this group of patients. We would like to thank all the authors for their efforts and the excellence of their contributions. We hope that as research into heart failure continues we will be able to call upon them in the future to fill in some of the many gaps that remain in our understanding of this devastating clinical problem and its treatment.

David B. Barnett
Hubert Pouleur
Gary S. Francis

Contents

Contributors

Elliott M. Antman, M.D. Director, Levine Cardiac Unit, Associate Professor of Medicine, Department of Medicine/Cardiology, Brigham and Women's Hospital and Harvard Medical School, Boston, Massachusetts

David B. Barnett, M.D., F.R.C.P. Professor of Clinical Pharmacology and Honorary Consultant Physician, Department of Pharmacology and Therapeutics, University of Leicester and Leicester Royal Infirmary, Leicester, United Kingdom

Ronald W. F. Campbell, M.B.Ch.B., F.R.C.P., F.E.S.C. Professor of Cardiology, Department of Academic Cardiology, University of Newcastle-Upon-Tyne, Newcastle-Upon-Tyne, United Kingdom

Cesare Casagrande Director, Cardiovascular Research Center, Zambon Research, Cormano, Milan, Italy

Jay N. Cohn, M.D. Professor of Medicine and Head, Cardiovascular Division, Department of Medicine, University of Minnesota Medical School, Minneapolis, Minnesota

Wilson S. Colucci, M.D. Associate Professor, Department of Medicine, Brigham and Women's Hospital and Harvard Medical School, Boston, Massachusetts

Michael K. Davies, M.D Senior Lecturer and Honorary Consultant Cardiologist, Department of Cardiovascular Medicine, Queen Elizabeth Hospital and University of Birmingham, Birmingham, United Kingdom

Eric J. Eichhorn, M.D. Associate Professor, Department of Medicine, University of Texas Southwestern and Dallas Veterans Administration Medical Centers, Dallas, Texas

Gary S. Francis, M.D. Professor of Medicine and Director, Acute Cardiac Care, Department of Medicine, University of Minnesota Hospital and Clinic, Minneapolis, Minnesota

Rekha Garg, M.D., M.S. Scientific Project Officer, Clinical Trials Branch, Division of Epidemiology and Clinical Applications, National Institutes of Health, National Heart, Lung and Blood Institute, Bethesda, Maryland

Peter Held, M.D., Ph.D. Associate Professor, Department of Medicine, Östra Hospital, University of Göteborg, Göteborg, Sweden

Spencer H. Kubo, M.D. Associate Professor of Medicine and Medical Director, Heart Failure–Heart Transplantation Program, Cardiovascular Division, Department of Medicine, University of Minnesota Medical School, Minneapolis, Minnesota

Gervasio A. Lamas, M.D. Director, Pacemaker Clinic, Cardiovascular Division and Assistant Professor of Medicine, Brigham and Women's Hospital, West Roxbury VAMC, and Harvard Medical School, Boston, Massachusetts

Joel S. Landzberg, M.D. Department of Medicine, Brigham and Women's Hospital and Harvard Medical School, Boston, Massachusetts

Kenneth M. McDonald, M.B., M.R.C.P.I. Assistant Professor of Medicine, Department of Medicine, Division of Cardiology, University of Minnesota Hospital and Clinic, Minneapolis, Minnesota

Marc A. Pfeffer, M.D., Ph.D. Associate Professor of Medicine, Cardiovascular Division, Brigham and Women's Hospital, West Roxbury VAMC, and Harvard Medical School, Boston, Massachusetts

Philip Alexander Poole-Wilson, M.D., F.R.C.P., F.E.S.C. Professor of Cardiology, Department of Cardiac Medicine, National Heart & Lung Institute, London, United Kingdom

Hubert Pouleur, M.D., Ph.D. Professor of Medicine, Department of Physiology and Pharmacology and Division of Cardiology, University of Louvain, Brussels, Belgium

Thomas S. Rector, Ph.D. Senior Research Associate, Cardiovascular Division, Department of Medicine, University of Minnesota Medical School, Minneapolis, Minnesota

B. Silke, M.D., F.R.C.P.I. Senior Lecturer in Therapeutics and Pharmacology and Consultant Physician, The Queen's University of Belfast, Belfast, Northern Ireland

Karl Swedberg, M.D., Ph.D., F.A.C.C., F.E.S.C. Associate Professor of Medicine and Head of Cardiology, Department of Medicine, Östra Hospital, University of Göteborg, Göteborg, Sweden

Marc D. Tischler, M.D. Director, Cardiac Ultrasound Laboratory, and Assistant Professor, University of Vermont College of Medicine, Burlington, Vermont

Douglas E. Vaughan, M.D. Assistant Professor of Medicine, Cardiovascular Division, Brigham and Women's Hospital, West Roxbury VAMC, and Harvard Medical School, Boston, Massachusetts

Derek G. Waller, B.Sc., D.M., F.R.C.P. Senior Lecturer, Clinical Pharmacology Group, Southampton General Hospital, Southampton, United Kingdom

Salim Yusuf, F.R.C.P., Ph.D. Director, Division of Cardiology, and Professor of Medicine, Department of Medicine, McMaster University, Hamilton, Ontario, Canada

Congestive Cardiac Failure

1

The Changing Face of Heart Failure

David B. Barnett
University of Leicester and Leicester Royal Infirmary, Leicester, United Kingdom

Hubert Pouleur
University of Louvain, Brussels, Belgium

Gary S. Francis
University of Minnesota Hospital and Clinic, Minneapolis, Minnesota

Despite a significant decline in mortality/morbidity rates due to heart disease in general in the United States and the United Kingdom, the incidence/prevalence of heart failure is on the increase. In some respects this apparent paradox is understandable on the basis of recent success in the management of ischemic heart disease. Thus, for example, a larger number of patients are surviving their first myocardial infarct and then potentially progressing to chronic pump dysfunction. Whatever the reason, there is good evidence from the United States that, overall, approximately 1% of the population suffers from heart failure (1). Prevalence figures for the United Kingdom are not readily available, although they are quite likely to be similar. However, evidence from prescription monitoring suggests that at any one time up to 2 million patients are receiving heart failure treatment in the U.K. In addition, the number of "new" prescriptions initiated in the U.K. for any drug for heart failure has been progressively increasing and is now in excess of 80,000 per annum (A. Cowley, Nottingham, England, personal communication). On this basis the U.K. "problem" is at least as great as that in the U.S. The importance of these observations relates not only to the size of the at-risk patient population but also to the size of the potential commercial pharmaceutical industry market in heart failure remedies.

It is therefore appropriate at this time to review the important developments in our understanding of the causes of heart failure and how these relate to the progress that has been made in treatment.

There have been many attempts to adequately define heart failure:

> A state in which the heart fails to maintain an adequate circulation for the needs of the body despite a satisfactory filling pressure.
>
> Paul Wood (1950)

> A pathophysiological state in which an abnormality of cardiac function is responsible for the failure of the heart to pump blood at a rate commensurate with the requirements of the metabolising tissues.
>
> Eugene Braunwald (1980)

> A clinical syndrome caused by an abnormality of the heart and recognised by a characteristic pattern of haemodynamic, renal, neural and hormonal responses. Ventricular dysfunction with symptoms.
>
> Phillip Poole-Wilson

None of these definitions can be considered to adequately represent the true nature of heart failure. Thus, in physiological terms, it is possible to establish criteria for heart failure based on assessment of central hemodynamics and measurement of absolute changes of pressure/output. However, most clinicians recognize heart failure as a syndrome of symptoms and physical signs and are usually prepared to treat the patient on this basis alone without the need for complex investigations.

In recent years, it has become apparent that viewing heart failure in a purely clinical context is no longer adequate and that an understanding of the mechanical and pathophysiological mechanisms underlying the clinical expression of disease is necessary to fully exploit the newer therapeutic regimes. This altered understanding, or "changing face," of heart failure can be considered under three headings.

1. *Epidemiology/etiology*. The incidence of clinical heart failure has gradually increased. This is due in part to the general aging of the population but also relates to a change in the major etiological factors. Although myocardial disease has remained the most significant pathology in congestive heart failure (CHF) in both the U.S. and the U.K., there have been important changes in underlying etiology. Thus, in the mid-1940s, at the time of the initiation of the Framingham studies, the principal cause of heart failure was hypertensive heart disease, whereas the recent data from the SOLVD study group indicate—perhaps not surprisingly—that ischemic heart disease is the major etiological factor (1,2). Within this framework our understanding of the definition of cardiac dysfunction has also changed. Thus, although in most cases of heart failure decreased cardiac output (reduced ejection fraction) and impairment of systolic function is

the principal problem, patients in overt heart failure may have "normal" systolic function but significant abnormalities of cardiac relaxation/diastolic function (3,4).

2. *Pathophysiology*. The emergence of a fuller understanding of the pathophysiological mechanisms of heart failure has had a major impact on the design of treatment regimens and the relative importance of different drugs. Thus, it is now well recognized that a variety of neurohumoral responses that are initially activated to support the gradually failing heart may eventually contribute to the progressive nature of the disease process and further reduce cardiac function. This has been termed the vicious circle of heart failure (Fig. 1). Targeting of drugs to break this downward spiral of worsening cardiac function followed by further activation of compensatory mechanisms leading to increasing load and strain on the already damaged heart—for example, with the use of vasodilators—has been very successful (5–8).

3. *Therapeutic end points*. The major therapeutic end point in heart failure treatment has been the control of symptoms, principally breathlessness and fatigue. This is often subsumed into the less readily defined goal of improvement in "quality of life," which takes account of the problems of adverse effects of therapy. It is only within the last decade that we

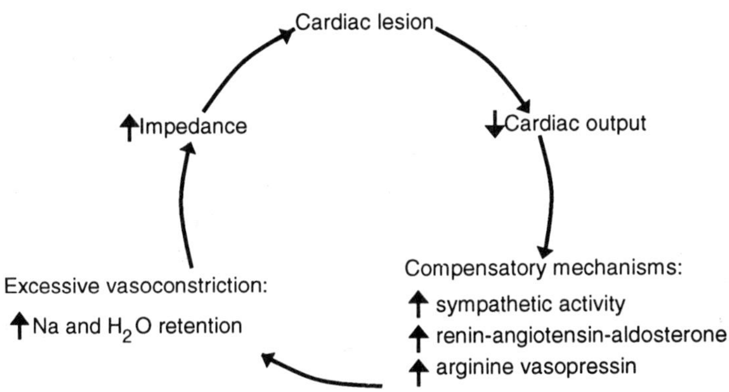

Figure 1 The vicious circle of heart failure. The development of depressed cardiac function from whatever cause is associated with the activation of neurohumoral compensatory mechanisms. These processes are a means whereby the heart and circulation are readjusted to cope with reduced output. Although initially of help, eventually the effect of these mechanisms causes excessive cardiac stimulation and additional mechanical load, which adds to the overall cardiac burden and actively contributes to further decline in function.

have seen a major change in these goals, with the emergence of strong evidence from clinical trials that improvements in longevity are also feasible with modern heart failure treatment.

These elements of change have resulted in a revolution in the clinical approach to heart failure. Most clinicians now recognize that symptom control is achievable in the short term for all but the very worst of their heart failure cases. Perhaps more important, it is also possible to favorably affect longevity in most patients irrespective of the degree of their incapacity.

We should not, however, be complacent about the present position. For example, it is apparent that life was extended a mere 9 months in the treatment arm of SOLVD and perhaps 18 months on average in VHeFT II (6,7). These improvements in survival, although statistically significant and clinically important, seem rather trivial when one considers the entire scope of heart failure from the asymptomatic phase until death. Moreover, neither SOLVD nor V-HeFT demonstrated any sustained improvement in quality of life, implying that all physicians really do is extend the amount of time that the patient must put up with the disability. Thus, symptomatic relief is still a problem for the more severe heart failure cases, and the long-term outlook for most patients is uncertain. Within the general community, heart failure continues to be a serious problem, and the need for research and the development of further drug treatments remains of paramount importance.

In addition, although the success of modern treatment is impressive as far as it goes, it still relates to those patients with heart failure who are identified on the basis of the original simple clinical definition as exhibiting characteristic symptoms and signs. Almost certainly these cases represent the tip of a large iceberg There is a substantial population of patients with preclinical or so-called compensated heart failure who are not receiving any of the potential benefits of our modern approach to the disease. Progressive deterioration in this group leads eventually to their identification and treatment as they present with clinical symptoms. Some of these persons will also die suddenly as a result of their preclinical disease and thus not be helped at all (Fig. 2). It is therefore necessary to identify this group and consider methods of treatment that may reduce the rate of disease progression, delay the onset of symptoms, and possibly even further increase longevity. The analogous situation exists with hypertension. A patient presenting for the first time with a cerebral hemorrhage secondary to undiagnosed/uncontrolled hypertension would be considered a very serious treatment failure, having suffered from a devastating and potentially preventable complication. On this basis the use of hypertension screening programs and the related education of clinicians and the general public is now considered an essential part of modern health care.

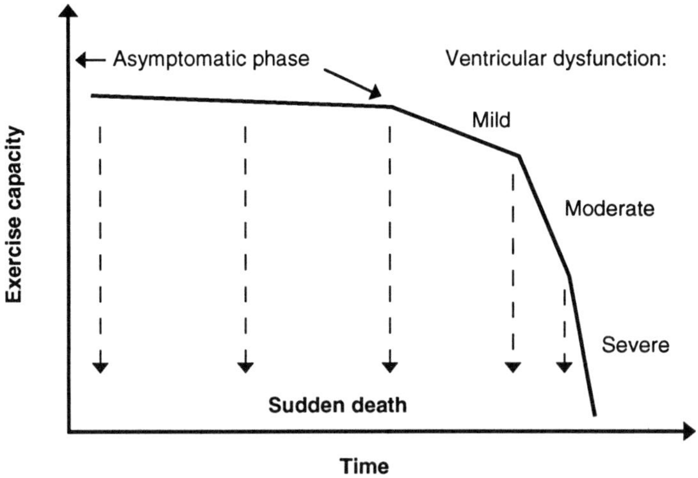

Figure 2 The progression of heart failure. Patients with symptoms of heart failure represent the tip of a potentially large iceberg. Asymptomatic individuals in so-called compensated heart failure may progress slowly for a number of years, during which compensatory mechanisms maintain heart function adequately for their needs. Eventually, usually in relation to an intercurrent problem (e.g., chest infection), "decompensation" will occur and symptoms will develop, bringing the patient to the attention of his medical adviser. From this point on, the progression of heart failure is almost inexorable, although it can be partially modified by modern therapy. Subjects with heart failure may also die suddenly at any time, even during the asymptomatic "compensated" phase and, under these circumstances, before receiving any potential benefit from drug therapy.

Can we identify this preclinical group of heart failure sufferers? There are some neurohumoral markers of the pathophysiological response to reducing cardiac output that can be measured and that may presage the onset of clinical symptoms. In this category is the activation of the sympathetic nervous system, which possibly represents the first early response of the body to the failing heart (9,10). This was first recognized in the Framingham study, where a rapid resting heart rate indicating high sympathetic tone was identified as an important risk factor associated with development of heart failure in asymptomatic subjects (1). Other markers of early heart failure should be identified and fully evaluated before a screening program for individuals at risk can be justified. If this is possible, a clinical trials program assessing the early use of drug therapy in these asymptomatic individuals will be the next step.

We have made some advances in recent years in identifying individuals potentially at risk. Thus, post-myocardial infarction left ventricular dilatation/remodeling in asymptomatic patients has been a target of investigation. Results so far are encouraging, suggesting that early intervention in this group—for example, with ACE inhibitor therapy—may reduce progressive ventricular dilatation and thus potentially the development of heart failure (11). However, more information is needed in this group of patients regarding heart failure morbidity and long-term outlook before we can adopt this strategy into routine clinical practice.

A number of recently reported international collaborative studies have shed more light on this aspect of preventive medicine. Of particular interest have been the results of trials undertaken by the SOLVD Investigators group, the CONSENSUS study group, and the SAVE study (12–14). These studies have evaluated the effects of ACE inhibitors, either captopril or enalapril, in patients with asymptomatic left ventricular dysfunction either discovered immediately following myocardial infarction (13,14) or as part of an ongoing evaluation of subjects with known heart disease (7). The results indicate significant effects of these drugs on progression of left ventricular dysfunction in this subgroup of patients which is associated with clinically important reduction in the incidence of heart failure and related hospitalizations. In addition, mortality due to major cardiovascular events is significantly reduced by the use of ACE inhibitors in this way. Although these results are very encouraging, there are still a number of unanswered questions. These include the correct timing of introduction of the ACE inhibitor following myocardial infarction. Thus the early use (within the first 24 h) of enalapril following infarction was not associated with significant effects on mortality in the treated patients compared to placebo (13). In addition, it will be important to discover what, if any, benefits accrue to the post-infarct patient who does not have initial evidence of left ventricular dysfunction. This latter question may be answered by the findings of the large ISIS4 study presently ongoing internationally, which hopes to finish recruitment of up to 50,000 patients by mid-1993.

In this volume we have brought together international opinion on the present state of our understanding of heart failure mechanisms and management. The individual contributors have been asked to give an overview of the subject, with particular emphasis on the relationship between mechanisms and treatment as well as, where possible, an indication of future directions. The text has been divided into two principal sections, the first dealing with the important developments in our understanding of pathophysiological mechanisms and the second with individual treatment approaches. In addition, there are contributions dealing with the epidemiology of heart failure and the assessment of response to treatment.

Modern therapy for heart failure is in a very exciting phase of development, with possibilities of further improvement in both morbidity and mortality on the horizon. We have seen a number of major changes in this area over the last two decades and can confidently expect that heart failure research will remain high on the agenda of important clinical investigation topics for the foreseeable future.

REFERENCES

1. Kannel, WB. Epidemiological aspects of heart failure. Cardiology Clinics 1989; 7(1):1–9.
2. Bangdiwala SI, Bourassa MG, Freisinger G, Weiner, DH et al. The studies of life ventricular dysfunction registry—rationale, design, methods and description of baseline characteristics. Am J Cardiol 1992. In press.
3. Marantz PR, Tobin JN, Wasserthiel-Smoller S, Steingart RM, et al. The relationship between left ventricular systolic function and congestive heart failure diagnosed by clinical criteria. Circulation, 1988; 77:607–612.
4. Packer M. Abnormalities of diastolic dysfunction as a potential cause of exercise intolerance in chronic heart failure. Circulation, 1990; 81((III)): p. 78–86.
5. Cohn JN, Archibald DG, Zeische S, Franciosa JA, et al. Effect of vasodilator therapy on mortality in chronic congestive heart failure. N Engl J Med, 1986; 314:1547–1552.
6. Cohn JN, Johnson G, Ziesche S, Cobb, F, et al. A comparison of enalapril with hydralazine-isosorbide dinitrate in the treatment of chronic congestive heart failure. N Engl J Med, 1991; 325:303–310.
7. SOLVD Investigators. Effect of enalapril on survival in patients with reduced left ventricular ejection fraction and congestive heart failure. N Engl J Med, 1991; 325:303–310.
8. The Consensus Trial Study Group. Effects of enalapril on mortality in severe congestive heart failure: Results of the Cooperative North Scandinavia Enalapril Survival Study (CONSENSUS). N Engl J Med, 1987; 316:1429–1435.
9. Bayliss J, Norell M, Canepa-Anson R, Sutton G, et al. Untreated heart failure; clinical and neuroendocrine effects of introducing diuretics. Br Heart J, 1987; 57:17–22.
10. Francis G, Benedict C, Johnstone, DE, Kirlin PC, et al. Comparison of neuroendocrine activation in patients with left ventricular dysfunction with and without congestive heart failure. A substudy of the studies of left ventricular dysfunction (SOLVD). Circulation, 1990; 82:1724–1729.
11. Sharpe NJ, Murphy J, Smith H, Hannon S. Treatment of patients with symptomless left ventricular dysfunction after myocardial infarction. Lancet, 1988; i:255–259.
12. SOLVD Investigators. Effect of enalapril on mortality and the development of heart failure in asymptomatic patients with reduced left ventricular ejection fractions. N Engl J Med. 1922; 327:685–691.

13. Swedberg K, Held P, Kjekshus J, Rasmussen K, et al. Effect of the early administration of enalapril on mortality in patients with acute myocardial infarction. N Engl J Med., 1992; 327:678–684.
14. Pfeffer MA, Braunwald E, Moye LA, Basta, L, et al. Effect of captopril on mortality and morbidity in patients with left ventricular dysfunction after myocardial infarction. N Engl J Med, 1992; 32:669–677.

2

Epidemiology of Congestive Heart Failure

Rekha Garg
National Institutes of Health,
National Heart, Lung and Blood Institute,
Bethesda, Maryland

Salim Yusuf
McMaster University, Hamilton,
Ontario, Canada

Despite major advances in the prevention and treatment of various cardiovascular diseases, as evidenced by a substantial decline in mortality rates due to acute myocardial infarction and strokes in the United States and several Western countries, national statistics from these countries indicate that the incidence and prevalence of congestive heart failure (CHF) have been increasing in recent years. Therefore, CHF remains a major cause of mortality and morbidity in most developed countries. This chapter will discuss the prevalence and incidence of CHF, risk factors and etiologic factors, the use of various drug treatments, and the prognosis of CHF.

PREVALENCE/INCIDENCE

In the United States, the prevalence of CHF is estimated to be 2.5 to 3.0 million, or about 1% of the population. Moreover, CHF is the only cardiovascular disorder that has been increasing in prevalence in the U.S. It is estimated that about 400,000 new cases of CHF occur each year. The incidence of CHF in the U.S. is based on extrapolation from the Framingham Heart Study of 5209 subjects who have been followed for 30 years. The incidence of CHF rises with age. The annual incidence was reported to be 3 per 1000 among men and women 35 to 64 years of age compared with 10 per 1000 among those 65 to 94 years (1). There is a slight male predominance in the incidence of CHF among those under the age of 65, due primarily to the high prevalence of coronary heart disease (CHD). Among those above age 75, more women develop CHF. In a survey conducted to assess the prevalence of CHF in three general practices in Northwest London, England, Sutton reported an overall prevalence of 0.4% (2). The prevalence was 2.8% among those over 65 years of age, compared to 0.06% among those under 65 years of age. In another population-based surveillance study, Remes et al. reported the age-adjusted incidence rate of heart failure among subjects aged 45 to 74 years to be 4.0 per 1000 men and 1.0 per 1000 women in eastern Finland (3).

The number of deaths in which CHF was listed on the death certificate as the underlying or contributing cause increased from 118,000 in 1970 to 230,000 in 1988 in the U.S. Although this increase is largely due to the aging of the population, the age-adjusted death rate also appeared to increase twofold over this 20-year period. In 1970, the age-adjusted death rate was 3.8 per 100,000, compared to 7.7 per 100,000 in 1988. Taking into account the change in coding of the International Classification of Diseases in 1978–1979, the increase in the CHF death rate is probably around 40% to 50%. There has been an increase in CHF mortality in both sexes and in all races (Fig. 1). The age-adjusted death rates are highest among black men followed by black women, then white men and white women. Death due to CHF is about 1.5 times more common in blacks and other racial groups than in whites (4). The increase in CHF among older individuals is most likely related to the substantial decrease in CHD death rates and the improved survival of patients with various heart diseases, such as those treated for hypertension, those hospitalized because of myocardial infarction, and those with other forms of coronary artery disease. In 1990, CHF was the primary discharge diagnosis for about 722,000 hospitalizations and constituted the leading "diagnostic related group" among hospitalized patients over 65 years of age (5,6). This reflects a threefold increase in hospitalization rates for CHF, from 82 hospitalizations per 100,000 in 1970 to 281 hospitalizations per 100,000 in 1990 in the U.S. National hospital discharge statistics for CHF from 1973 to 1986 indicated that, on average, the rate of hospitalization was 33% higher among nonwhite men than among white men (7) (Fig. 2). The rate of hospitalization was 50% higher among nonwhite women than among white women. The hospitalization rates also increased sharply among those over 55 years of age, while they remained constant or decreased among those younger than 55 years.

This increase in CHF hospitalization rates is seen not only in the U.S. but also in several other Western countries. In a study done by Eriksson and Svardsudd in Gothenburg, Sweden, hospitalization rates for cardiac

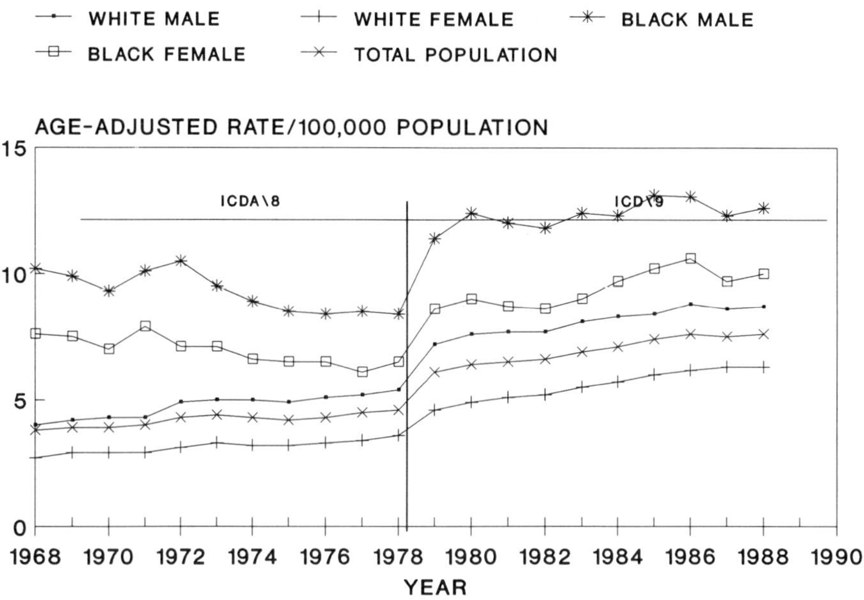

Figure 1 Age-adjusted annual death rates for heart failure by race and sex, United States, 1968–1988.

failure among women have been steadily increasing from 1970 to 1986 (8). In particular, women 75 years of age and older have had the most marked increase in hospitalizations for cardiac failure, from about 165 per 100,000 in 1970 to 500 per 100,000 in 1986. Although similar patterns are reported among elderly men in Sweden, the current rates of hospitalization are still higher among women than among men. In another survey of admissions for heart failure at a community hospital in England, conducted from October 1987 to March 1988, Sutton reported 140 admissions over a 6-month period (2). Extrapolation of these data to a 1-year period would yield 280 admissions from a population of 155,000, or approximately 180 hospitalizations per 100,000.

In 1989, the Heath Care Financing Agency estimated the costs related to CHF hospitalizations to be over 6.4 billion U.S. dollars, while the total costs associated with the care of CHF patients (including hospitalization, physician and other professional services, medication costs, and nursing home care) were estimated to be about 8.9 billion U.S. dollars.

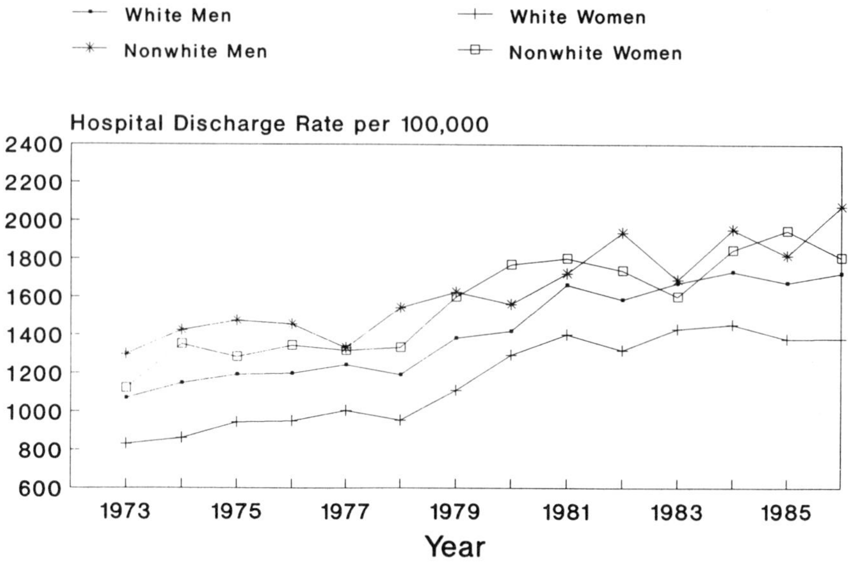

Figure 2 Age-adjusted annual hospital discharge rates for heart failure by race and sex, United States, 1973–1986. Source: Ref. 7.

ETIOLOGY/RISK FACTORS

The presence of long-standing hypertension has generally been considered to be the major predisposing risk factor for developing CHF. In the Framingham study, over 75% of the individuals who developed CHF had blood pressures greater than or equal to 160/95 mm Hg (1). Although a history of CHD was found in 46% of the men and 27% of the women, the vast majority of these patients also had hypertension (1) (Table 1). The incidence of CHF increased across all ages with increasing levels of systolic blood pressure. This relationship was stronger at higher ages, particularly among those 65 years of age and older. Similar patterns were observed for diastolic blood pressure; however, the risk of developing CHF appears to be more strongly related to systolic than to diastolic blood pressure.

Although hypertension was considered to be the most common cause of CHF among the Framingham cohort, this has not been seen in other recent studies of patients with CHF. However, most of these studies are based on recruitment of patients admitted to the hospital. In the Studies of Left Ventricular Dysfunction (SOLVD) Registry, patients were enrolled if they had an ejection fraction (EF) < 0.45 or had radiologic evidence of CHF (with no restriction on the EF) (9). Among the patients with an EF

Table 1 Prevalence of Etiologic Factors Among Persons with CHF in Four Studies

Etiologic factor	Framingham[a] N = 485		SOLVD Registry[b]		DIG Study[c]		Sutton[d]
	Men	Women	EF < 45 N = 4853	CHF N = 1327	EF < 45 N = 5050	EF > 45 N = 649	N = 140
Ischemic heart disease	45.8	27.4	74.3	48.4	70.8	55.5	41.0
Hypertensive heart disease	76.4	79.1	4.2	18.2	7.9	21.3	6.0
Valvular heart disease	2.4	3.2	6.4	10.3	1.4	7.4	9.0
Idiopathic cardiomyopathy	—	—	11.4	17.4	14.5	11.2	1.0
Specific cardiomyopathy	—	—	3.5	3.5	3.5	1.8	—
Other	11.9	16.8	0.2	0.2	1.6	1.7	7.0
Unknown	—	—	—	—	—	—	36.0

[a]Framingham study is a cohort of 5209 subjects followed for over 3 decades. The etiologies for this study are not mutually exclusive. Valvular heart disease was due to rheumatic heart disease. The other category includes mostly cardiomyopathy.
[b]SOLVD Registry enrolled patients who had either an ejection fraction (EF) <0.45 or had radiological evidence of CHF without any restriction on the ejection fraction.
[c]The DIG study is an ongoing trial of patients with clinical heart failure, in sinus rhythm and EF ≤0.45. Patients with an EF >0.45 are entered into a parallel but separate ancillary study.
[d]Sutton conducted a survey of community hospitals for all admissions for heart failure in London from October 1987 to March 1988.

< 0.45, the overwhelming majority (74%) had ischemic heart disease (IHD) as the primary cause of CHF, while among those with radiologic evidence of CHF, 48% had IHD and 18% had hypertension as the primary cause. This is supported by the ongoing Digitalis Investigation Group (DIG) study of patients with clinical heart failure, in sinus rhythm and with an EF $\leq$ 0.45. Patients with heart failure and an EF > 0.45 are entered into a parallel but separate ancillary study. At present, about 4200 patients have been enrolled, with an overall goal of about 7500 to 8000 patients. Among patients with an EF ≤ 0.45, 71% had IHD and 8% had hypertension listed as the primary cause of heart failure, whereas among those with an EF $>$ 0.45, 56% had IHD and 21% had hypertension. In the separate survey conducted by Sutton of patients admitted to a community hospital for CHF, the following were listed as the primary causes of CHF: 41% had IHD, 36% had no known etiology, 9% had valvular disease, 6% had hypertension, and the remaining 8% had other etiologies (2). Therefore, the SOLVD Registry, the DIG Study, and the Sutton survey suggest that IHD is the commonest cause of CHF in the 1990s; this finding differs from that of the Framingham study, initiated in 1949, which suggested that hypertension was the commonest cause of CHF. It also appears that those with a lower EF are more likely to have IHD, while those with hypertension are more likely to develop CHF with a relatively preserved EF, indicating a higher incidence of diastolic dysfunction in the latter group.

Other predisposing risk factors for development of CHF are electrocardiographic signs indicative of left ventricular hypertrophy (ECG-LVH) or radiographic evidence of cardiac enlargement (Table 2). In the Framingham study, the incidence of CHF increased markedly among those with ECG-LVH; the age-adjusted rate was 71 per 1000 among men aged 35 to 64 years with ECG-LVH, compared to 3 per 1000 among those without ECG-LVH (1). The presence of cardiac enlargement on an x-ray also increases the risk of developing CHF. The combination of radiographic evidence of cardiac enlargement and ECG-LVH results in a substantial increase in the risk of developing CHF.

Diabetes is another important risk factor in the development of CHF. Part of the risk is due to increased coronary atherosclerosis and hypertension in diabetics. However, these do not account for the entire excess risk of CHF in diabetics. In the Framingham study, both men and women with diabetes have at least a fourfold increased risk of developing CHF compared to nondiabetics (1). In addition, among nondiabetics with impaired glucose tolerance, there was a two- to sevenfold increased risk of CHF, with the greatest relative risk among women and those under 65 years of age. It has been suggested that, in addition to accelerated coronary atherosclerosis of the medium-sized arteries, microangiopathy of the smaller

Table 2 Risk of Cardiac Failure by ECG-LVH According to X-Ray-LVH Status. Framingham Study, 32-Year Follow-Up

	Age-adjusted biennial rate per 1000			
	35–64		65–94	
ECG-LVH	X-ray LVH absent	X-ray LVH present	X-ray LVH absent	X-ray LVH present
Men				
Absent	3	16	14	56
Present	71	128	102	135
Women				
Absent	2	17	12	21
Present	16	83	89	89

ECG-LVH = electrocardiogram-left ventricular hypertrophy.
Source: Ref. 1.

vessels similar to that seen in the skin, retina, and kidney among diabetics may be responsible for the higher incidence of CHF (10). This suggests that some specific form of diabetic cardiomyopathy may exist, especially among insulin-dependent diabetic patients.

A rapid resting heart rate and reduced vital capacity are two markers that possibly reflect deteriorating myocardial function even before the development of overt CHF. In the Framingham study, these two factors were strongly associated with increased risk of developing CHF (1). The incidence of CHF increased progressively with increases in resting heart rate (Fig. 3). Even after adjustment for blood pressure, diabetes, and smoking, this relationship remains significant in men but not in women. Before the development of overt CHF, patients may have a reduction of their vital capacity reflecting subclinical pulmonary congestion. The decrease in vital capacity is associated with an increased risk of CHF and has been reported

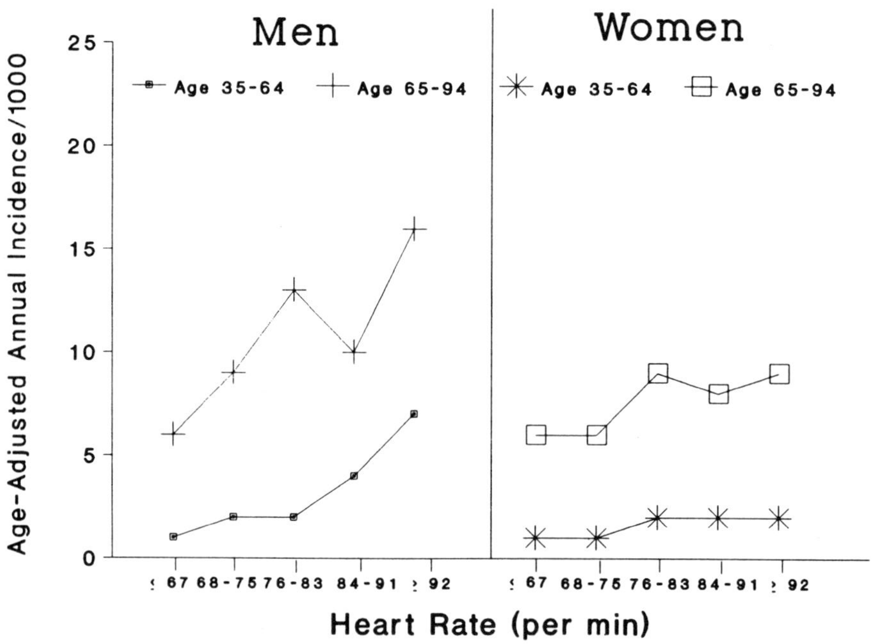

Figure 3 Age-adjusted annual incidence of congestive heart failure by heart rate. Framingham study, 30-year follow-up.

to remain statistically significant after other cardiovascular factors are taken into account (Fig. 4). Among patients with both low vital capacity and rapid heart rate, the risks are especially high.

Valvular heart disease was considered to be the cause of heart failure in 7.3% of patients in the SOLVD Registry and 2.7% in the DIG trial (9). Among older subjects, aortic valve disease due to aortic sclerosis can often present with CHF. In many developing countries, rheumatic valvular disease is likely to be a more common cause of CHF, particularly among younger individuals.

PREVENTION OF CONGESTIVE HEART FAILURE

Several randomized trials of drug treatment of hypertension have indicated a substantial reduction in the risk of CHF (4,11,12). The benefit appears

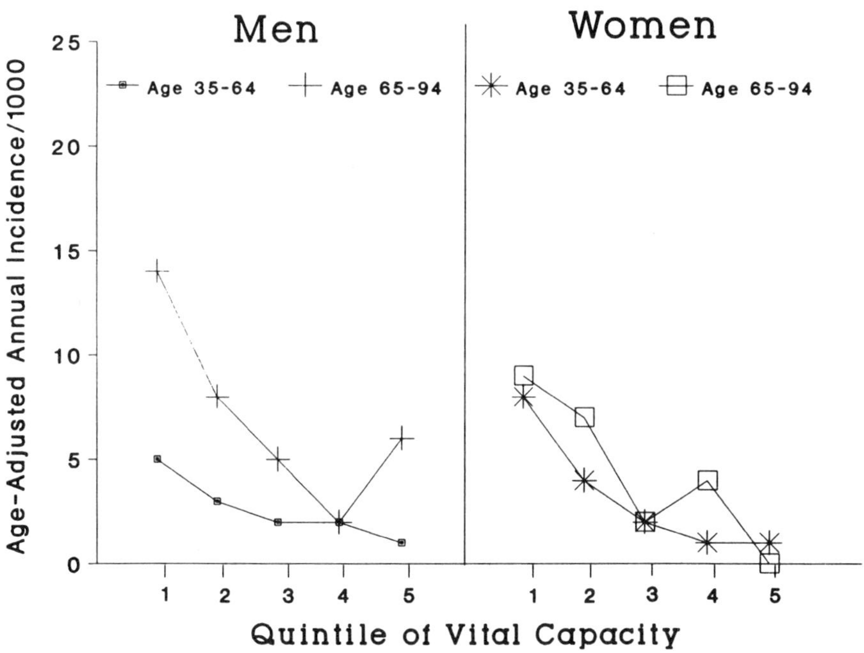

Figure 4 Age-adjusted annual incidence of congestive heart failure by quintile of vital capacity. Framingham study, 30-year follow-up.

to be most marked among those with severe hypertension, the elderly, and those with end organ damage. In an overview of nine randomized trials of antihypertensive agents, Yusuf et al. reported a 52% risk reduction (95% CI = 33% to 66%, $p < 0.001$) in the incidence of heart failure (4) (Table 3). The benefit of using diuretics to prevent the development of CHF among elderly patients with isolated systolic hypertension has recently been confirmed (11). In the Systolic Hypertension in the Elderly Program (SHEP), a multicenter, randomized clinical trial, 4736 men and women with isolated systolic hypertension (systolic blood pressure > 160 mm Hg and diastolic blood pressure < 90 mm Hg) were randomized to either low-dose chlorthalidone or placebo. This trial reported a 54% risk reduction (95% CI = 35% to 66%, $p < 0.001$) for the development of left ventricular failure among the active-treatment group compared to the placebo group. Similar results are reported by the Swedish Trial in Old Patients with Hypertension (STOP-Hypertension), which is a randomized, double-blind trial of 1627 patients at 116 centers in Sweden (12). This study compared an antihypertensive regimen (three beta-blockers and one diuretic) to placebo among hypertensive men and women aged 70 to 84 years. This trial reported a 51% reduction (95% CI = 17% to 71%, $p < 0.01$) in heart failure among the active-treatment group compared to the placebo group. Therefore, it appears that the overall impact of antihypertensive agents is to reduce the incidence of CHF by about 50% (95% CI = 40% to 61%, $p < 0.001$). In the SOLVD Prevention Trial, 4228 patients with an EF ≤ 0.35 not requiring therapy for CHF were randomized to receive the angiotensin converting enzyme (ACE) inhibitor enalapril or placebo (13). Treatment with enalapril reduced the risk of developing CHF by 37% (95% CI = 28% to 44%, $p < 0.001$) and hospitalization for CHF by 36% (95% CI = 22% to 46%, $p < 0.001$). There was also a nonsignificant trend toward lower cardiovascular mortality. Greater benefit of treatment on all outcomes was observed among those patients with lower EF. The benefits of treatment were observed irrespective of underlying etiology, age, sex, or other drugs used (14).

MEDICATIONS USED IN PATIENTS WITH CONGESTIVE HEART FAILURE

Most patients with CHF are prescribed multiple medications. Some of these medications are for the relief of congestion and other symptoms, whereas other medications are to treat associated conditions such as angina or diabetes. In the SOLVD Registry of about 6000 patients with an EF < 45% or clinical heart failure from 18 centers in the U.S., Canada, and Belgium, over 60% of the patients were on diuretics, 45% were on digitalis,

Table 3 Incidence of Congestive Heart Failure in Randomized Trials of Antihypertensive Drugs and Angiotensin Converting Enzyme Inhibitors

	Events/# of patients		Odds reduction (%)	95% confidence interval	*p*-value
	Active	Control			
Antihypertensive Drug					
Yusuf, Thom & Abbott (4)	46/3526	96/3533	52	33,66	< 0.001
SHEP (11)	48/2365	102/2371	54	35,66	< 0.001
STOP (12)	19/812	39/815	51	17,71	< 0.01
Total	113/6703	237/6719	52	40,61	< 0.001
Use of ACE-I in Low Ejection Fraction					
SOLVD Prevention Trial (13)	438/2111	640/2117	37	28,44	< 0.001

ACE-I = angiotensin converting enzyme inhibitors.

33% were on ACE inhibitors, and about 37% were on calcium channel antagonists (15) (Fig. 5). The pattern of drug use for the treatment of CHF is similar in other developed countries. A survey of four European countries (Italy, France, Germany, and the United Kingdom) reported that diuretics and digoxin are the most commonly used drugs in all four of these countries (16). The proportion of patients on ACE inhibitors ranged from 15% to 35% and that of patients on calcium channel antagonists from 25% to 35% in the above survey. It is interesting that such a large proportion of patients are on a calcium channel antagonist despite the lack of proven benefit in CHF patients. Indeed, several studies indicate that the calcium channel antagonists exacerbate heart failure in patients with poor ventricular function (17,18). By contrast, ACE inhibitors have been shown not only to improve symptoms and exercise tolerance, but also to decrease the risk of mortality and morbidity (19–22). The role of digitalis in improving exercise tolerance and reducing symptoms has been evaluated in several small, short-term randomized trials (23–34). Several of these studies suggest that a small increase in exercise time, a reduction in symptoms, and an increase in ejection fraction occur. However, the impact of digitalis on mortality and morbidity is not known and is currently being evaluated in the DIG

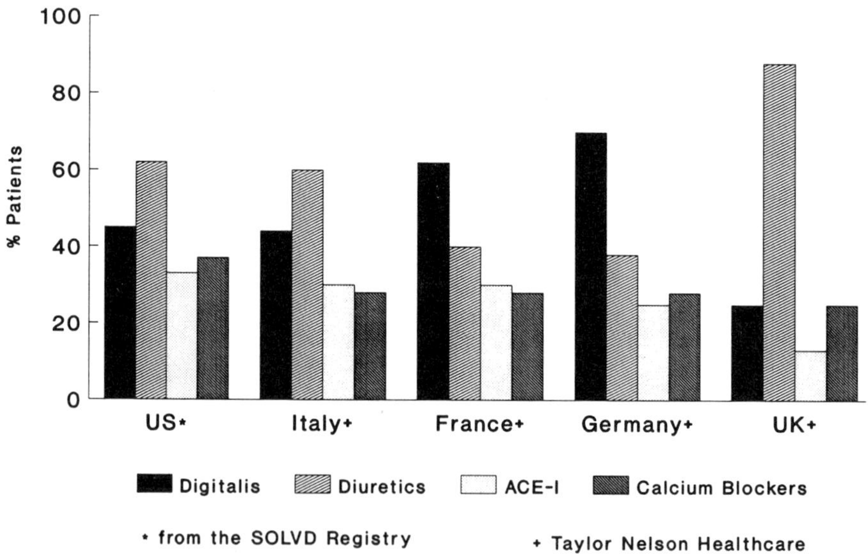

Figure 5 Medication used in the treatment of patients with congestive heart failure from the SOLVD Registry (*) and a survey conducted by Taylor Nelson Healthcare in Europe (+).

study, a large randomized trial of 7500 patients cosponsored by the U.S. National Heart, Lung and Blood Institute and the Department of Veterans Affairs.

PROGNOSIS AFTER DEVELOPMENT OF CONGESTIVE HEART FAILURE

In patients with left ventricular dysfunction, the development of CHF increases the risk of death substantially. For example, in the SOLVD Prevention Trial, the 1-year risk of death was 4.8 times greater than among those who did not develop CHF (13). The annual mortality rate of patients with CHF is approximately 10% (1). The increase in death rates among patients with CHF compared to those without CHF but with similar levels of left ventricular dysfunction is due to higher rates of both cardiovascular and noncardiovascular mortality (19). Among patients with low ejection fraction and CHF, 90% of the deaths were due to cardiovascular causes (19). Of the cardiovascular deaths, 25% were due to progressive pump failure, 25% were sudden without worsening heart failure, and 25% were due to progressive pump failure with a terminal event that was presumed to be arrhythmic. The remaining 25% of the cardiovascular deaths were due to myocardial infarction, pulmonary embolism, strokes, and other cardiovascular causes.

The rates of hospitalization among patients with CHF are also high. For example, at 1 year after diagnosis, 40% of patients are hospitalized at least once and about 15% are hospitalized multiple times (SOLVD Registry, unpublished data). Three-quarters of the hospitalizations are for cardiovascular reasons. Of these, half are for worsening CHF. The remaining cardiovascular reasons for hospitalization include arrhythmias, unstable angina, myocardial infarction, thromboembolic events, cardiac surgery, and others.

The degree of left ventricular dysfunction (EF), the severity of symptoms (New York Heart Association [NYHA] class), and the functional capacity as measured on a simple 6-minute walk test are the strongest independent predictors of 1-year mortality and hospitalization rates in the SOLVD Registry (35). Of the neurohormones measured in this study, the levels of atrial natriuretic peptide and plasma renin were also strong predictors of survival; plasma norepinephrine levels were moderately related to survival, whereas arginine vasopressin levels were not related to outcome (36). However, neurohormone levels were weaker risk predictors than EF, NYHA classification, or the 6-minute walk test. The relationship between ventricular arrhythmia and prognosis is unclear. Some studies have claimed to demonstrate a relationship, whereas others have demonstrated no association after corrections for other risk factors such as the degree of left ventricular dysfunction (37).

Of the various drugs used in the treatment of patients with CHF, ACE inhibitors have been shown to reduce mortality and hospitalization rates (13,19–22). By contrast, trials of inotropic agents—both phosphodiesterase inhibitors and those with β_1-agonist properties—suggest an increase in mortality (38,39). Despite the use of ACE inhibitors, mortality and hospitalization rates remain high. Therefore, additional means of reducing mortality and morbidity are required. Current trials are evaluating the role of digitalis, flosequinan (a direct-acting vasodilator), amiodarone, and beta-blockers in CHF. Other promising interventions include oral magnesium supplementation, angiotensin-2 antagonists, and some of the newer calcium channel antagonists. However, careful evaluation of the risk-benefit profile of all these agents is essential to establish their appropriate role in heart failure.

One can conclude from these epidemiological data that CHF remains a major clinical and public health problem and accounts for a significant part of health care costs. The incidence of CHF and its associated hospitalization and morality rates have been markedly increasing over the past two decades. Given the increase in CHF mortality and morbidity, the goals of therapy should be to prevent CHF, relieve symptoms, improve quality of life, prevent hospitalizations, and improve survival. Attainment of these goals remains a major challenge for future clinical research in the area of CHF and left ventricular dysfunction.

REFERENCES

1. Kannel, WB. Epidemiological aspects of heart failure. Cardiology Clinics 1989; 7(1):1–9.
2. Sutton GC. Epidemiologic aspects of heart failure. Am Heart J 1990; 120:1538–1540.
3. Remes J, Reunanen A, Aromaa A, Pyorala K. Incidence of heart failure in eastern Finland: a population-based surveillance study. Eur Heart J 1992; 13:588–593.
4. Yusuf S, Thom T, Abbott RD. Changes in hypertension treatment and in congestive heart failure mortality in the United States. Hypertension 1989; 13(Suppl I):I-74–I-79.
5. Graves EG. National Hospital Discharge Survey, Annual Summary 1990, National Center for Health Statistics. Vital Health Stat 13; 112:1992
6. Hospital Care Statistics Branch, National Center for Health Statistics, 1990. (unpublished)
7. Ghali JK, Cooper R, Ford E. Trends in hospitalization rates for heart failure in the United States, 1973–1986. Arch Intern Med 1990; 150:769–773.

8. Eriksson H, Wilhelmsen L, Caidahl K, Svardsudd K. Epidemiology and prognosis of heart failure. Z Kardiol 1991; 80:(Suppl 8):1–6.
9. Bangdiwala SI, Bourassa MG, Friesinger G, Weiner DH, Yusuf S for the SOLVD Investigators. The Studies of Left Ventricular Dysfunction Registry—rationale, design, methods and description of baseline characteristics. Am J Cardiol 1992; 70:347–353.
10. Smith WM. Epidemiology of congestive heart failure. Am J Cardiol 1985; 55:3A–8A.
11. SHEP Cooperative Research Group. Prevention of stroke by antihypertensive drug treatment in older persons with isolated systolic hypertension—final results of the Systolic Hypertension in the Elderly Program (SHEP). J Am Med Assoc 1991; 265:3255–3264.
12. Dahlof B, Lindholm LH, Hansson L, Schersten B, Ekbom T, Wester PO. Morbidity and mortality in the Swedish Trial in Old Patients with Hypertension (STOP-Hypertension). Lancet 1991; 338:1281–1285.
13. SOLVD Investigators. Effect of enalapril on mortality and the development of heart failure in asymptomatic patients with reduced left ventricular ejection fraction. N Engl J Med 1992; 327(10):685–691.
14. Pitt B, Yusuf S for the SOLVD Investigators. Studies of Left Ventricular Dysfunction (SOLVD): subgroup results. J Am Coll Cardiol. 1992; 19(3):215A.
15. Young JB, Weiner DH, Yusuf S, Pratt CM, Kostis JB, Weiss MB, Schroeder E, Guillote M for the SOLVD Investigators. Contemporary patterns of medication use in patients with left ventricular dysfunction or congestive heart failure—a report from the Registry of Studies of Left Ventricular Dysfunction. Submitted for publication.
16. Taylor Nelson Healthcare Survey.
17. Elkayam U, Amin J, Mehra A, Vasquez J, Weber L, Rahimtoola SH. A prospective randomized, double blind crossover study to compare the efficacy and safety and chronic nifedipine therapy with that of isosorbide dinitrate and their combination in the treatment of chronic heart failure. Circulation 1990; 82:1954–1961.
18. Goldstein RE, Boccuzzi SJ, Cruess D, Nattel S, the Averse Experience Committee and the Multicenter Diltiazem Postinfarction Research Group. Diltiazem increases late-onset congestive heart failure in postinfarction patients with early reduction in ejection fraction. Circulation 1991; 83:52–60.
19. SOLVD Investigators. Effect of enalapril on survival in patients with reduced left ventricular ejection fraction and congestive heart failure. N Engl J Med 1991; 295:293–302.
20. Cohn JN, Johnson G, Ziesche S, Cobb F, Francis G. Tristani F, Smith R, Dunkman WB, Loeb H, Wong M, Bhar G, Goldman S, Fletcher RD, Doherty J, Hughes CV, Carson P, Cintron G, Shabetai R, Haakenson C. A comparison of enalapril with hydralazine–isosorbide dinitrate in the treatment of chronic congestive heart failure. N Engl J Med 1991; 325:303–310.
21. Furberg CD, Yusuf S. Effect of drug therapy on survival in chronic congestive heart failure. Am J Cardiol 1988; 62(2):41A–45A.

22. The CONSENSUS Trial Study Group. Effects of enalapril on mortality in severe congestive heart failure: results of the Cooperative North Scandinavian Enalapril Survival Study (CONSENSUS). N Engl J Med 1987; 316:1429–1435.
23. Starr J, Luchi RJ. Blind study on the action of digitoxin on elderly women. Am Heart J 1969; 78:740–751.
24. Kirsten E, Rodstein M., Iuster Z. Digoxin in the aged. Geriatrics 1973; (I):95–101.
25. Dobbs SM, Kenyon WI, Dobbs RJ. Maintenance digoxin after an episode of heart failure: placebo-controlled trial in outpatients. Br Med J 1977; 1:749–752.
26. Lee DC, Johnson RA, Bingham JB. Heart failure in outpatients. N Engl J Med 1982; 306:699–705.
27. Fleg JL, Gottlieb SH, Lakatta EG. Is digoxin really important in treatment of compensated heart failure? Am J Med 1982; 73:244–250.
28. Taggart AJ, Johnston GD, McDevitt DG. Digoxin withdrawal after cardiac failure in patients with sinus rhythm. Cardiovasc Pharm 1983; 5:229–234.
29. Guyatt GH, Sullivan MJJ, Fallen EL, et al. A controlled trial of digoxin in congestive heart failure. Am J Cardiol 1988; 61:371–375.
30. Pugh SE, White NJ, Aronson JK, Grahame-Smith DG, Bloomfield JG. Clinical, hemodynamic, and pharmacologic effects of withdrawal and reintroduction of digoxin in patients with heart failure in sinus rhythm after long term treatment. Br Heart J 1989; 61:529–539.
31. Captopril-Digoxin Group. Comparative effects of therapy with captopril and digoxin in patients with mild to moderate heart failure. J Am Med Assoc 1988; 259:539–544.
32. Xamoterol Group. Double blind placebo-controlled comparison of digoxin and xamoterol in chronic heart failure. Lancet 1988; i:489–493.
33. Di Bianco R, Shabetai R, Kostuk W, Moran J, Schlant RC, Wright R, for the Milrinone Multicenter Trial Group. A comparison of oral milrinone, digoxin, and their combination in the treatment of patients with chronic heart failure. N Engl J Med 1989; 320:677–683.
34. Fleg JL, Rothfeld B, Gottlieb SH, Wright J. Effect of maintenance digoxin therapy on aerobic performance and exercise left ventricular function in mild to moderate heart failure due to coronary artery disease: a randomized placebo-controlled crossover trial. J Am Coll Cardiol 1991; 17:743–757.
35. Bittner V, Rogers WJ, Weiner DH, Schroder E, Kostis JB, Kronenberg MW, Woods P, Gregory JJ, Kohn RM, Bangdiwala S, Gosselin G, Yusuf S. The six-minute walk test predicts morbidity and mortality in patients with left ventricular dysfunction (abstr). Circulation 1991; 84(4):(Suppl II):6.
36. Nicklas JM, Benedict C, Johnstone DE, Kay R, Kirlin PC, Weiner D, Bourassa MG, Yusuf S. Relationship between neurohormonal profile and one year mortality in patients with CHF and/or LV dysfunction (abstr). Circulation 1990; 82(4):(Suppl II):469.

37. deSoyza N, Bennett FA, Murphy ML, Bissett JK, Kane JJ. The relationships of paroxysmal ventricular tachycardia complicating the acute phase and ventricular arrhythmia during the late hospital phase of myocardial infarction to long term survival. Am J Med 1978; 64:377–381.
38. Yusuf S, Teo KK. Inotropic agents increase mortality in patients with congestive heart failure (abstr). Circulation 1990; 82(4):III-197.
39. Packer M, Carver JR, Rodeheffer RJ, Ivanhoe RJ, DiBianco R, Zeldis SM, Hendrix GH, Bonner WJ, Elkayam U, Kukin ML, Mallis GI, Sollano JA, Shannon J, Tandon PK, DeMets DL, for PROMISE Study Research Group. Effect of oral milrinone on mortality in severe chronic heart failure. N Engl J Med 1991; 325:1468–1475.

PATHOPHYSIOLOGY

3

The Sympathetic Nervous System and Myocardial Adrenoceptor Function and Regulation in Cardiac Failure

David B. Barnett
University of Leicester and Leicester Royal Infirmary, Leicester, United Kingdom

INTRODUCTION

There is general agreement that in chronic cardiac failure (CCF) the sympathetic nervous system (SNS) is activated as part of the neurohumoral response to declining cardiac output. However, there remains considerable controversy regarding the role of this autonomic response in modifying both the presentation and the progression of the pathophysiological and clinical abnormalities in heart failure. Thus there is a balance between the role of the SNS in supporting the failing heart and the potential deleterious effects of excess catecholamines, both on the circulation and directly on the myocardium (Table 1), that might contribute to the progression of the disease process. This balance of good and evil may vary at different stages of the development of CCF, and, therefore, the potential benefit of therapeutic strategies designed to modify the activity of the SNS may also be variably effective. Other compensatory humoral responses, including activation of the renin-angiotensin system and increased secretion of vasopressin, are associated with the development of CCF and are dealt with in more detail elsewhere in this volume. In this chapter I will concentrate on the evidence for and the consequences of the increased activity of the SNS in heart failure.

Table 1 Cardiovascular Consequences of Activating the Sympathetic Nervous System

Useful	Detrimental
↑ Contractile force	↑ Vasoconstriction
↑ Diastolic relaxation	↑ Myocardial oxygen consumption
↑ Venous return	Tachycardia/arrhythmias
	Calcium overload
	Tachyphylaxis

SYMPATHETIC NERVOUS SYSTEM ACTIVATION IN CHRONIC CARDIAC FAILURE

In CCF, levels of plasma catecholamines, principally noradrenaline, are increased, reflecting the increased output of the SNS (1,2). Absolute levels of noradrenaline appear to correlate with the degree of failure as judged by hemodynamic variables, suggesting a close relationship between increasing cardiac decompensation and the degree of activation of the SNS (3). Conversely, levels of plasma adrenaline and renin do not correlate with degree of heart failure as defined by hemodynamic or clinical parameters. Activation of the SNS occurs early on in the development of CCF. Thus, plasma noradrenaline levels are significantly elevated in asymptomatic patients with evidence of left ventricular dysfunction on the basis of reduced left ventricular ejection fraction only (4,5). In these subjects there is no significant increase in plasma renin activity. In addition, moderately symptomatic heart failure patients (New York Heart Association [NYHA] class II–III) prior to diuretic treatment have elevated plasma noradrenaline levels at rest and on exercise but normal plasma renin activity (6). After 1 month's therapy with loop diuretics these same patients exhibit symptomatic improvement but now have elevated plasma renin both at rest and on exercise. It therefore seems likely that activation of the SNS is important as a primary compensatory mechanism in CCF, while other neurohumoral responses are secondary phenomena, possibly occurring as a response to therapy rather than as a result of the disease process itself.

The level of plasma noradrenaline at the time of clinical presentation also correlates well with prognosis (7). Thus, those subjects with the highest plasma levels have the worst long-term outlook (Fig. 1). Although this does not prove that the absolute levels of noradrenaline are the cause of the poor outcome, this index of sympathetic overactivity is more closely related to prognosis than other deranged humoral or hemodynamic variables.

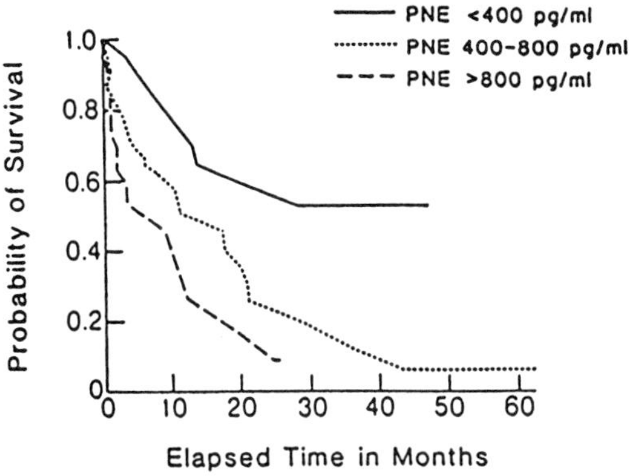

Figure 1 Life table analysis of survival among patients with congestive heart failure according to tercile, based on the level of plasma noradrenaline (PNE) at presentation. Group 1 (< 400 pg/m/), n = 27; Group 2 (400–800 pg/m/), n = 49; Group 3 (> 800 pg/m/), n = 30. The probability of survival in each group is significantly different from the probabilities of survival in the other two groups. (From Ref. 7.)

Why then should SNS activity, which initially plays an important supportive compensatory role in early heart failure, become an excessive and potentially deleterious factor as the disease progresses? One possible explanation is a progressive reduction in the sensitivity of the baroreflexes and cardiopulmonary reflexes that normally act to "restrain" sympathetic tone. There are several pieces of evidence that support this altered sensitivity of circulatory reflexes in CCF. In dogs with experimental heart failure, deactivation of the carotid baroreceptors by common carotid occlusion is accompanied by a smaller pressor response than in normal animals (8). In CCF patients, plasma catecholamine response to exercise is excessive as compared to normal controls (1), and the heart rate and catecholamine responses to modification of blood pressure by injection of vasoactive drugs are reduced—for example, following infusion of sodium nitroprusside (9). Response to changes in right atrial filling pressure is also impaired in CCF. Thus, experimental induction of small degrees of lower-body negative pressure leading to modest reduction in venous return causes reflex forearm vasoconstriction in normal subjects but not in patients with severe left ventricular dysfunction (10). In addition, plasma noradrenaline response to assumption of the upright posture is markedly reduced in these CCF patients when they are examined using a tilt table (11). Finally, in the later stages of heart failure there may also be positive interactions between the SNS and the renin-angiotensin system. The SNS plays a major role in directly stimulating release of renin from the kidney. In addition, it is now well recognized that angiotensin II stimulates the SNS at various central and peripheral sites (12,13).

Thus, major reflexes restraining the SNS become deactivated in CCF, and this, combined with the possible reciprocal potentiation of the SNS by angiotensin II, leads to progressive uncontrolled increase in sympathetic activity as heart failure worsens. The consequences of this excessive activity both beneficial and adverse can be seen in the general circulation and the myocardium.

THE SYMPATHETIC NERVOUS SYSTEM AND THE CIRCULATION IN HEART FAILURE

One of the principal symptoms in heart failure is fatigue and diminished exercise capacity. This is related to reduction in total voluntary muscle blood flow during exertion. However, in the early stages of CCF muscle blood flow is relatively well preserved in comparison to other tissues, including splanchnic and renal. Thus, although in absolute terms exercise-induced increase in muscle blood flow is blunted in CCF, the proportion of blood flow to other tissues is reduced to a much greater extent as a large part of their share of the cardiac output is redistributed to the exercising muscles (14) (Table 2).

A number of different factors as well as the SNS are important in modulating vascular resistance and hence organ blood flow in CCF. These include lactate production during exercise, local hormones (e.g., prostaglandins), and endothelium-derived relaxing and constricting factors. The role of these individual factors and their interaction with the SNS remains controversial. As heart failure progresses, increasing arterial vasoconstric-

Table 2 Reduction of Cardiac Output and Regional Blood Flow in Heart Failure at Rest and During Exercise*

	Rest	Exercise
Cardiac output	70	55
Renal	59	33
Splanchnic	57	31
Skin	40	50
Skeletal muscle	73	70

*All figures are percentages of expected values obtained in normal subjects (modified from Ref. 14).

tion occurs. This causes a generalized increase in peripheral vascular resistance leading to loss of the circulation's ability to respond to changing tissue requirements and to increasing impedance to left ventricular emptying. This increased resistance to flow leads to further reduction in cardiac output and to the well-recognized vicious circle and downward spiral seen in progressive heart failure. There is a considerable body of evidence indicating that this increase in systemic vascular resistance can be significantly reduced by alpha-blocking agents such as prazosin and phentolamine. However, the absolute vasodilatory effect of prazosin on leg (principally muscle) blood flow at rest in CCF patients is small, reflecting a modest contribution of the SNS to altered vascular resistance of muscle. On exercise, this vasoconstrictor effect is virtually abolished (15). Conversely, forearm blood flow, which proportionately reflects flow to tissues other than muscle, can be increased by administration of phentolamine in CCF patients. Angiotension converting enzyme (ACE) inhibitors (e.g., captopril) do not reduce forearm vascular resistance unless SNS activity has been blocked by prior administration of phentolamine (14). These findings suggest that at rest the SNS is the principal overall modulator of blood flow and that the effects of ACE inhibition are apparent only after its removal. A specific vasodilatory abnormality has also been demonstrated in exercising muscles in CCF patients, one that is independent of the SNS and may be related to local hormonal and metabolic effects (16).

In summary, therefore, although systemic vascular resistance is generally increased in CCF as a result of overactivity of the SNS, this is unlikely to be the principal reason for decreased blood flow to muscles or for poor exercise performance. The original concept of maldistribution of the cardiac output in CCF away from exercising muscles is less likely, and in fact the proportional distribution of blood flow to muscle is reasonably appropriate as compared to normal (Table 2). The problem seems to be simply related to the absolute reduction in cardiac output, which is not sufficient to meet all the body's requirements.

MYOCARDIAL ADRENOCEPTOR FUNCTION AND REGULATION IN CHRONIC CARDIAC FAILURE

Chronic agonist stimulation leads in a number of receptor systems to desensitization or tachyphylaxis of response, which may be associated with loss of functional cell surface receptors known as "down-regulation." Reduction of agonist stimulation either by withdrawal of the agonist or by the administration of a specific competitive antagonist leads to recovery or "up-regulation" of the receptors, with return of cell responsiveness (17). The progressively increasing levels of circulating catecholamines found in

CCF are therefore a potential cause of densitization and down-regulation of myocardial adrenoceptors (ADR). These changes in receptor sensitivity may represent protection of the myocardium from overstimulation but may also contribute to the decline in cardiac function.

In recent years there has been increasing interest in the function and regulation of myocardial ADR in CCF. In order to appreciate fully the relevance of the changes that have been described, it will be necessary to review briefly the function of normal myocardial ADR.

Myocardial Adrenoceptors in Normal Heart

β-*Adrenoceptors*

It is now well recognized that both β_1- and β_2-ADR subtypes coexist in the human heart. Radioligand binding studies have demonstrated the presence of both subtypes in all four chambers of the normal human heart, but in varying proportions (18,19). In the majority of studies using radioligand binding techniques, predominance of the β_1 subtype has been demonstrated in ventricular tissue, whereas approximately equal proportions of both subtypes have been found in atrial myocardium. The first evidence that both subtypes produced positive inotropic effects was provided by Ablad et al. (20) in studies of isolated, electrically driven human right atria. They found that β_1-selective antagonists inhibited the positive inotropic action of noradrenaline more potently than that of adrenaline, although there was no difference in the inhibition of stimulation for both agonists produced by the nonselective antagonist propranolol. Since that time, numerous authors have reported in vitro studies supporting this duality of response using various combinations of selective and nonselective agonists and antagonists (21). Taken overall, the functional studies definitively demonstrate that activation of either β-ADR subtype can produce positive inotropic and chronotropic effects in the human heart, and that the results of receptor activation will depend on their location and whether the stimulating agent is adrenaline or noradrenaline.

Stimulation of either β-ADR subtype increases contractile force through a final common biochemical pathway, namely, activation of adenylate cyclase (AC) and the production of cyclic AMP. The extent to which each subtype contributes to AC activation remains controversial. Thus, early studies in human right atrium suggested that only β_2-ADR stimulation was responsible for AC activation (22). It now seems likely that β_1-ADR stimulation will also activate AC, although to a lesser extent than β_2-ADR, but there remains an apparent discrepancy between these results and the predominant role of β_1-ADR in mediating the inotropic effects of catecholamines in vitro (23).

The action of β-ADR agonists on contractile function is quite different from that of other inotropes (e.g., digoxin) in that both force of contraction (positive inotropic effect) and rate of relaxation (positive lusitropic effect) of cardiac muscle are enhanced (Fig. 2). These paradoxical effects are related to the action of cyclic AMP–dependent protein kinase on the transfer of calcium across the cell membrane, as well as the rate of binding and release of calcium from both the sarcoplasmic reticulum and the contractile proteins (24) (Fig. 3). These biochemical events are the basis of the normal physiological response to catecholamines on myocardial β-ADR. Thus, activation of the sympathetic nervous system increases cardiac output by increasing stroke volume and heart rate. As heart rate increases there is a progressive reduction of diastolic filling time. The "compensatory" effect of catecholamines in shortening the time of relaxation therefore extends the effectiveness of heart rate as a mechanism for increasing cardiac output. In heart disease, when the myocardium becomes less compliant, this mechanism may become even more relevant.

α-Adrenoceptors

α-Adrenoceptors have been found in the myocardium of most mammalian species. There is, however, considerable species variation in the density of α-ADR assessed by radioligand binding in cardiac tissue (25,26). Thus,

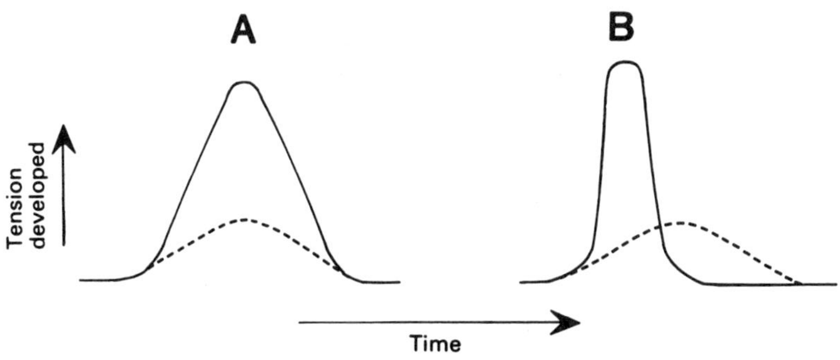

Figure 2 Diagrammatic representation of the effects of different inotropic stimuli on the contraction of isolated ventricular muscle strips. Solid line represents the effect of the agonist compared to control contraction (dotted line). (A) cyclic AMP *independent* mechanism; e.g., digoxin or α_1-adrenoceptor agonist stimulation. (B) cyclic AMP *dependent* mechanism; e.g., β-adrenoceptor agonist stimulation. Note overall shortening of the time scale of the contractile event in B as compared with A, despite equivalent increase in force of contraction (positive inotropic effect). This is due to increased rate of relaxation of muscle fibers in B (positive lusitropic effect).

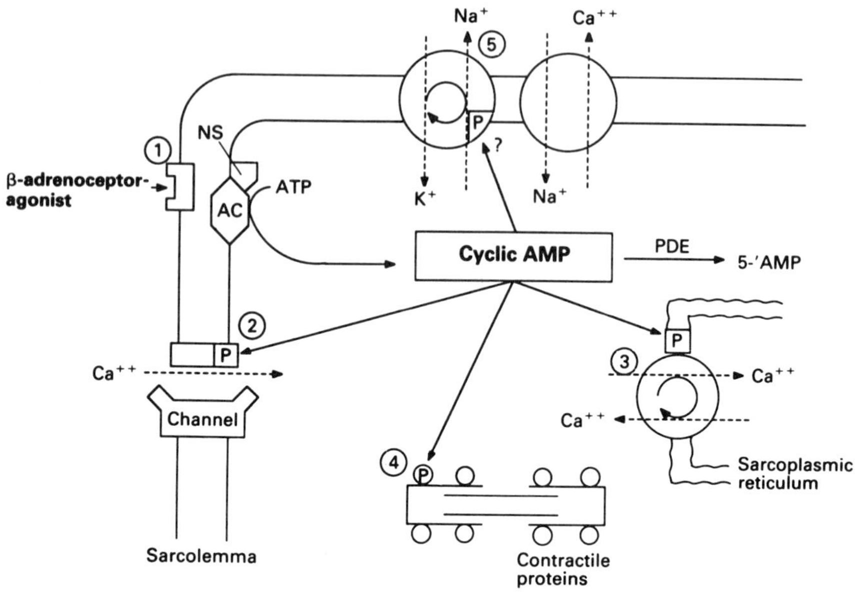

Figure 3 Biochemical basis of β-adrenoceptor activation of myocardial contraction and relaxation. (1) Stimulation of myocardial β-adrenoceptors leads to increased intracellular cyclic AMP production, which via activation of specific protein kinase causes phosphorylation (P) of a number of proteins influencing Ca^{2+} transport and binding. Positive inotropic response (increased force of contraction) is produced by increasing the availability of free intracellular Ca^{2+} by increased transmembrane flux of Ca^{2+} via the voltage-dependent calcium channels (2) and by enhanced release of Ca^{2+} from the sarcoplasmic reticulum (3). Positive lusitropic response (increased rate of relaxation) is produced by increased dissociation of Ca^{2+} from the contractile proteins (4), in particular troponin I, which regulates the interaction between actin and myosin. In addition, Ca^{2+} reuptake into the sarcoplasmic reticulum is also enhanced (3). Protein kinase stimulated Na^+ pump activation via Na^+/K^+ ATPase may also occur (5), leading to increased transmembrane Na^+ gradient and acceleration of Ca^{2+} efflux via the $Na^+{:}Ca^{2+}$ exchange mechanism. (Reproduced in part from Br J Pharmacol 1989; 27:527–537.)

as a proportion of total ADR density (β plus α), α_1-ADR predominate in rat and rabbit hearts but represent only 2% to 15% of total ADR in the normal human heart (26,27). That cardiac α_1-ADR activation is associated with a positive inotropic but little or no chronotropic effect has been demonstrated in a number of mammalian species (28,29) as well as human myocardium (30,31). There is, however, an important qualitative difference in alpha and beta inotropic responses, in that α_1 stimulation leads to an increased force of contraction without the characteristic shortening of the overall contractile event due to enhanced rate of relaxation seen following β-ADR stimulation (Fig. 2). In clinical terms these differences in functional response would translate into the absence of lusitropic effect following α-adrenergic stimulation. The biochemical basis of α_1-ADR inotropic response is not dependent on cyclic AMP generation and almost certainly involves an alternative second messenger pathway associated with hydrolysis of plasma membrane inositol phosphates in both animal (29,32) and human (33) myocardium. Thus, although these mechanisms are only partly verified in human cardiac tissue, it seems likely that α_1-ADR activation leads to the production of two intracellular breakdown products of the inositol phosphates, inositol trisphosphate and diacylglycerol. These by-products in turn enhance the release of intracellular calcium from the sarcoplasmic reticulum as well as inward flux via the slow calcium channel and increase in the calcium sensitivity of the contractile proteins (29,32) (Fig. 4). The role of this alternative inotropic pathway in normal and diseased human myocardium is still uncertain. It remains possible that α-ADR–mediated cardiac effects may be relevant in situations of reduced β-adrenergic responsiveness, as for example during treatment with β-ADR blocking drugs or in CCF (see later). In addition, the effect of α_1-ADR stimulation on myocardial electrophysiology (i.e., the increase in the magnitude and delay in the decay of the slow inward calcium current) may be relevant to the production of serious rhythm disturbances at times of increased catecholamine production associated with ischemia and CCF (34).

Myocardial Adrenoceptors in Heart Failure

β-*Adrenoceptors*

Chronic cardiac failure is associated with significant alterations in myocardial β-ADR density. Reduced density of β-ADR in ventricular myocardium obtained from heart transplant recipients in severe end-stage CCF as compared to normal controls was first demonstrated by Bristow et al. (35) using radio ligand binding techniques. This down-regulation was correlated with reduced contractile response of ventricular muscle strips and of cyclic AMP generation to β-ADR agonists. The effect was receptor-specific in that no change in response to histamine acting at myocardial H_2 receptors coupled to adenylate cyclase was found in the same tissue.

Since then, other studies have shown that this loss of β-ADR is likely to be a progressive phenomenon and not simply an incidental finding in severely damaged hearts, and also that β_1-ADR are probably more affected

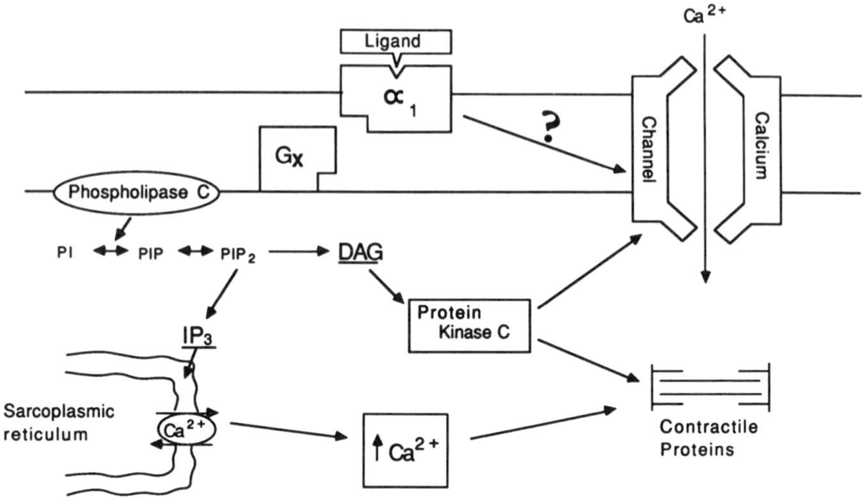

Figure 4 Proposed biochemical basis of α_1-adrenoceptor–mediated inotropic effects. Stimulation of the myocardial α_1-adrenoceptors activates phospholipase-C, probably via a guanine nucleotide binding protein (Gx), leading to the hydrolysis of membrane polyphosphoinositides and the production of inositol trisphosphate (IP_3) and diacyglycerol (DAG). IP_3 enhances the release of CA^{2+} from intracellular stores by interaction with IP_3 receptors on the sarcoplasmic reticulum. DAG activates protein kinase C, which in turn by protein phosphorylation may lead to enhanced calcium sensitivity of the contractile proteins and increased influx of extracellular Ca^{2+} via the voltage-dependent calcium channels. Activation of calcium channels may also occur as a direct consequence of α_1-adrenoceptor stimulation (?). These processes lead to the characteristic myocardial response of α_1-adrenoceptor stimulation, i.e., increased force of contraction without change in the overall time course of the contractile event.

than β_2-ADR. Thus Fowler et al. (36) demonstrated a relationship between the density of β-ADR in right ventricular endomyocardial biopsies and the degree of impairment of cardiac function measured by left ventricular ejection fraction (LVEF) in patients at various stages of CCF. They showed that total β-ADR density was reduced by approximately 58% as compared to normal controls in severe failure ($LVEF < 0.25$) and by only 38% in subjects less severely affected ($LVEF > 0.25$ and < 0.5). In addition, some of the subjects studied were given graded infusions of either dobutamine (to assess β-adrenergic response) or calcium gluconate (to assess non-receptor-mediated inotropism) in order to evaluate in vivo inotropic response. Dobutamine-induced inotropism was reduced in CCF, while the calcium response was unchanged. In addition, the proportional reduction in dobutamine response correlated well with both the decrease in LVEF and the reduction in β-ADR density. Despite uncertainties about the representative nature of right ventricular biopsy material, these studies give considerable support to the possible pathophysiological relationship between progressive CCF and reduced β-ADR density and function.

In another study, using larger fragments of left ventricular myocardium obtained from explanted hearts from transplant recipients, Bristow et al. (37) examined the relative proportions of β-ADR subtypes. They found that the ratio of β_1- to β_2-ADR in severely failing hearts (60/40) was markedly different from that of normal controls (75/25). This was apparently due to significant down-regulation of β_1-ADR alone, with no significant change in the β_2 subtype. These studies were extended to show that this relative "sparing" of the β_2-ADR was also seen in the inotropic responsiveness to selective agonists of strips of isolated myocardium obtained from the same subjects. However, β_2-agonist–stimulated muscle contraction and adenylate cyclase activity in failing human myocardium is still reduced by approximately 30% as compared to control (38). Since β_2-ADR density is not significantly reduced in severe CCF, these findings suggest that a small proportion of the β_2-ADR are "uncoupled" from adenylate cyclase. Thus, in end-stage CCF β-adrenergic responsiveness may be impaired because of reduced density principally of β_1-ADR and a degree of uncoupling of β_2-ADR from adenylate cyclase. Despite this major loss of responsiveness, the β-adrenergic pathway in CCF is still capable of mediating effective inotropic support in response to infused β-agonists in the intact patient, this effect being greater in absolute terms than the nonspecific effects of calcium infusion (36).

It seems likely that, as in other tissues, myocardial β_2-ADR are situated extrajunctionally and are noninnervated "hormonal" receptors responding principally to circulating adrenaline, whereas the postsynaptic β_1-ADR are closely associated with the noradrenergic nerve terminal and neuronally released noradrenaline (39). The observations that have been made regarding β-ADR function in CCF are compatible with the hypothesis that the myocardial β_1-ADR receives the major direct effects of neuronally released noradrenaline, with increasing sympathetic nervous stimulation during the development of CCF leading to selective β_1-ADR down-regulation and relative β_2-ADR sparing. It is possible that as heart failure progresses the β_2-ADR becomes increasingly more important as a target for catecholamines maintaining inotropic support for the myocardium. Conversely, the loss of β_1-ADR response to sympathetic stimulation may be an important pathophysiological mechanism of CCF, and the preservation of this inotropic pathway could influence the rate of progression of cardiac decompensation. Studies of myocardial β-ADR subtype densities in earlier stages of heart failure will be important in the further evaluation of this hypothesis.

The "selective" loss of myocardial β_1-ADR in CCF may not be universal in all forms of the disease but may relate principally to patients with idiopathic dilated cardiomyopathy, who form the vast majority of subjects used in the studies described so far. Other investigations indicate that irrespective of the underlying pathology, all patients with CCF show a direct relationship between increasing stage of heart failure and increasing "loss" of total myocardial β-ADR. However, subjects with CCF secondary to ischemic heart disease exhibit concomitant reduction in both β-ADR subtypes (40). The situation in valvular heart disease is a little more complicated. Thus, patients with mitral valve disease and severe CCF show reduced densities of both β-ADR subtypes, whereas those with aortic valve disease exhibit selective loss of the β_1 subtype only (41,42). Finally, patients with CCF due to Fallot's tetralogy have reduced β-ADR density as compared to normal adult hearts but with a normal β_1/β_2 ratio (40). The lack of sufficient age-matched control data for the congenital heart disease group reduces the significance of these latter observations. These interesting differences may relate to the earlier stage of heart failure in some of the subjects studied, in particular patients with congenital and aortic valve disease from whom samples of myocardium were obtained during corrective surgery. This was not true for the subjects with ischemic heart disease, in which case myocardium was obtained from explanted hearts prior to transplantation. In addition, the patients with mitral valve disease were all in NYHA grade III–IV heart failure, and biopsy material was obtained during valve surgery. It therefore remains possible that there is a difference in the pathophysiological mechanisms of β-ADR subtype regulation in CCF that is disease-specific and may have important therapeutic implications.

α-Adrenoceptors

Studies of the density and function of α-ADR in CCF are less numerous and have produced conflicting results. Bristow et al. (26) found no change in α_1-ADR density in ventricular myocardium from explanted failing hearts as compared with normal controls, although β-ADR density was reduced in the same samples, as in previous studies. In addition, the effect of noradrenaline on phosphoinositide hydrolysis was not significantly different in failing and nonfailing hearts. Conversely, Vago et al. (27) found significant up-regulation of α_1-ADR in a similar group of patients with CCF. Finally, Bohm et al. (43) studied receptor density and contractile function using papillary muscles from patients with end-stage CCF compared to those undergoing mitral valve replacement (hence not "normal" hearts). These authors found the characteristic down-regulation of β-ADR but no change in α_1-ADR density in the severely failing hearts. In addition, although, as was expected, the inotropic effect of isoprenaline on muscle strips was significantly reduced in the same tissue, there was no difference in the effect of α_1 stimulation when muscle strips were exposed to phenylephrine in the presence of propranolol.

Myocardial Guanine Nucleotide Regulatory Proteins in Heart Failure

Membrane receptors constitute the first component in the pathway of regulation of cell function by hormones/neurotransmitters. Within the cell membrane, guanine nucleotide regulatory (G) proteins occupy a key role in transducing the process of receptor stimulation to activation of second messenger production. This process of transduction has been extensively characterized for a large number of different receptor systems in numerous tissues and species. The G proteins are a family of proteins that bind guanosine triphosphate (GTP) and share a striking molecular similarity, being composed of α, β, and γ subunits. It is now well established that the stimulatory effects of catecholamines on β-ADR are linked to adenylate cyclase via a membrane transducing G protein called G_s. Conversely, inhibitory effects on adenylate cyclase (e.g., muscarinic and β_2-ADR agonists and adenosine) involve an alternative protein G_i. These two proteins are made up of the three subunits, two of which (β and γ) are common to G_s and G_i. The third subunit differs between the two G proteins (α_s and α_i) and probably accounts for their differing functions (Fig. 5). G proteins can be studied by the use of various bacterial toxins. Two toxins, those derived from *Vibrio cholerae* and *Bordetella pertussis*, are particularly useful. With the use of radiolabeled nicotinamide adenine dinucleotide (NAD) and either cholera or pertussis toxin, it is possible to tag and identify α_s and α_i respectively and enable quantification of these subunits on electrophoretic gels. In addition, the various functional components of the transducing system can be evaluated by assessment of adenylate cyclase activity and cyclic AMP production following stimulation with various chemical agonists (see Fig. 5 legend).

Reduction of β-ADR–stimulated adenylate cyclase activity in failing myocardium was first described by Bristow and colleagues (35). More recently, Denniss et al. (44) have extended these observations in order to probe the various components of the G protein transducing system in membranes from failing left ventricles from explanted hearts. Their results

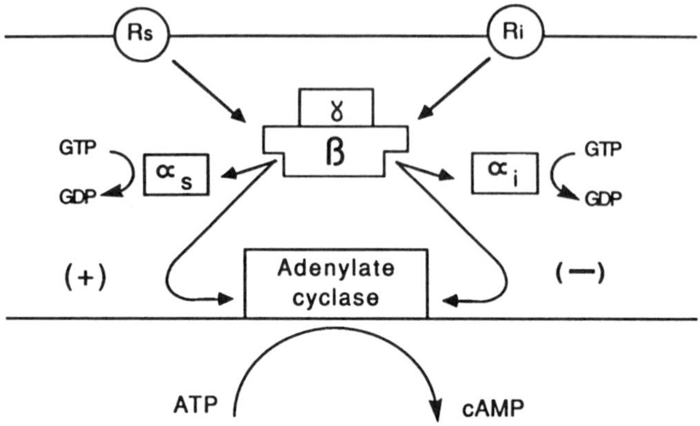

Figure 5 Coupling of cell membrane receptors to adenylate cyclase via the G-protein complex. Receptors that stimulate (Rs) or inhibit (Ri) the production of cyclic AMP are coupled to adenylate cyclase via the G-protein complex, which comprises three subunits: α, β, and γ. The β and γ subunits are common to both Rs and Ri interactions. The α subunit is a distinctive protein that differs in molecular weight between stimulatory (+) and inhibitory (−) receptor functions (α_s and α_i, respectively). The α subunit interacts with the receptor and regulates adenylate cyclase activity via the binding and hydrolysis of guanosine triphosphate (GTP) to guanosine diphosphate (GDP). The various components of the transducing mechanism can be studied by the evaluation of the generation of cyclic AMP following occupation of Rs or Ri with a specific agonist or via direct stimulation of the α subunit or adenylate cyclase using GTP or forskolin, respectively. The relative concentrations of α_s and α_i can be evaluated using the bacterial toxins derived from *Vibrio cholerae* and *Bordetella pertussis*, respectively. The toxins covalently modify the respective α subunit in the presence of adenine diphosphate (ADP) and nicotinamide adenine dinucleotide (NAD). In the case of α_s this so-called ADP ribosylation allows the subunit to become persistently active in stimulating adenylate cyclase. In the case of α_i, inhibition of the function of the subunit is produced by the addition of pertussis toxin. Using radiolabeled NAD and either cholera or pertussis toxin, it is possible to tag α_s or α_i and to identify and quantify the proteins on electrophoretic gels.

indicated that adenylate cyclase activity in these membranes is markedly reduced when assessed by isoprenaline stimulation via the β-ADR (presumably secondary to receptor down-regulation) or by stimulating the G_s/cyclase interaction using GTP (i.e., bypassing the β-ADR). However, maximal direct stimulation of adenylate cyclase by forskolin was not significantly different from normal control, indicating no change in total cyclase activity but rather a qualitative change in G protein transducing function in CCF.

It is possible that changes in the absolute quantities or the relative proportions of myocardial G proteins may be the cause of these observed abnormalities in adenylate cyclase activity and may contribute to the adrenergic dysfunction in CCF. Thus, the functional changes observed in CCF outlined above (i.e., reduction of β-ADR–mediated inotropism) could be related to either a decrease in G_s, an increase in G_i, or both.

In a canine model of CCF, a 59% reduction in the quantity of G_s in the failing left ventricle compared with normal control has been demonstrated (45). However, this model of heart failure involves pressure overload by aortic banding and, unlike the human situation, is associated with a significant increase in β-ADR density. In human myocardium obtained from severely failing hearts, a significant increase in G_i has been observed associated with no change in G_s (46,47). Horn et al. (48) found an 80% reduction in G_s from circulating lymphocytes in patients with CCF compared to normal controls, and this was partially reversed by treatment with ACE inhibitors. These authors also demonstrated a correlation between total levels of G_s in lymphocytes and cardiac tissue in end-stage CCF patients undergoing cardiac transplantation. Conversely, Maisel et al. (49) were unable to demonstrate any quantitative alteration in G proteins in circulating mononuclear leukocytes in CCF patients as compared to age-matched normal controls. However, these latter authors showed that treatment of intact leukocytes with pertussis toxin (to inhibit G_i) followed by subsequent stimulation of cyclic AMP generation revealed a tonic inhibition of cyclic AMP production in these cells from the CCF patients, suggesting a qualitative alteration in G protein function in these subjects. However, it is unclear how well dynamic changes in lymphocyte G proteins reflect those in cardiac tissue during early heart failure and the response to therapy.

The reported changes in G proteins may not be the same for all causes of CCF, as has been similarly shown for the relative susceptibility of the β-ADR subtypes to down-regulation (see above). Thus Bohm et al. (50) showed that there was a 37% increase in G_i in myocardial membranes obtained from explanted hearts of patients with idiopathic dilated cardiomyopathy but no change in those with ischemic heart disease. This difference between the pathological conditions was also evident when basal and GTP-stimulated adenylate cyclase activity was measured, indicating reduced activity in the idiopathic cardiomyopathy group only. There was also a marked reduction in inotropic response to isoprenaline in muscle strips obtained from all the hearts studied, but this was more pronounced in the idiopathic cardiomyopathy cases, although the total β-ADR density was similarly reduced in both groups. More recently, Reithman et al. (51) studied the effect of chronic noradrenaline stimulation on G protein subunits in rat myocardial cells in cell culture. They demonstrated that the treated cells were desensitized to catecholamines in that isoprenaline stimulation of adenylate cyclase was significantly (52%) reduced. This was associated with a significant increase in the quantity of G_i in the cell membranes, suggesting that the increase in G_i was responsible for the desensitization of adenylate cyclase response.

At present, the role of quantitative or qualitative G protein abnormalities in CCF is uncertain. In addition, it is impossible to state whether the changes reported are primary or secondary phenomena related to chronic noradrenaline stimulation of the β-ADR or to a change in the genetic expression of various G protein subunits (52). However, the results so far indicate that the myocardial G proteins are potentially an important therapeutic target in CCF, and their investigation remains an active area of research.

CONCLUSIONS

It is now well established that the SNS is progressively activated during the development and progression of CCF. Recent evidence also suggests that stimulation of the SNS may be the first of the various neurohumoral compensatory mechanisms to be activated. Although at first this stimulation of the heart and circulation is beneficial, it is apparent that in the longer term the effects of the SNS are deleterious and may contribute to the progressive decline in cardiac function. Alterations in the distribution of the circulation to various organs and the damaging effects of the increased afterload, due to peripheral vasoconstriction, on the left ventricle are significant factors in the progression of heart failure. Recently, however, there has been increasing interest in the role of the adverse effects of excess catecholamine stimulation on myocardial adrenoceptor function. Studies in a number of laboratories have been directed toward elucidating the alterations in the adrenergic pathways in failing myocardium. The results of these investigations indicate that there is a specific and progressive abnormality of myocardial β-ADR function in heart failure related to alteration in receptor density and probably the process of coupling, via the G proteins, of the β-ADR to adenylate cyclase.

It remains uncertain whether the changes in beta ADR function that have been described are critical determinants of prognosis in heart failure or merely an epiphenomenon marking the extent of SNS activation and the severity of the hemodynamic disturbance. There is, however, a dynamic two-way interaction between the SNS and the myocardium in heart failure.

Reduction in pump function is associated with increased activity of the SNS, and conversely, increased SNS activity is associated with reduction in functional performance of myocardial β-ADR. These interactions are potentially of great importance in the understanding of the pathophysiology and pharmacology of heart failure. Thus, agents that alter the activity of the SNS or interfere with the function of the myocardial β-ADR will affect cardiac performance and are of potential therapeutic value in heart failure.

REFERENCES

1. Chidsey CA, Harison DC, Braunwald E. Augmentation of the plasma norepinephrine response to exercise in patients with congestive heart failure. N Engl J Med 1962; 267:650–654.
2. Thomas JA, Marks BH. Plasma norepinephrine in congestive heart failure. Am J Cardiol 1978; 41:233–243.
3. Levine BT, Francis GS, Goldsmith SR, Simon AB, Cohn JN. Activity of the sympathetic nervous system and renin angiotensin system assessed by plasma hormone levels and their relation to haemodynamic abnormalities in congestive heart failure. Am J Cardiol 1982; 49:1659–1666.
4. Francis GS. Differences in neurohumoral activation in patients with left ventricular dysfunction with and without heart failure. J Am Coll Cardiol 1989; 13(2):246A.
5. Francis GS, Benedict C, Johnstone DE, Kirlin PC, Nicklas J, Liang C, Kubo SH, Rudin-Toretsky E, Yusuf S. Comparison of neuroendocrine activation in patients with left ventricular dysfunction with and without congestive heart failure. Circulation 1990; 82:1724–1729.
6. Bayliss J, Norell M, Canepa-Anson R, Sutton G, Poole-Wilson P. Untreated heart failure: clinical and neuroendocrine effects of introducing diuretics. Br Heart J 1987; 57:17–22.
7. Cohn JN, Levine TB, Olivari MT, Garberg V, Lura D, Francis GS, Simon AB, Rector T. Plasma norepinephrine as a guide to prognosis in patients with congestive heart failure. N Engl J Med 1984; 311:28–35.
8. Higgins CB, Vatner JF, Eckberg DL, Braunwald E. Alterations in baroreceptor reflex in conscious dogs with heart failure. J Clin Invest 1972; 51:715–724.
9. Olivari MT, Levine TB, Cohn JN. Abnormal neurohumoral response to nitroprusside infusion in congestive heart failure. J Am Coll Cardiol 1983; 2:411–417.
10. Ferguson DW, Abboud FM, Mark AL. Selective impairment of baroreceptor mediated vasoconstrictor responses in patients with ventricular dysfunction. Circulation 1984; 69:451–460.
11. Levine TB, Francis GS, Goldsmith SR, Cohn JN. The neurohumoral and haemodynamic response to orthostatic tilt in patients with congestive heart failure. Circulation 1983; 67:1070–1075.

12. Zanchetti A, Stella A. Neural control of renin release. Clin Sci Mol Med 1975; 48:215–223.
13. Mancia G, Gainnattasio G, Grassi G, Morganti A, Zanchetti A. Reflex control of the circulation and ACE inhibition in man. J Hypertension 1988; 6:545–549.
14. Dargie H. Sympathetic activity and regional blood flow in heart failure. Eur Heart J 1990; 11(suppl A):39–43.
15. Wilson JR, Ferraro N, Weiner DH. Effect of the sympathetic nervous system on limb circulation and metabolism during exercise in patients with heart failure. Circulation 1985; 72:72–78.
16. Le Jemtel T, Maskin CS, Lucido D, Chadwick BS. Failure to augment maximal limb blood flow in response to one leg versus two leg exercise in patients with severe heart failure. J Clin Invest 1986; 74:245–252.
17. Lefkowitz RJ, Caron MG, Stiles GL. Mechanisms of membrane receptor regulation. N Engl J Med 1984; (i):1570–1579.
18. Brodde OE. Cardiac beta adrenergic receptors. ISI Atlas of Science: Pharmacology. 1987; 107–112.
19. Summers RJ, Molenaar P, Russel F, Elnatan J, Jones CR, Buxton BF, Chang V, Hambley J. Coexistence and localisation of $beta_1$ and $beta_2$ adrenoceptors in the human heart. Eur Heart J 1989; 10(suppl B):11–21.
20. Ablad B, Carlsson B, Carlsson E, Dahlof C, Ek L, Hultberg E. Cardiac effects of beta adrenergic antagonists. Adv Cardiol 1974; 12:290–302.
21. Jones CR, Molenaar P, Summers RJ. New views of human cardiac beta adrenoceptors. J Moll Cell Cardiol 1989; 21:519–535.
22. Waelbrook M, Taton G, Delhaye M, Chatelain P, Camus JC, Pochet R, Leclerc JL, De Smet JM, Robberecht P, Christophe J. The human heart beta adrenergic receptors. Mol Pharmacol 1983; 24:174–182.
23. Kaumann AJ, Hall JA, Murray KJ, Wells FC, Brown MJ. A comparison of the effects of adrenaline and noradrenaline on the human heart: the role of $beta_1$ and $beta_2$ adrenoceptors in the stimulation of adenylate cyclase and contractile force. Eur Heart J 1989; 10(suppl B):29–37.
24. Katz AM. Cyclic adenosine monophosphate effects on the myocardium: A man who blows hot and cold with the same breath. J Am Coll Cardiol 1983; 2:143–149.
25. Mukherjee A, Haghani Z, Brady J, Bush L, McBride W, Buja LM, Willerson JT. Differences in myocardial alpha and beta adrenergic receptor numbers in different species. Am J Physiol 1983; 245:H957–H961.
26. Bristow MR, Minobe W, Rasmussen R, Hershberger RE, Hoffman BB. $Alpha_1$ adrenergic receptors in the non failing and failing human heart. J Pharmacol Exp Ther 1988; 247:1039–1045.
27. Vago T, Bevilacqua M, Norbiatom G, Baldi G, Chebat E, Bertora P, Baroldi G, Accini R. Identification of $alpha_1$ adrenergic receptors on sarcolemma from normal subjects and patients with idiopathic dilated cardiomyopathy: characteristics and linkage to GTP-binding protein. Circ Res 1989; 64:474–481.

28. Benfey BG. Cardiac alpha adrenoceptors. Can J Physiol 1980; 58:1145–1157.
29. Scholz J, Schaefer B, Schmitz W, Scholz H, Steinfath M, Lohse W, Schwabe U, Purunen J. $Alpha_1$ adrenoceptor mediated positive inotropic effect and inositol triphospate increase in mammalian heart. J Pharmacol Exp Ther 1988; 245:327–335.
30. Skomedal T, Aass H, Osnes J, Fjeld N, Klingen G, Langslet A, Semb G. Demonstration of an alpha adrenoceptor mediated inotropic effect of norepinephrine in human atria. J Pharmacol Exp Ther 1985; 233:441–446.
31. Aass H, Skomedal T, Osnes J, Fjeld N, Klingen G, Langslet A, Svennevig J, Semb G. Noradrenaline evokes an alpha adrenoceptor mediated inotropic effect in human ventricular myocardium. Acta Pharmacol Toxicol 1986; 58:88–90.
32. Otani H, Das DK. $Alpha_1$ adrenoceptor mediated phosphoinositide breakdown and inotropic response in rat left ventricular papillary muscles. Circ Res 1988; 62:8–17.
33. Kohl C, Schmitz W, Scholz H, Scholz J. Evidence for the existence of inositol tetrakisphosphate in mammalian heart. Circ Res 1990; 66:580–583.
34. Davey MJ. Alpha adrenoceptors—an overview. J Moll Cell Cardiol 1968; 18(suppl 5):1–15.
35. Bristow MR, Ginsburg R, Minobe W, Cubiciotti RS, Scott-Sageman W, Lurie R, Billingham ME, Harrison DC, Stinson EB. Decreased catecholamine sensitivity and beta adrenergic receptor density in failing human hearts. N Engl J Med 1982; 307:205–211.
36. Fowler MB, Laser JA, Hopkins GL, Minobe W, Bristow MR. Assessment of the beta adrenergic pathway in the intact failing human heart: Progressive receptor down regulation and subsensitivity to agonist response. Circulation 1986; 74:1290–1302.
37. Bristow MR, Ginsburg R, Umans V, Fowler M, Minobe W, Rasmussen R, Zera P, Menlove R, Shah P, Jamieson S, Stinson EB, $Beta_1$ and $beta_2$ adrenergic receptor subpopulations in non failing and failing human ventricular myocardium: coupling of both receptor subtypes to muscles contraction and selective $beta_1$ receptor downregulation in heart failure. Circ Res 1986; 59:297–309.
38. Bristow MR, Hershberger RE, Pole JD, Rasmussen R. $Beta_1$ and $beta_2$ adrenergic receptor mediated adenylate cyclase stimulation in non failing and failing human ventricular myocardium. Mol Pharm 1989; 35:295–303.
39. Ariens EJ. The classification of beta adrenoceptors. Trends Pharmacol Sci 1981; 2:170–172.
40. Brodde OE, Zerkowski HR, Borst HG, Maier W, Michel MC. Drug and disease induced changes of human cardiac $beta_1$ and $beta_2$ adrenoceptors. Eur Heart J 1989; 10(suppl B):38–44).
41. Brodde OE, Zerkowski HR, Doetsch H, Motomura S, Khamssi M, Michel MC. Myocardial beta adrenoceptor changes in heart failure: concomitant reduction of $beta_1$ and $beta_2$ adrenoceptor function related to the degree of

heart failure in patients with mitral valve disease. J Am Coll Cardiol 1989; 14:323–331.
42. Michel MC, Maisel AS, Brodde OE. Mitigation of beta$_1$ and/or beta$_2$ adrenoceptor function in human heart failure. Br J Clin Pharm 1990; 30(suppl 1):37S–42S.
43. Bohm M, Diet F, Feiler G, Kemkes B, Erdmann E. Alpha adrenoceptors and alpha adrenoceptor mediated positive inotropic effects in failing human myocardium. J. Cardiovasc Pharmacol 1988; 12:357–364.
44. Dennis AR, Colucci WD, Allen PD, Marsh JD. Distribution and function of human ventricular beta adrenoceptors in congestive heart failure. J Moll Cell Cardiol 1989; 21:651–660.
45. Longbaugh JP, Vatner DE, Vatner SF, Homey CJ. Decreased stimulatory guanosine triphosphate binding protein in dogs with pressure overload left ventricular failure. J Clin Invest 1988; 81:420–424.
46. Feldman AM, Cates AE, Veezey WB, Hershberger RE, Bristow MR, Baughman KL, Baumgartner WA, Van Dop C. Increase of the 40,000 molecular weight pertussis toxin substrate (G-protein) in the failing human heart. J Clin Invest 1988; 82:189–197.
47. Neumann J, Scholz H, Doring V, Schmitz W, Meyernick L, Kalmar P. Increase in myocardial Gi protein in heart failure. Lancet 1988; ii:936–937.
48. Horn EM, Corwin SJ, Steinberg SF, Chow YK, Neuberg GW, Cannon PJ, Powers ER, Bilezikian JP. Reduced lymphocyte stimulatory gaunine nucleotide regulatory protein and beta adrenergic receptors in congestive heart failure and reversal with angiotensin converting enzyme inhibitor therapy. Circulation 1988; 78:1373–1379.
49. Maisel AS, Michel MC, Insel PA, Ziegler MG, Phillips C. Pertussis toxin treatment of whole blood: a novel approach to assess G protein function in congestive heart failure. Circulation 1990; 81:1198–1204.
50. Bohm M, Gierschik P, Jakobs KH, Pieske B, Schnabel P, Ungerer M, Erdmann E. Increase in Gi alpha in human hearts with dilated but not ischaemic cardiomyopathy. Circulation 1990; 82:1249–1265.
51. Reithmann C, Gierschik P, Sidiropoulos D, Werden K, Jakobs KH. Mechanism of noradrenaline induced heterologous desensitisation of adenylate cyclase stimulation in rat heart muscle cells: increase in the level of inhibitory G-protein alpha subunits. Eur J Pharmacol 1989; 172:211–221.
52. Feldman AM, Cates AE, Bristow MR, Van Dop C. Expression of the alpha Gi gene in the failing heart. J Mol Cell Cardiol 1988; 20:17–22.

4

Pathophysiology of Heart Failure: Neuroendocrine Factors

Kenneth M. McDonald and Gary S. Francis
University of Minnesota Hospital and Clinic, Minneapolis, Minnesota

INTRODUCTION

Congestive cardiac failure is characterized by activation of several distinct neuroendocrine systems (1). Increased activity of the sympathetic nervous system has been well demonstrated in this syndrome (2) and, along with the renin-angiotensin system (3) and arginine vasopressin (4), helps to maintain systemic perfusion in the setting of poor ventricular function. To counterbalance the intense vasoconstriction and sodium retention associated with these systems, the production of a number of vasodilator substances, such as atrial natriuretic peptide (5) and prostaglandins, is increased. As heart failure progresses, the effects of the vasoconstrictor systems predominate, contributing to further deterioration in ventricular function.

Neuroendocrine substances may play a further role in left ventricular dysfunction other than the control of systemic hemodynamics and salt and water retention. Recent data have demonstrated that vasoconstrictor substances stimulate cell growth (6–9). Specifically, angiotensin II (6,9) and norepinephrine (8) have been associated with myocyte growth as well as growth of the cardiac interstitium (10,11). Endogenous vasodilators, however, such as atrial natriuretic peptide, inhibit cell growth (12). It is possible, therefore, that these vasomotor compounds also influence myocardial and vascular remodeling following myocardial damage.

This chapter will review the available data on neuroendocrine system activity in heart failure. Specific attention will be given to the renin-angiotensin system, arginine vasopressin, and atrial natriuretic peptide. Data regarding the sympathetic nervous system have been presented elsewhere in this book.

RENIN-ANGIOTENSIN SYSTEM

Increased activity of the systemic renin-angiotensin system (RAS) in congestive heart failure has been documented for many years. Almost 50 years ago Merrill and colleagues demonstrated elevated plasma renin activity in this syndrome (13). More recent experimental data have shown progressive increase in the activation of this system with worsening hemodynamic function in a canine model of heart failure (14). Riegger and colleagues, using the pacing model of heart failure, demonstrated a close relationship between plasma renin activity and hemodynamic abnormalities. Moreover, on cessation of pacing, plasma renin activity normalized along with hemodynamic function (14).

There are many potential stimuli for the activation of the RAS in heart failure (15,16). Decreased renal perfusion and a reduction in the renal-tubular concentrations of sodium and chloride ions around the macula densa can activate the RAS. Increased activity of the sympathetic nervous system also can stimulate renin production.

While a close relationship exists between activation of the RAS and severity of heart failure in experimental models (14), a similar relationship does not exist in humans. Low, normal, and high levels of plasma renin activity have been demonstrated in patients with heart failure (15,17). This variability has been described even in untreated patients (15). The response of plasma renin activity to diuretics in patients with heart failure has also been variable, with low values increasing and high values decreasing (15). While this variability may suggest a less direct relationship between the RAS and heart failure in humans, it is more likely that these findings reflect the sensitivity of plasma renin activity to a large number of variables prominent in heart failure. Included among these are drugs used in the management of heart failure, in particular diuretics (18,19) and vasodilators (20), and also the effect of variable sodium dietary intake. Such factors have almost certainly influenced the plasma renin activity levels when assessed in humans, whereas analysis in experimental animals is not affected by such variables. While estimation of plasma renin activity may not correlate with the severity of heart failure in humans, there does appear to be a relationship between the acute hemodynamic response to an angiotensin converting enzyme (ACE) inhibitor and the level of renin activity in the plasma (17). Patients with significantly elevated baseline levels of plasma renin activity show an impressive reduction in systemic vascular resistance following the administration of an ACE inhibitor, whereas those with normal or modestly increased levels of renin activity show a less marked response (17).

Because levels of plasma renin activity are so variable, it is difficult to causally link the activation of the RAS to prognosis in heart failure. However, peripheral vasoconstriction is likely to play an important part in the progression of this syndrome (21). Angiotensin II is a powerful vasoconstrictor and is almost certainly an important factor in the increased left ventricular impedance characteristic of heart failure (3). The marked beneficial effect of the ACE inhibitors on symptoms (22–24) and survival (25,26) in this syndrome supports a close association between activation of this system and progression of the disease. Converting enzyme inhibitors improve symptoms in all grades of heart failure (22–24). Moreover, when prescribed in patients with moderate and severe heart failure, ACE inhibitors are capable of improving survival (25–27) and in this regard appear to be superior to hydralazine-nitrate combination (26), the other prognosis-improving vasodilator regimen in heart failure (28).

These described benefits of ACE inhibitors may not all be due to the inhibition of angiotensin II formation. The preservation of bradykinin and increased production of vasodilatory prostaglandins may also have a beneficial hemodynamic effect (29,30). The development of angiotensin II receptor antagonists may help clarify the relative importance in heart failure of the varied pharmacologic effects of ACE inhibitors (31). Initial results with an angiotensin II type 1 receptor blocking agent (DuP 753) have shown that this agent produces a hemodynamic effect in this syndrome similar to that of the ACE inhibitor enalapril (32). Raya and colleagues demonstrated in the rat model of myocardial infarction that DuP 753 prevented the increase in left ventricular end-diastolic pressure that was observed in the control group in the early period following infarctions (32). Moreover, this agent also displayed an antiremodeling effect, as evidenced by a smaller end-diastolic volume index after 2 weeks of therapy. While far more experience with angiotensin II receptor antagonists is required, these preliminary data suggest that the hemodynamic effect of ACE inhibitors in heart failure is primarily due to their inhibition of angiotensin II formation.

Depletion of body stores of potassium (33), magnesium (34), and sodium (18) is a characteristic feature of heart failure, and depletion of each of these elements has been associated with a reduced survival in this syndrome

(34,35). Rendering of the myocardium more susceptible to arrhythmia most likely explains this association. These electrolyte abnormalities represent another means by which heightened activity of the RAS could influence prognosis in heart failure. Angiotensin II is an important stimulant of aldosterone and vasopressin secretion, thereby promoting hyponatremia (18) and loss of potassium (33) and magnesium (34). Angiotensin converting enzyme inhibitor therapy improves potassium (33) and magnesium (36) homeostasis and helps reverse hyponatremia (18). Whether these effects are instrumental in the improved prognosis associated with ACE inhibitors in this condition is unknown.

Tissue Renin-Angiotensin System

For many years the RAS was perceived as a circulating endocrine system. Recently, as a result of major advances in molecular biology, it has become clear that the basic elements of the RAS are synthesized in extrarenal tissue, including the heart, giving rise to the concept of the tissue-bound RAS (37,38). Data indicating local synthesis of the components of the RAS, the presence of appropriate receptors, and evidence that the elements of the system respond to modulating factors suggest that the tissue-bound RAS is distinct from the circulating RAS.

Cardiac angiotensinogen gene expression has been documented in various experimental models (39,40). Expression of this gene is modified by dietary sodium intake (41) and ACE inhibitor therapy (42). Nephrectomy, however, while affecting the expression of the angiotensinogen gene in various tissues, does not alter its expression in the myocardium, suggesting that the cardiac RAS is indeed an independent system (39). Marked increases in myocardial angiotensinogen have been documented in pressure overload ventricular hypertrophy (43). Preliminary data from a rat infarct model demonstrate increased expression of the gene in viable myocardium following infarction (44).

Renin gene expression has also been identified in myocardial tissue (45). Quantitatively, the expression of the renin gene is less marked than that of angiotensinogen, suggesting that renin may be the rate-limiting enzyme in this local tissue system (40). Like angiotensinogen, renin production would appear to be modified by various factors including dietary sodium intake (46) and various drugs (41).

Converting enzyme (CE) activity is most prominent in the lungs, but like angiotensinogen and renin, it has also been identified in the heart (47). Increased expression of the gene encoding for the CE protein has been recognized in experimental left ventricular overload (48) and ischemic heart failure (49). The importance of converting enzyme in the formation of angiotensin II is variable and may be species-dependent. In the rat, angiotensin II formation is primarily dependent on CE activity. However, in hamster and human cardiomyopathy, enzymes other than the angiotensin converting enzyme are primarily involved in the formation of angiotensin II (50). Similar findings have been noted in vascular tissue, where enzymes such as cathepsin and elastin are capable of converting angiotensin I to angiotensin II (51).

That the documentation of local synthesis of components of the RAS reflects a functionally integrated and independent RAS system is further supported by two other lines of evidence. First, in nephrectomized rats, where circulating angiotensins are undetectable, myocardial levels of angiotensin I are noted to be increased (52). Second, specific angiotensin II receptors have been identified on cardiac myocytes, coronary blood vessels, and sympathetic nerves in the myocardium, confirming the potential for an autocrine or paracrine effect of a local RAS (53).

What is the potential clinical relevance of a tissue-bound RAS in heart failure? As yet no direct evidence has linked the activity of this system to the regulation of cardiac function. However, the local RAS may play a role in ventricular remodeling following myocardial damage. Ventricular remodeling consists of several distinct pathological events including infarct expansion, myocyte slippage, eccentric and concentric hypertrophy of the remaining viable myocytes, and growth of the cardiac interstitium (54). The resultant increase in chamber size has been associated with a reduced short-term (55) as well as long-term prognosis (56). Inhibition of ventricular remodeling has been consistently achieved by ACE inhibitor therapy (57,58) and has been associated with an improvement in ventricular function and survival in an experimental model (59,60). Response to other vasodilators has been less consistent (61–63). While these data do not exclude nonspecific load reduction as the mechanism of benefit, it is possible that the tissue-bound RAS has a specific impact on these processes. Supporting a role for the local RAS are data associating angiotensin II with cardiocyte hypertrophy (9) and fibroblast proliferation (10,64). Moreover, preliminary data have demonstrated an increase in mRNA for angiotensinogen in cardiac tissue following infarction (44). Furthermore, in models of ventricular overload nonhypotensive doses of ACE inhibitors have caused regression of left ventricular mass or prevented an increase in left ventricular mass, suggesting a role for locally generated angiotensin II (65,66). Therefore, it is possible that angiotensin II has a direct effect on myocardial growth, including both cardiac myocyte hypertrophy and proliferation of the interstitial tissue. Immediately following myocardial damage the RAS may have an important role in tissue repair. Continued and unrestrained activity of this system in this period, however, may dispose to excessive and deleterious remodeling. While both experimental and clinical data have shown that ACE inhibitors can retard or prevent remodeling (57–60), the important question of the timing of this intervention remains unanswered. Delayed intervention (i.e., beyond 1 week following infarction) appears to be both safe and effective (57,58). While the data on acute intervention are scarce, work by Gay suggests that early intervention with captopril (within 2 h of infarction) has no advantage over delayed intervention, beginning at 21 days (67). This important question of when to intervene with inhibitors of the RAS in an effort to attenuate ventricular remodeling following myocardial infarction requires further study (68). The recent preliminary data from CONSENSUS II indicate no apparent survival benefit over a 6-month follow-up period from early ACE inhibitor therapy in patients with acute myocardial infarction.

It must be pointed out that bradykinin shares some of the actions of angiotensin II, including chronotropy and inotropy. Converting enzyme inhibition results in enhanced local concentration of bradykinin. The effect of bradykinin on myocyte and fibroblast growth is unclear. However, cyclic guanosine monophosphate-generating compounds, other than bradykinin, have been shown to have a direct antiproliferative effect on several tissues in vitro (12,69). It is possible, though unproven, that bradykinin may have an antigrowth effect on myocardial issue, which might partially explain the antiremodeling effect of ACE inhibitors. Future experiments using the angiotensin II and bradykinin receptor blocking agents will help elucidate the specific role of these agents in myocardial growth and remodeling.

ATRIAL NATRIURETIC PEPTIDE

Atrial natriuretic peptide (ANP) is a naturally occurring hormone first isolated in 1981 by deBold and colleagues (70). Since then, many workers have demonstrated the varied activities of ANP including diuresis, natriuresis, and vasodilation as well as inhibition of aldosterone, renin, and vasopressin release (71–74). Elevated levels of ANP have been documented in several pathological states including systemic hypertension (75) and congestive heart failure (70,71), where it is thought to have a counter-regulating influence on the activities of vasoconstrictor substances in these syndromes. Several different molecular forms of ANP have been isolated (76–78). Alpha-ANP represents the major circulatory form in humans. Beta-ANP is also found in human plasma and has a more prolonged duration of action than alpha-ANP. Conversion of beta-ANP to the alpha form can occur in the plasma. The major storage form for ANP is gamma-ANP. Its conversion to the circulatory forms of this hormone occurs either at the cellular level or immediately following secretion. Gel chromatographic analysis of atrial tissue from rats with severe heart failure reveals a predominance of alpha-ANP. This suggests that heightened conversion to the alpha form occurs at the tissue level in severe heart failure, a feature not seen in the milder forms of the disease.

Synthesis of ANP occurs predominantly in the atria. Northern blot analysis has identified mRNA for the ANP precursor (gamma-ANP) in atrial tissue (78). Moreover, a positive correlation exists between the amount of mRNA for ANP precursor found in atrial tissue and right atrial pressure (79). These data suggest that right atrial pressure or stretch is an important determinant of ANP production. Atrial myocytes, however, are not the sole source of ANP. This peptide has been identified in several other tissues including ventricular myocardium (80,81). In several of these tissues (brain, eye, and kidney) the amount of ANP is extremely low, and its presence is probably the result of binding of circulating hormone. While the concentration of ANP in the ventricular myocardium is 300 times less than in the atria, it is significantly higher than in other tissues, suggesting local synthesis of the peptide. This is consistent with the data demonstrating intracellular dense granules in ventricular myocytes in early embryonic life in several species (82). It appears that expression of the ANP gene is markedly suppressed in late embryonic life and after birth. Recent experiments suggest that this repressed genetic expression is unmasked in several pathological states associated with ventricular overload (80,81,83–85). In hypertrophied rat ventricles increased tissue levels of ANP and its mRNA have been identified (81,86). In fact, ventricular muscle ANP is an excellent marker for hypertrophy. Similar findings have been observed in experimental (87) and human (88) cardiomyopathies, where a significant correlation has been found between tissue ANP levels and increased pulmonary capillary wedge pressure. The reemergence of the fetal capacity of adult ventricular tissue to synthesize ANP in the setting of ventricular overload and hypertrophy probably represents an attempt to maintain volume homeostasis. Whether the increased capacity of the ventricle to synthesize ANP contributes to the plasma level of ANP is unknown. Data from Yasue and colleagues (88) showed a significant "step-up" in plasma ANP in the cardiac interventricular vein in patients with dilated cardiomyopathy, suggesting a contribution from the ventricle to the plasma level. Conversely, however, data from Roman et al. suggest that ventricular hypertrophy secondary to aortic valve regurgitation does not increase plasma ANP levels (80). The difference between these two studies may be explained by the difference in animal models of ventricular overload and type of hypertrophy. The failure to increase plasma ANP levels, however, does not exclude a local paracrine effect of ANP in ventricular myocardium.

As previously mentioned, increased plasma levels of ANP are present in heart failure and tend to correlate with right atrial and pulmonary capillary pressure (71). Mild increases in plasma ANP have recently been described in patients with left ventricular dysfunction but no overt heart failure (89). The cardiovascular and renal effects of ANP probably act to counterbalance the various vasoconstrictor systems activated in congestive heart failure. Accordingly, the administration of exogenous ANP would seem to be an attractive approach to the management of this syndrome. Studies have demonstrated that exogenously administered ANP can improve cardiac function (71) and inhibit aldosterone secretion in patients with heart failure in a manner similar to other vasodilators. However, the renal effects of this substance appear to be attenuated in the setting of heart failure. The preservation of the extrarenal effects of ANP argues against a generalized receptor down-regulation to explain the loss of renal responsiveness. Increased intrarenal enzymatic degradation of ANP by neutral endopeptidases (NEP) may explain the diminished diuretic and natriuretic effect of exogenously administered ANP in heart failure. Neutral endopeptidase is highly concentrated at the proximal tubule brush border of the kidney. Attenuation of this enzyme by a synthetic NEP inhibitor has been shown to significantly increase the renal effects of ANP, as evidenced by increased diuresis, natriuresis, and urinary production of cyclic guanosine monophosphate (90,91). The acute hemodynamic effects of NEP inhibitors are minimal, but their long-term effects are poorly defined. This enzyme inhibitor may possibly provide a useful approach to the management of heart failure, and clinical trials are currently under way.

The potent cardiovascular, renal, and neurohumoral effects of ANP have been well defined. Recent in vitro work additionally suggests that this substance may also have a moderating effect on cell growth. Atrial natriuretic peptide has an antiproliferative effect on renal mesangial cells, smooth muscle cells, and endothelial cells (92–94). Contradictory results, however, have been documented with zona glomerulosa cells (95,96). It is possible, therefore, that ANP, like some other endogenous and exogenous vasodilators, may have a direct antigrowth effect distinct from its vasomotor action. The significance of these in vitro findings needs to be further clarified. It is interesting to speculate that the increased expression of mRNA for ANP in ventricular myocardium in the setting of increased workload may represent an attempt to prevent the hypertrophic process from becoming excessive.

ARGININE VASOPRESSIN (ANTIDIURETIC HORMONE)

Increased activity of the sympathetic nervous system and the RAS contributes to the elevated systemic vascular resistance that is characteristic of congestive heart failure. The role of the human antidiuretic hormone arginine vasopressin (AVP) in this setting is less clear. It is known that AVP is a potent vasoconstrictor (97,98). Plasma levels of this hormone can be elevated in heart failure (99), but this is not a uniform finding (100). Elevated levels of this hormone have also been documented in patients with left ventricular dysfunction but no overt heart failure (89). Moreover, hemodynamic improvement has been associated with lowering of AVP levels in those patients with very elevated basal AVP levels (101). The synthesis and release of AVP from the posterior hypothalamus in normal and pathological states is regulated by osmotic and nonosmotic stimuli (102,103). Osmotic stimuli include hyponatremia, while excessive diuresis and hypotension, reflex control mechanisms, and angiotensin II act as nonosmotic stimuli (102,103). The primary stimulus for increased AVP in heart failure is probably nonosmotic in nature, but this issue remains unresolved. It is possible that increased angiotensin II levels stimulate the release of AVP from the posterior pituitary. In heart failure, drugs other than diuretics can influence plasma AVP levels. Digitalis, for example, may actually reduce AVP levels through sensitizing of cardiac baroceptors (104). The physiological effects of AVP are mediated through activation of so-called V_1 and V_2 receptors. The V_1 receptors are found mainly in vascular tissue, where they subserve vasoconstriction. The renal-tubular effects of AVP are mediated via the V_2 receptors, which are coupled to cAMP production. V_2 receptors may also be found in vascular tissue, where they subserve vasodilation in response to high concentrations of AVP, and V_2 receptors are also involved in the sensitization of arterial baroreceptors (105).

Elevated levels of AVP are most commonly found in patients who have severe heart failure. Moreover, increased pituitary gland mRNA for the prehormone for AVP has been documented in heart failure in the rat (106). Increased plasma levels of AVP have, however, not been a consistent feature of this syndrome (99,100,107). Goldsmith and colleagues demonstrated a significant average increase in plasma AVP in heart failure patients compared with normal individuals (99). The level of AVP did not correlate with serum sodium, plasma norepinephrine, or any hemodynamic variable. There was a weak correlation with plasma renin activity. Creager and colleagues could document an increase in plasma AVP in only three of ten patients with heart failure (107). In the presence of similar degrees of ventricular dysfunction and neuroendocrine activation, this variability in plasma AVP is unexplained.

The recent development of an AVP antagonist has helped ascertain the pathophysiological role of AVP in heart failure. In a rat model of heart failure a specific V_1 receptor antagonist reduced mean arterial pressure and increased venous capacitance (108). The mean AVP level in these rats was significantly greater than in normal controls (18.6 ± 3.2 vs 3.5 ± 0.9 pg/ml, $p = 0.001$). Nicod and colleagues examined the effect of the same compound in humans with moderate to severe heart failure (109). Only one of ten patients in this group responded favorably. The remaining nine showed no significant change in mean arterial pressure or ventricular filling pressures. The mean AVP level in the nonresponders was 2.3 pg/ml, which is not significantly increased above normal. The one responder in this experiment had an AVP level of 55 pg/ml. A similar finding has been documented by Creager and colleagues (107). Three of ten patients had elevated plasma levels of AVP. These patients were the only ones in this group who responded to the AVP antagonist by demonstrating a significant drop in systemic vascular resistance. These data suggest that elevated AVP levels may have only a limited role in the genesis of increased systemic vascular resistance in heart failure. However, in those patients with an elevated AVP level, use of a specific V_1 antagonist (e.g., OPC-21268) may be of at least short-term hemodynamic benefit.

ENDOTHELIAL VASOACTIVE SUBSTANCES

Over the last 10 years intense research interest has focused on the role of the endothelium in the control of vascular tone (110). Two important moieties, endothelium-derived relaxation factor (EDRF) and endothelin, have been identified and have been demonstrated to possess significant effects on vascular tone. Endothelium-derived relaxation factor mediates vasodilatation by stimulating the production of cyclic guanosine monophosphate via a short-acting (second) mediator, nitric oxide (NO). A variety of signals, including acetylcholine, thrombin, AVP, and changes in blood flow can stimulate the release of EDRF. Endothelin, on the other hand, is one of the most potent vasoconstrictors known to man (111). Its mechanism of action is less clear than that of EDRF, but preliminary data suggest that endothelin acts via a receptor to activate the inositol triphosphate (IP_3) and diacylglycerol (DAG) pathways (111). Specific defects in EDRF activity have been identified in an experimental model of heart failure in a setting where the response to nonspecific vasodilators is preserved (112). Preliminary data from human subjects with heart failure suggest a similar defect in endothelially mediated vasodilatation (113). Forearm blood flow response to methacholine, a muscarinic agonist that stimulates EDRF release, was attenuated in heart failure subjects compared with normal controls. Patients maintained a normal response to non-EDRF-mediated vasodilatation, as evidenced by the blood flow response to nitroprusside (113).

In an experimental canine model of heart failure produced by rapid ventricular pacing, plasma endothelin levels were significantly elevated in comparison with a group of normal dogs (114). Moreover, endothelin levels were correlated with left and right ventricular filling pressures. Endothelin levels in plasma are also elevated in clinical heart failure (115). Hiroe and colleagues have demonstrated an association between plasma endothelin levels and New York Heart Association functional classification and left ventricular fractional shortening as assessed by echocardiography (115). Apart from its potent vasoconstrictor properties endothelin, like other endogenous vasoconstrictors, may be a growth-promoting substance. In vitro work has demonstrated that endothelin can stimulate smooth muscle cell growth (116). Clinical studies demonstrating increased endothelin levels in patients with atherosclerosis (117) and pulmonary hypertension (118) suggest that endothelin may have a role in vascular remodeling. Its influence on myocardial remodeling has not been investigated. The pathophysiologic relevance of endothelin in heart failure and other conditions will be further clarified by the use of antiendothelin antibodies and further experiments.

NEUROPEPTIDE Y

The 36-amino-acid peptide neuropeptide Y (NPY) is an important part of the sympathetic nervous system and is secreted along with norepinephrine from central and peripheral neurons (119). Neuropeptide Y is a known vasoconstrictor (120), but, unlike the catecholamines, this peptide exerts a negative inotropic and chronotropic effect on the myocardium (121). It acts through a receptor that is coupled to the inhibitory guanosine triphosphate binding protein (G_i)and IP_3 and DAG. Elevated levels of this neuropeptide have been documented in heart failure (122) and are correlated with plasma norepinephrine levels. It is possible that NPY contributes to the deterioration in ventricular function in end-stage heart failure by inhibiting cAMP, especially as the function of G_i, which mediates the action of neuropeptide Y (123), is augmented in myocardial tissue of patients with severe heart failure (124).

β-ENDORPHIN

Elevated levels of plasma β-endorphin have been documented in heart failure and are correlated with the severity of the disease and with exercise tolerance (125). Antagonists to this opiate, which is primarily released from the pituitary, have been shown to improve hemodynamic function in a canine model of heart failure (126,127) and to improve abnormalities in reflex control mechanisms. The hemodynamic effect of opiate antagonists in clinical heart failure has not been clearly defined, but they have been shown to increase cardiac output and reduce systemic vascular resistance in various forms of shock (127). Further study of this neurohormone is required to clarify its prognostic impact and effects on ventricular function (128).

CALCITONIN GENE-RELATED PEPTIDE

Recently the effects of calcitonin gene-related peptides (CGRP) on myocardial function have been described in experimental and clinical heart failure (129). While the data are still limited, the initial work suggests a potential role for CGRP in this syndrome. These substances have been identified in the central and peripheral nervous system as well as in the myocardium and vasculature (130,131). They exert receptor-mediated cardiovascular effects in humans and several animal species that result in marked systemic vasodilatation, tachycardia, and positive inotropy, though the contractile influence of CGRP may be species-dependent (132). These effects are not influenced by adrenergic, histaminergic, or prostaglandin-synthesis blockade. Elevated levels of CGRP have been identified in human heart failure (129), but as with many other neurohormones there is a wide variation in values and poor correlation with hemodynamic status. Exogenously administered CGRP produces a dose-dependent vasodilator effect in clinical heart failure, with low doses demonstrating a predominant arterial dilator effect and larger doses behaving as a mixed vasodilator (129). The preferential effect on the arterial circulation is in agreement with earlier data on the effect of CGRP on forearm blood flow in normal humans (133). Systemic vasodilation was associated with an increase in stroke volume index, which probably does not reflect a positive inotropic action of this substance (129). Calcitonin gene-related peptides also produced a beneficial hemodynamic effect in an animal model of heart failure, one that was associated with an improvement in renal blood flow (129).

Further work is needed to identify the importance of CGRP in the pathogenesis of heart failure and its potential role in the management of this condition.

OTHER SUBSTANCES

Several other neuropeptides have been isolated. Whether these substances have a role in congestive heart failure is unclear. Other members of the ANP family have been discovered, including brain natriuretic peptide (BNP). Urodilatin may be the major form of this group of compounds in the urine

(134). The role of BNP and urodilatin in the regulation of sodium fluid homeostasis in heart failure requires further study. Vasoactive intestinal peptide (VIP) and substance P (SP) also both affect cardiovascular function. Vasoactive intestinal peptide immunoreactive neurons have been identified in mammalian heart tissue, including humans. They are more prominent in atrial and conduction tissue as compared with ventricular tissue. Vasoactive intestinal peptide possesses positive chronotropic (135,136) and inotropic effects (136,137), facilitates atrioventricular conduction in animal models, (138) and vasodilates the coronary and systemic vasculature (139). Substance P, which co-localizes with CGRP, also demonstrates vasodilatory potential and induces tachycardia (140). Because of these cardiovascular activities, the role of these substances in heart failure warrants investigation.

SUMMARY

Congestive cardiac failure is characterized by the activation of an array of neurohumoral systems. Many of these systems interact with each other. The hemodynamic effects of several of these substances have now been well defined. Further research to determine whether they contribute importantly to vasoconstriction or vasodilatation in heart failure will be required. Future research may provide further important data on the potential proliferative and antiproliferative effects of many of these neurohormones, and should help clarify whether such neurohormonal factors have a role in controlling myocardial remodeling following damage.

REFERENCES

1. Francis GS. Neuroendocrine activity in congestive heart failure. Am J Cardiol 1990; 66(suppl D):33D–39D.
2. Cohn JN, Levine TB, Olivari MT, Garberg V, Lira D, Francis GS, Simon AB, Rector T. Plasma norepinephrine as a guide to prognosis in patients with congestive heart failure. N Engl J Med 1984; 311:819–823.
3. Cody RJ. Angiotensin II-mediated vasoconstriction in chronic congestive heart failure, and response to to converting enzyme inhibition. Am J Med 1984; 77:71–77.
4. Goldsmith SR, Francis GS, Cowley AW, Levine TB, Cohn JN. Increased plasma arginine vasopressin levels in congestive heart failure. J Am Coll Cardiol 1983; 1:1385–1390.
5. Gottlieb SG, Kukin ML, Ahern D, Packer M. Prognostic importance of atrial natriuretic peptide in patients with chronic heart failure. J Am Coll Cardiol 1989; 13:1534–1539.

6. Geisterfer AAT, Peach MJ, Owens GK. Angiotensin II induces hypertrophy, not hyperplasia, of cultured rat aortic smooth muscle cells. Circ Res 1988; 62:749–756.
7. Geisterfer AAT, Owens GK. Arginine vasopressin-induced hypertrophy of cultured rat aortic smooth muscle cells. Hypertension 1989; 14:413–420.
8. Simpson P. Norepinephrine-stimulated hypertrophy of cultural rat myocardial cells is an $alpha_1$ adrenergic response. J Clin Invest 1983; 72:732–738.
9. Baker KM, Aceto JF. Angiotensin II stimulation of protein synthesis and cell growth in chick heart cells. Am J Physiol 1990; 259:H610–H618.
10. Weber KT, Brilla CG. Pathological hypertrophy and cardiac interstitium: Fibrosis and the renin-angiotensin-aldosterone system. Circulation 1991; 83:1849–1865.
11. Boucek RJ, Noble WL. Histamine, norepinephrine and bradykinin stimulation of fibroblast growth and modification of serotonin response. Proc Soc Exp Biol Med 1973; 144:929–933.
12. Itoh H, Pratt RE, Dzau VJ. Atrial natriuretic polypeptide inhibits hypertrophy of vascular smooth muscle cells. J Clin Invest 1990; 86:1690–1697.
13. Merrill AJ, Morrison JL, Brannon ES. Concentration of renin in renal venous blood in patients with chronic heart failure. Am J Med 1946; 1:468–472.
14. Riegger GAJ, Liebau G, Holzschah M, Witkowski D, Steilner H, Kochsiek K. Role of the renin-angiotensin system in the development of congestive heart failure in the dog as assessed by chronic converting enzyme inhibition. Am J Cardiol 1984; 53:614–618.
15. Brown JJ, Davies DL, Johnson VW, Lever AF, Robertson JIS. Renin relationships in congestive heart failure, treated and untreated. Am Heart J 1970; 80:329–342.
16. Davis JO, Freeman RH. Mechanisms regulating renin release. Physiol Rev 1976; 56:1–56.
17. Curtiss C, Cohn JN, Vrobel T, Franciosa JA. Role of the renin-angiotensin system in the systemic vasoconstriction of chronic congestive heart failure. Circulation 1978; 58:763–769.
18. Levine TB, Franciosa JA, Vrobel T, Cohn JN. Hyponatremia as a marker for high renin heart failure. Br Heart J 1982; 47:161–166.
19. Schaer GL, Covit AB, Laragh JH, Cody RJ. Association of hyponatremia with increased renin activity in chronic congestive heart failure: Impact of diuretic therapy. Am J Cardiol 1983; 51:1635–1638.
20. Colucci WS, Willimas GH, Alexander RW, Braunwald E. Mechanisms and implications of vasodilator tolerance in the treatment of congestive heart failure. Am J Med 1981; 71:89–97.
21. Cohn JN. Vasodilator therapy for heart failure: the influence of impedance on left ventricular performance. Circulation 1973; 48:5–8.
22. Dzau VJ, Colucci WS, Williams GH, Curfman G, Meggs L. Sustained effectiveness of converting enzyme inhibition in patients with severe congestive heart failure. N Engl J Med 1980; 302:1373–1379.

23. Levine TB, Franciosa JA, Cohn JN. Acute and long-term response to an oral converting-enzyme inhibitor, captopril, in congestive heart failure. Circulation 1980; 62:35–41.
24. Captopril-Digoxin Multicenter Research Group. Comparative effects of therapy with captopril and digoxin in patients with mild to moderate heart failure. JAMA 1988; 259:539–544.
25. CONSENSUS Trial Study Group. Effects of enalapril on mortality in severe congestive heart failure: results of the Cooperative North Scandinavian Enalapril Survival Study (CONSENSUS). N Engl J Med 1987; 316:1429–1435.
26. Cohn JN, Johnson G, Ziesche S, Cobb F, Francis GS, Tristani F, Smith R, Dunkman WB, Loeb H, Wang M, Bhat G, Goldman S, Fletcher RD, Doherty J, Hughes CV, Carson P, Cintron G, Shabetai R, Haakenson C. A comparison of enalapril with hydralazine-isosorbide dinitrate in the treatment of congestive cardiac failure. N Engl J Med 1991; 325:303–310.
27. The SOLVD Investigators. Effect of enalapril on survival in patients with reduced left ventricular ejection fractions and congestive heart failure. N Engl J Med 1991; 325:293–302.
28. Cohn JN, Archibald DG, Ziesche S, Franciosa JA, Harston WE, Tristani FE, Dunkman WB, Jacobs W, Francis GS, Flohr KH, Goldman S, Cobb FR, Shah PM, Saunders R, Fletcher KD, Loeb HS, Hughes VC, Barker B. Effect of vasodilator therapy on mortality in chronic congestive heart failure. N Engl J Med 1986; 314:1547–1552.
29. Packer M. Interaction of prostaglandins and angiotensin II in the modulation of renal function in congestive heart failure. Circulation 1988; 77(suppl 1): 64–73.
30. Zusman RM. Renin and non-renin mediated antihypertensive action of converting enzyme inhibition. Kidney Int 1984; 25:969–983.
31. Timmermans PBMWM, Cairni DJ, Chiu AT, Duncia JV, Price WA, Wells GJ, Wong PC, Johnson AL, Wexler RR. The discovery of a new class of highly specific nonpeptide angiotensin II receptor antagonists. Am J Hypertension 1991; 4(suppl 2):275–281.
32. Raya TE, Fonker SJ, Lee RW, Daughterty S, Goldman S, Wang PC, Timmermans PBMWM, Morkin E. Hemodynamic effects of direct angiotensin II blockade compared to converting enzyme inhibition in a rat model of heart failure. Am J Hypertension 1991; 4(suppl 2):334S–340S.
33. Dargie HJ. Interrelation of electrolytes and renin-angiotensin system in congestive heart failure. Am J Cardiol 1990; 65:28E–32E.
34. Gottlieb SG, Baruch L, Kukin ML, Bernstein JL, Fisher ML, Packer M. Prognostic importance of the serum magnesium concentration in patients with congestive heart failure. J Am Coll Cardiol 1990; 16:827–831.
35. Cleland JGF, Dargie HJ, Ford I. Mortality in heart failure: Clinical variables of prognostic value. Br Heart J 1987; 58:572–582.
36. Stevenson RN, Keywood C, Amadi AA, Davies JR, Patterson DLH. Angiotensin converting enzyme inhibition and magnesium conservation in patients with congestive heart failure. Br Heart J 1991; 66:19–21.

37. Dzau VJ. Circulating versus local renin-angiotensin system in cardiovascular homeostasis. Circulation 1988; 77(suppl 1):1–4.
38. Lindpainter K, Garten D. The cardiac renin-angiotensin system. An appraisal of present experimental and clinical evidence. Circ Res 1991; 68:905–921.
39. Campbell DJ, Habener JF. The angiotensinogen gene is expressed and differently regulated in multiple tissues of the rat. J Clin Invest 1986; 78:31–39.
40. Dzau VJ, Ellison KE, Brody T, Ingelfinger J, Pratt R. A comparative study of the distribution of renin and angiotensinogen messenger ribonucleic acids in rat and mouse tissues. Endocrinology 1987; 120:2334–2338.
41. Dzau VJ. Cardiac renin-angiotensin system: Molecular and function aspects. Am J Med 1988; 84:22–27.
42. Li C, Prakash O, Re RN. Altered regulation of angiotensin gene expression in the left ventricle of the hypertensive rat (abstr). Circulation 1989; 80:II-450.
43. Baker KM, Chernin MI, Wixson SK, Aceto JF. Renin-angiotensin system involvement in pressure overload cardiac hypertrophy in rats. Am J Physiol 1990; 2593:H324–H332.
44. Drexler H, Lindpainter K, Lu W, Schieffer B, Ganten D. Transient increase in the expression of cardiac angiotensinogen in a rat model of myocardial infarction and failure (abstr). Circulation 1989; 80:II–459.
45. Dzau VJ, Re RN. Evidence for the existence of renin in the heart. Circulation 1987; 75(suppl 1):134–136.
46. Dzau VJ, Ingelfinger JR, Pratt RE. Regulation of tissue renin and angiotensinogen gene expression. J Cardiovasc Pharmacol 1986; 8:S11–S16.
47. Cushman DW, Cheung HS. Concentrations of angiotensin converting enzyme in tissues of the rat. Biochem Biophys Act 1971; 250:261–265.
48. Lorell BH, Schunkert H, Grice WN, Tang SS, Apstein CS, Dzau VJ. Alteration in cardiac converting enzyme activity in pressure overload hypertrophy (abstr). Circulation 1989; 80:II–297.
49. Fabris B, Jackson B, Kohzuki M, Perich R, Johnston CI. Increased cardiac angiotensin-converting enzyme in rats with chronic heart failure. Clin Exp Pharmacol Physiol 1990; 17:309–314.
50. Urata H, Healy B, Stewart RW, Bumpus FM, Husain A. Angiotensin-II forming pathways in normal and failing human hearts. Circ Res 1990; 66:883–890.
51. Dzau VJ. Possible prorenin activating mechanisms in the blood vessel wall. J Hypertension 1987; 5(suppl 2):15–18.
52. Unger T, Ganten D, Long SE. Tissue converting enzyme and cardiovascular actions of converting enzyme inhibitors. J Cardiovasc Pharmacol 1986; 8(suppl):75–81.
53. Urata H, Healy B, Stewart RN, Bumpus FM, Husain A. Angiotensin II receptors in normal and failing human hearts. J Clin Endocardial Metab 1989; 69:54–66.

54. Pfeffer MA, Braunwald E. Ventricular remodeling after myocardial infarction. Experimental observations and clinical implications. Circulation 1990; 81:1161–1172.
55. Pirolo JS, Hutchins GM, Moore JW. Infarct expansion: pathologic analysis of 204 patients with a single myocardial infarct. J Am Coll Cardiol 1986; 7:349–354.
56. Hammermeister KE, DeRouen TA, Dodge HT. Variables predictive of survival in patients with coronary disease. Circulation 1979: 59:421–430.
57. Pfeffer MA, Lamas GA, Vaughan DE, Parisi AF, Braunwald E. Effect of captopril an progressive ventricular dilatation after anterior myocardial infarction. N Engl J Med 1988; 319:80–86.
58. Sharpe N, Murphy J, Smith H, Hannan S. Preventive treatment of asymptomatic left ventricular dysfunction following myocardial infarction. Eur Heart J 1990; 11(suppl B):147–156.
59. Pfeffer JM, Pfeffer MA, Braunwald E. Influence of chronic captopril therapy on the infarcted left ventricle of the rat. Circ Res 1985; 57:84–95.
60. Pfeffer JM, Pfeffer MA, Steinberg C, Finn P. Survival after an experimental myocardial infarction: beneficial effects of long-term therapy with captopril. Circulation 1985; 72:406–412.
61. Raya TE, Gay RG, Aguire M, Goldman S. Importance of venodilatation in prevention of left ventricular dilatation after chronic large myocardial infarction in rats: a comparison of captopril and hydralazine. Circ Res 1989; 64:336–337.
62. McDonald KM, Francis GS, Matthews J, Carlyle PF, Hauer K, Wennburg P, Hunter D, Cohn JN. The effect of $alpha_1$ adrenoceptor blockade on ventricular remodeling in the dog (abstr). Circulation 1990; 82(suppl III):48.
63. McDonald KM, Francis GS, Matthews J, Hunter DW, Cohn JN. Oral nitrate therapy prevents early left ventricular mass increase following left ventricular damage. J Am Coll Cardiol (in press).
64. Weber KT, Janicki JS. Angiotensin and the remodeling of the myocardium. Br J Clin Pharmacol 1989; 28:141S–150S.
65. Baker KM, Chernin MI, Wilson SK, Aceto JF. Renin-angiotensin system involvement in pressure-overload cardiac hypertrophy in rats. Am J Physiol 1990; 259:H324–H332.
66. Linz W, Scholkens BA, Ganten D. Converting enzyme inhibition specifically prevents the development and induces regression of cardiac hypertrophy in rats. Clin Exp Hyper Theory Practice 1989; AII(7):1325–1350.
67. Gay RG. Early and late effects of captopril treatment after large myocardial infarction in rats. J Am Coll Cardiol 1990; 16:967–977.
68. Nabel EG, Topol EJ, Galeana A, Ellis SG, Bates ER, Werns SW, Walter JA, Maller DW, Schwanger M, Pitt B. A randomized placebo-controlled trial of combined early intravenous captopril and recombinant tissue type plasminogen activator therapy in acute myocardial infarction. J Am Coll Cardiol 1991; 17:467–473.

69. Garg UC, Hassid A. Nitric-oxide generating vasodilators and 8-Bromo-cyclic guanosine monophosphate inhibit mitogenesis and proliferation of cultured rat vascular smooth muscle cells. J Clin Invest 1989; 83:1774–1777.
70. deBold AJ, Borenstein HB, Veress AT, Sonnenberg H. A rapid and potent natriuretic response to intravenous injection of atrial myocardial extract in rats. Life Sci 1981; 28:89–94.
71. Cody RJ, Atlas SA, Laragh JH, Kubo SH, Covit AB, Ryman KS, Shaknovich A, Pondolfino K, Clark M, Camargo MJF, Scarborough RM, Lewicki JA. Atrial natriuretic factor in normal subjects and heart failure patients. J Clin Invest 1986; 78:1362–1374.
72. Saito Y, Nakao K, Nishimura K, Sugawara A, Okumura K, Obata K, Sonoda R, Ban T, Yasue H, Imura H. Clinical application of atrial natriuretic polypeptide in patients with congestive heart failure: beneficial effects on left ventricular function. Circulation 1987; 76:115–124.
73. Maack T, Marion DN, Camargo MJF, Kleinert HD, Laragh JH, Vaughan ED, Atlas SA. Effects of auriculin (atrial natriuretic factor) on blood pressure, renal function and the renin-aldosterone system in the dog. Am J Med 1984; 77:1069–1075.
74. Samson WK. Atrial natriuretic factor inhibits dehydration and hemorrhage-induced vasopressin release. Neuroendocrinology 1985; 40:277–279.
75. Sugawara A, Nakao K, Sakamoto M, Morii N, Yamada T, Itoh H, Shiono S, Imura H. Plasma concentration of atrial natriuretic polypeptide in essential hypertension. Lancet 1985; 2:1426–1427.
76. Bloch KD, Scott JA, Zisfien JB, Fallon JT, Margolis MN, Seidma CE, Matsueda GR, Homcy CJ, Graham RM, Seidman JG. Biosynthesis and secretion of proatrial natriuretic factor by cultured rat cardiocytes. Science 1985; 230:1168–1171.
77. Sugawara A, Nakao K, Morii N, Yamada T, Itoh H, Shiono S, Saito Y, Mukoyama M, Arai H, Nishimura K, Obata K, Yasue H, Ban T, Imura H. Synthesis of atrial natriuretic polypeptide (ANP) in human failing hearts evidence for altered processing of ANP precursors and augmented synthesis of beta-human ANP. J Clin Invest 1988; 81:1962–1970.
78. Imura H, Nakao K. Atrial natriuretic peptide in heart failure: altered gene expression and processing and possible pathophysiological significance. In: Dollery CT, Sherwood LM, eds. Cardiac and Renal Failure: An Expanding Role for ACE Inhibitors. Philadelphia: Hanley and Belfus, 1989; 129–142.
79. Cantin M, Genest J. The heart and the atrial natriuretic factor. Endocr Rev 1985; 6:107–127.
80. Roman MJ, Devereux RB, Atlas SA, Pini R, Ganau A, Hochreiter C, Niles NW, Borer JS, Laragh JH. Relationship of atrial natriuretic factor to left ventricular volume and mass. Am Heart J 1989; 118:1236–1242.
81. Matsubara H, Yamamoto J, Hirata Y, Mori Y, Oikawa S, Inada M. Changes of atrial natriuretic peptide and its messenger RNA with development and regression of cardiac hypertrophy in renovascular hypertensive rats. Circ Res 1990; 66:176–184.

82. Kikuchi K, Nakao K, Hayaski R, Morii N, Sugawara A, Sakamoto M, Imura H, Midawa H. Ontogeny of atrial natriuretic polypeptide in human heart. Acta Endocrinol 1987; 115:211–217.
83. Day ML, Schwartz D, Wiegand RC, Stockman PT, Brunnert SR, Tolunay E, Currie MS, Standaert DG, Needleman P. Ventricular atriopeptide. Unmasking of messenger RNA and peptide synthesis by hypertrophy or dexamethasone. Hypertension 1987; 9:485–491.
84. Drexler H, Hanze J, Finckh M, Lu W, Just H, Lang RE. Atrial natriuretic peptide in a rat model of cardiac failure. Circulation 1989; 79:620–633.
85. Edwards BS, Ackerman DM, Lee ME, Reeder GS, Wold LE, Burnett JC Jr. Identification of atrial natriuretic factor within ventricular tissue in hamsters and humans with congestive heart failure. J Clin Invest 1988; 81:82–86.
86. Arai H, Nakao K, Saito Y, Morii N, Sugawara S, Yamada T, Itoh H, Shiono S, Mukoyama M, Ohkubo H, Nakanishi S, Imura H. Augmented expression of atrial natriuretic polypeptide (ANP) gene in ventricles of spontaneously hypertensive rats (SHR) and SHR-stroke prone rats. Circ Res 1988; 62:926–930.
87. Riegger GAJ, Elsner D, Kromer EP, Daffner C, Forssmann WG, Muders F, Pascher EW, Kochsiek K. Atrial natriuretic peptide in congestive heart failure in the dog: plasma levels, cyclic guanosine monophosphate, ultrastructure of atrial myoendocrine cells and hemodynamic, hormonal and renal effects. Circulation 1988; 77:398–406.
88. Yasue H, Obata K, Okumura K, Kurose M, Ogawa H, Matsuyama K, Nakao K, Imura H. Increased secretion of atrial natriuretic peptide from the left ventricle in patients with dilated cardiomyopathy. J Clin Invest 1989; 83:46–51.
89. Francis GS, Benedict C, Johnstone DE, Kirlin PC, Nicklas J, Liang C-S, Kubo SH, Ruder-Toretsky E, Yusuf S. Comparison of neuroendocrine activation in patients with left ventricular dysfunction with and without congestive heart failure: a substudy of the studies of left ventricular dysfunction (SOLVD). Circulation 1990; 82:1724–1729.
90. Granger JP. Inhibitors of ANF metabolism. Circulation 1990; 82:313–315.
91. Cavero PG, Margulies KB, Winaver J, Seymour M, Delaney NG, Burnett JC Jr. Cardiorenal actions of neutral endopeptidase inhibition in experimental congestive heart failure. Circulation 1990; 82:196–201.
92. Johnson A, Lermioglu F, Garg UC, Morgan-Boyd R, Hassid A. A novel biological effect of atrial natriuretic hormone: inhibition of mesangial cell mitogenesis. Biochem Biophys Res Commun 1988; 152:893–897.
93. Itoh H, Pratt RE, Dzau VJ. Atrial natriuretic polypeptide inhibits hypertrophy of vascular smooth muscle cells. J Clin Invest 1990; 86:1690–1697.
94. Itoh H, Pratt RE, Dzau VJ. A novel action of atrial natriuretic polypeptide (ANP) as an anti-growth factor of endothelial cells (abstr). Clin Res 1991; 39:286.

95. Mazzocchi G, Rebuffat P, Nussdorfer GG. Atrial natriuretic factor (ANF) inhibits the growth and the secretory activity of rat adrenal zona glomerulosa cells in vivo. J Steroid Biochem 1987; 28:643–646.
96. Horiba N, Nomura K, Saito Y, Demura H, Shizune K. Rat atrial natriuretic polypeptide stimulation of adrenal zona glomerulosa cell growth. Biochem Biophys Res Commun 1985; 132:261–263.
97. Mantani JP, Liard JF, Schoun J, Mohring J. Hemodynamic effects of exogenous and endogenous vasopressin at low plasma concentration in conscious dogs. Circ Res 1980; 47:346–355.
98. Aisenbrey G, Handelman WA, Arnold P, Manning M, Schrier R. Vascular effects of arginine vasopressin during fluid deprivation in the rat. J Clin Invest 1981; 67:961–968.
99. Goldsmith SR, Francis GS, Cowley AW, Levine TB, Cohn JN. Increased plasma arginine vasopressin levels in patients with congestive heart failure. J Am Coll Cardiol 1983; 1:1385–1390.
100. Anand IS, Rerrari R, Kalra GS, Wahi PL, Poole-Wilson PA, Harris PC. Edema of cardiac origin. Circulation 1989; 80:299–305.
101. Bichet DG, Kortas C, Mettauer B, Manzini C, Marc-Aureli J, Rouleau JL, Schrier RW. Modulation of plasma and platelet vasopressin by cardiac function in patients with heart failure. Kidney Int 1986; 29:1188–1196.
102. Schrier RW, Berl T, Anderson RJ. Osmotic and nonosmotic control of vasopressin release. Am J Physiol 1979; 236:F321–F332.
103. Schrier RW. Pathogenesis of sodium and water retention in high-output and low-output cardiac failure, nephrotic syndrome, cirrhosis and pregnancy. N Engl J Med 1988; 319:1058–1064 (Part 1) and 1127–1134 (Part 2).
104. Thames MD, Waickman CA, Abboud FM. Sensitization of cardiac receptors (vagal afferents) by intracoronary acetylstrophanthidin. Am J Physiol 1980; 239:H628–H635.
105. Cowley AW, Switzer S, Guinn M. Evidence and quantification of the vasopressin arterial pressure control system in dogs. Cir Res 1980; 46:58–67.
106. Kim JK, Michel JB, Soubrier F, Durr J, Corvol P, Schrier RW. Arginine vasopressin gene expression in chronic cardiac failure in rats. Kidney Int 1990; 38:818–822.
107. Creager MA, Faxon DP, Cutter SS, Kohlmann O, Tyan TJ, Gavras H. Contribution of vasopressin to vasoconstriction in patients with congestive heart failure: Comparison with the renin-angiotensin system and the sympathetic nervous system. J Am Coll Cardiol 1986; 7:758–765.
108. Raya TE, Gay RG, Goldman S. Selective vasopressin inhibition in rats with heart failure decreases afterload and results in venodilatation. J Pharm Exp Ther 1990; 255:1015–1020.
109. Nicod P, Waeber B, Bussien JP, Goy JJ, Turini G, Wassberger J, Hofbauer KG, Brunner HR. Acute hemodynamic effect of a vascular antagonist of vasopressin patients with congestive heart failure. Am J Cardiol 1985; 55:1043–1047.

110. Furchgott RF. The role of endothelium in the response of vascular smooth muscle to drugs. Annu Rev Pharmacol Toxicol 1984; 31:186–194.
111. Yanagisawa M, Kurihara H, Kimura S, Tomoke Y, Kobayaski M, Mitsui Y, Yazaki Y, Goto K, Masaki T. A novel potent vasoconstrictor peptide produced by vascular endothelial cells. Nature 1988; 332:411.
112. Kaiser L, Spickard RC, Oliver NB. Heart failure depresses endothelium-dependent responses in canine femoral artery. Am J Physiol 1989; 256:H962.
113. Kubo SH, Rector TS, Williams RE, Bank AJ, Heifetz SM. Endothelium dependent vasodilation is attenuated in patients with heart failure. Circulation 1991; 84:1589–1596.
114. Margulies KB, Hildebrand FL, Lerman A, Perrella MA, Burnett Jr JC. Increased endothelin in experimental heart failure. Circulation 1990; 82:2226–2230.
115. Hiroe M, Hirata Y, Fujita N, Umezawa S, Hiroshi I, Tsujino M, Koike A, Nogami A, Takamoto T, Marumo F. Plasma endothelin levels in idiopathic dilated cardiomyopathy. Am J Cardiol 1991; 68:1114–1115.
116. Dubin D, Pratt RE, Cooke JP, Dzau VJ. Endothelin, a potent vasoconstrictor, is a vascular smooth muscle mitogen. J Vasc Med Biol 1989; 1:150–154.
117. Lerman A, Edwards BS, Hallett JW, Heublein DM, Sandberg SM, Burnett JC Jr. Circulating and tissue endothelin immunoreactivity in advanced atherosclerosis. N Engl J Med 1991; 325:997–1001.
118. Stewart DJ, Levy RD, Cernacek P, Langleben D. Increased plasma endothelin-1 in pulmonary hypertension: marker or mediator of disease: Ann Intern Med 1991; 114:464–469.
119. Tatemoto K. Neuropeptide Y. Complete amino acid sequence of the brain peptide. Proc Natl Acad Sci USA 1982; 79:5485–5489.
120. Rioux F, Bachelard H, Mortel J-C, St. Pierre S. The vasoconstrictor effect of neuropeptide Y and related peptides in the guinea pig isolated heart. Peptides 1986; 7:27–31.
121. Zukowska-Grojec Z, Marks ES, Haass M. Neuropeptide Y is a potent vasoconstrictor and cardiopressant in the rat. Am J Physiol 1987; 251: H1234–H1239.
122. Maisel AS, Scott NE, Motulsky HJ, Michel MC, Boublik JH, Rivier JE, Ziegler M, Allen RS, Brown MR. Elevation of plasma neuropeptide Y levels in congestive heart failure. Am J Med 1989; 86:43–48.
123. Kassis S, Olasmaa M, Terenius L, Fishman P. Neuropeptide Y inhibits cardiac adenylate cyclase through a pertussis toxin sensitive G-protein. J Biol Chem 1987; 262:3429–3431.
124. Feldman AM, Cates AE, Veazey WB et al. Increase of the 40,000 molecular weight pertussis toxin substrate (G protein) in the failing human heart. J Clin Invest 1987; 82:189–197.
125. Kawashima S, Fukutake N, Nishian K, Asakuma S, Iwasaki T. Elevated plasma beta-endorphin levels in patients with congestive heart failure. J Am Coll Cardiol 1991; 17:53–58.

126. Liang CS, Imai N, Stone CK, Woolf PD, Kawashima S, Tuttle RR. The role of endogenous opioids in congestive heart failure: Effects of nalmefene on systemic and regional hemodynamics in dogs. Circulation 1987; 75:443–451.
127. Sakamoto S, Stone CK, Woolf PD, Liang CS. Opiate receptor antagonist in right-sided congestive heart failure: naloxone exerts salutary hemodynamic effects through its action on the central nervous system. Circ Res 1989; 65:103–114.
128. Johnson MW, Mitch WE, Wilcox CS. The cardiovascular actions of morphine and the endogenous opiate peptides. Prog Cardiovasc Dis 1985; 27:435–450.
129. Anand IS, Garder J, Wander GS, O'Gara P, Harding SE, Ferrari R, Cornacchiari A, Panzali A, Purshotam LW, Poole-Wilson PA. Cardiovascular and hormonal effects of calcitonin gene-related peptide in congestive heart failure. J Am Coll Cardiol 1991; 17:208–217.
130. Tschopp FA, Tobler PH, Fischer JA. Calcitonin gene-related peptide in the human thyroid, pituitary and brain. Mol Coll Endocrinol 1984; 36:53–57.
131. Mulderry PK, Ghatei MA, Rodrigo J, Allen JM, Rosenfeld MG, Polak JM, Bloom SR. Calcitonin gene-related peptide in cardiovascular tissues of the rat. Neuroscience 1985; 14:947–954.
132. Franco-Cereceda A, Gennari C, Nami R, Agnusdei D, Pernon J, Lundberg JM, Fischer JA. Cardiovascular effects of calcitonin gene-related peptides I and II in man. Circ Res 1987; 60:393–397.
133. McEwan JR, Merjanin N, Larkin S, Fuller RW, Dollery CT, MacIntyre I. Vasodilatation by calcitonin gene-related peptide and substance P: a comparison of their effects on resistance and capacitance vessels of human forearms. Circulation 1988; 77:1072–1080.
134. Saxenhofer H, Raselle A, Wudmann P, Forssmann W-G, Bub A, Ferrari P, Shaw SG. Urodilatin, a natriuretic factor from kidneys, can modify renal and cardiovascular function in men. Am J Physiol 1990; 259:F832–F838.
135. Rigel DF. Effects of neuropeptides on heart rate in dogs. Comparison of VIP, PHI, NPY, CGRP and NI. Am J Physiol 1988; 255:H311–H317.
136. Karasawa Y, Furikawa Y, Ren L-M, Takei M, Murakami M, Narita M, Oniba A. Cardiac response to VIP and VIP-ogic-cholinergic ineraction in isolated dog heart preparations. Eur J Pharm 1990; 187:9–17.
137. Rigel DF, Grupp IL, Balasubramanian A, Grupp G. Contractile effects of cardiac neuropeptides in isolated canine atrial and ventricular muscles. Am J Physiol 1989; 257:H1082–H1087.
138. Rigel DF, Lathrop DA. Vasoactive intestinal polypeptide facilitates atrioventricular nodal conduction and shortens atrial and ventricular refractory period in conscious and anesthesized dogs. Circ Res 1990; 67:1323–1333.
139. Smitherman TC, Popma JJ, Said SI, Krejs GJ, Dehmer GJ. Coronary hemodynamic effects of intravenous vasoactive intestinal peptide in humans. Am J Physiol 1989; 257:H1254–H1262.
140. Fuller RW, Maxwell DL, Dixon DMS, McGregor GP, Barnes VF, Bloom SR, Barnes PJ. The effect of substance P on cardiovascular and respiratory function in normal subjects. Appl Physiol 1987; 62:1473–1481.

5

Left Ventricular Remodeling

Douglas E. Vaughan, Gervasio A. Lamas, and Marc A. Pfeffer
Brigham and Women's Hospital, West Roxbury VAMC, and Harvard Medical School, Boston, Massachusetts

INTRODUCTION

Regional alterations in left ventricular systolic function are the hallmarks of an acute myocardial infarction. Infarcted territory generally exhibits an abnormal contraction pattern during systole that can be categorized as decreased (hypokinetic), absent (akinetic), or paradoxical (dyskinetic). These regional alterations in left ventricular function can be apparent in the hyperacute period. Some infarct survivors are also prone to further progressive alterations in the shape of the left ventricle, a process that has been termed "remodeling." Remodeling is defined as an alteration in the geometry of the ventricular cavity that occurs independently of changes in the distending pressure (Fig. 1). These geometrical alterations can be quantified both morphologically (in terms of the left ventricular contour) and volumetrically (in terms of the left ventricular end-systolic and end-diastolic volumes). Although a component of left ventricular remodeling appears to represent an adaptive process serving to preserve stroke volume and cardiac output following myocardial injury, the enlargement process may have deleterious long-term effects on global left ventricular function and on clinical prognosis. Indeed, it seems likely that remodeling of the left ventricle contributes to the transition from asymptomatic left ventricular dysfunction to the development of overt congestive heart failure. Fortu-

Left ventricular remodeling \ ***n***: Alteration in the contour or volume of the ventricular cavity that is not attributed to acute changes in distending pressure

Figure 1 Definition of left ventricular remodeling.

nately, recent experimental and clinical evidence indicates that ventricular remodeling and its accompanying deleterious consequences may be favorably modified.

RELATIONSHIP BETWEEN VENTRICULAR SIZE AND PROGNOSIS

Ventricular dilation following a myocardial infarction is an important manifestation of systolic dysfunction, and is viewed as a homeostatic response directed at preserving stroke volume. If the process were self-limited and not accompanied by adverse prognostic features, ventricular remodeling would not merit much clinical or investigative attention. The reality is that cardiac enlargement after a myocardial infarction is associated with distinctly reduced survival. Roentgenographic evidence of cardiac enlargement is associated with a threefold increase in mortality for survivors of myocardial infarction (1). This portentous finding has been confirmed by other investigators using contrast left ventriculography as a means of quantitating ventricular size. Hammermeister and colleagues (2) demonstrated that left ventricular size is one of the most powerful predictors of survival in patients with coronary artery disease. More recently, White and colleagues (3) found that survival after myocardial infarction correlated directly with ejection fraction and inversely with end-systolic and end-diastolic volumes. In their study, the end-systolic volume was the most powerful predictor of death, with 25 ml increments associated with exponentially increasing mortality rates. The relative risk of mortality was increased nearly 2.5-fold by an end-systolic volume of 75 ml, and fivefold by an end-systolic volume of 125 ml (normal 30–55 ml). In both of these ventriculographic studies, multivariate analysis indicated that angiographic left ventricular volume is the most powerful predictor of reduced survival, even more powerful than the extent of coronary artery disease.

Ventricular enlargement following infarction is also associated with shape distortion. The shape of the left ventricle appears to correlate with exercise capacity in patients following an anterior myocardial infarction (4). Using a "sphericity index" obtained by biplane ventriculography (calculated as volume observed/volume of a sphere using the long axis as diameter, and illustrated in Fig. 2), infarct survivors with more spherical ventricles had greater left ventricular volumes, lower ejection fractions, and more extensive wall motion abnormalities than individuals with a more preserved left ventricular shape. Preservation of normal left ventricular shape is a powerful correlate of exercise capacity in these patients, while greater shape distortion (sphericity) corresponds with increasing cardiovascular disability.

LEFT VENTRICULAR REMODELING: IDENTIFICATION OF HIGH-RISK SUBGROUPS

Although nearly all infarct survivors will manifest some degree of left ventricular dysfunction, only certain individuals appear to be at risk for left ventricular remodeling and dilation. In general, ventricular dilation after myocardial infarction reflects the severity of myocardial necrosis induced by the infarction. Global contractile performance, as defined by the left ventricular ejection fraction, declines in tandem with the extent of histological damage, both in animals (5) and in humans (6). In contrast, stroke volume in infarct survivors does not consistently decline postinfarction, nor does it necessarily correlate with the contractile dysfunction. Several different mechanisms contribute to the preservation of pump function following the abrupt loss of contractile tissue. Adrenergic receptor stimulation can increase inotropic and chronotropic activity, while in-

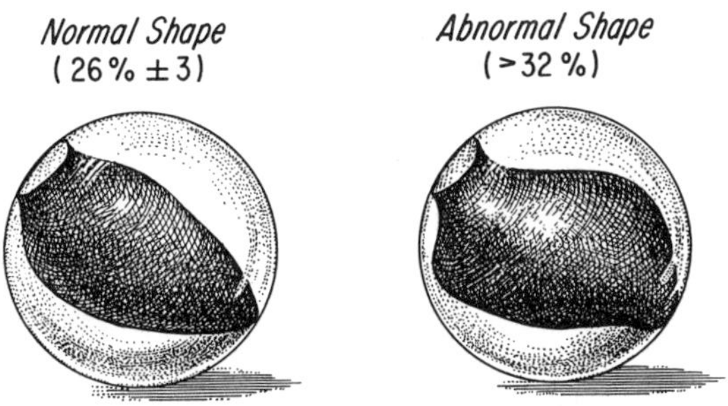

Figure 2 Left ventricular sphericity. The extent of left ventricular shape abnormality produced by the remodeling process can be graded using a sphericity index. The sphericity index consists of the biplane end-diastolic volume divided by the volume of a sphere with the same diameter. A normal ventricle is represented in the left panel; a remodeled, more spherical ventricle with a sphericity index outside the normal range [mean ±2 (SD)] is shown in the right panel.

creased filling pressures can promote the operation of the Frank-Starling mechanism. However, if the noncontractile region involves ≥20% of the left ventricular circumference, these compensatory mechanisms generally are inadequate to maintain cardiac output (7). Under these more difficult circumstances, stroke volume can be maintained by left ventricular dilatation. The extent of left ventricular remodeling that occurs after a myocardial infarction is predicated on the extent, depth, and location of the infarction (8,9), and individuals with large transmural anterior infarctions are apparently at highest risk.

TEMPORAL ASPECTS OF LEFT VENTRICULAR SHAPE ALTERATION

The pathological basis for changes in left ventricular geometry that underlie the remodeling process are complex and incompletely understood at the present time. It is clear that these morphological alterations originate in both infarcted and noninfarcted myocardium.

The infarcted territory is susceptible to forces that induce thinning and dilation over the short term (hours to weeks); this process has been termed "infarct expansion" (8). Infarct expansion is an important complication of acute myocardial infarction and is associated with increased mortality (8). Infarct expansion, by definition, involves the acute dilation and thinning of an area of infarction not explained by additional myocardial necrosis. The histological basis for infarct expansion has been extensively reviewed (10), and several processes probably contribute to wall thinning in the infarcted zone, with slippage between myocyte bundles and stretch and loss of intracellular space likely the predominant ultrastructural factors.

Infarct expansion is clinically detectable by echocardiography in patients as lengthening of a noncontractile region in the absence of evidence of reinfarction (11). Serial echocardiographic examinations permit the identification of infarct expansion, and, in the absence of comparable studies for a given patient, the length of akinetic or dyskinetic segments can be compared to normals.

Infarct expansion seems to be more common in patients experiencing transmural infarctions involving the anteroapical surface (8). This region appears to be most vulnerable because it is the thinnest and has the greatest curvature (12). Patients exhibiting infarct expansion are more likely to experience congestive heart failure, aneurysm formation, and myocardial rupture (11,13,14).

The noninfarcted territory is also susceptible to forces that induce morphological alterations and dilation over the long term. Theroux and colleagues (15) studied the sequential alterations in left ventricular function in dogs after permanent coronary artery ligation. These investigators noted a progressive increase in the end-diastolic length in the noninfarcted zone, which was remote from the area damaged by coronary ligation. These findings have been extended to humans in several studies. Using echocardiographic techniques, Erlebacher et al. (16) reported that patients with infarct expansion also manifested dilation of noninfarcted territory as a function of time. McKay and colleagues (17) demonstrated that ventricular enlargement occurs within 2 weeks of an acute myocardial infarction. This enlargement met the strict definition of remodeling because enlargement was observed even as filling pressures declined at 2 weeks. This remodeling was shown to involve both infarcted and noninfarcted regions of the left ventricle. In this study, the extent of systolic wall motion abnormality (akinesis plus dyskinesis) correlated with the magnitude of left ventricular cavity enlargement 2 weeks postinfarction. In chronic infarct survivors with isolated LAD disease, marked increases in left ventricular volumes (both end-diastolic and end-systolic) appear to correlate with the extent of wall motion abnormality (18). Again, these reported increases in volume appear to represent true left ventricular remodeling since they were detected in the absence of an increased filling pressure.

In the rat model of myocardial infarction, the size of a myocardial infarction predicts both ventricular function and survival (19). In long-term studies, left ventricular volume correlates with the extent of histological damage and time after infarction. Since ventricular volumes can be compared at a constant common distending pressure in the model, it lends itself well to studies of left ventricular morphology. Importantly, left ventricular cavity enlargement continues long after infarct healing is complete in this model, and, in fact, left ventricular volume increases progressively over time in relation to the initial extent of histological damage (20).

PATHOGENETIC MECHANISMS UNDERLYING LATE VENTRICULAR REMODELING

Wall Stress

As discussed previously, following the abrupt loss of contractile myocardium, the usual compensatory mechanisms are unable to maintain stroke volume when the noncontractile region exceeds 20% of the left ventricular circumference (6). Stroke volume can be preserved by augmenting the cavity size but at significant cost. According to the Laplace principle, as the left ventricular chamber enlarges (Fig. 3), wall stress increases. Furthermore, this increased wall stress must be borne by the residual viable

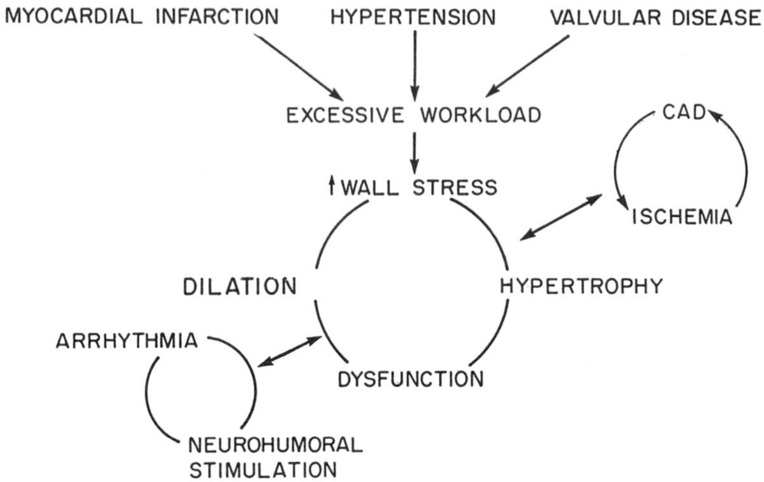

Figure 3 Central role of increased wall stress in promoting left ventricular remodeling. In this theoretical construct, increased wall stress promotes a cycle of hypertrophy and dilation in a damaged ventricle, leading to the development of congestive heart failure.

myocardium and likely serves as a stimulus for compensatory regional myocardial hypertrophy. If this compensatory hypertrophy were capable of matching volume increase and preserving the mass/volume ratio of the ventricle, this process might be self-limited. However, it appears that the degree of cellular hypertrophy in the viable myocardium initiated by the infarction is not capable of fully compensating for infarcted tissue (21). This compensatory hypertrophy appears to occur most prominently in the periinfarct "border" zones (22), which are precisely the regions that demonstrate the greatest shape change in the chronic phase after myocardial infarction (23). The failure of the residual myocardium to compensate adequately for the increased volume and wall stress following a large infarction also provides us with a potential explanation as to why this process is progressive in nature. Following the initial dilation of the left ventricular chamber associated with infarct expansion, the increased wall stress in the "internally" loaded ventricle begets additional dilation, inadequate hypertrophy, and persistent wall stress, which eventually produces a dysfunctional ventricle in which the expected decrease in wall stress coincident with ejection is no longer observed (24).

This hypothesis is supported by experimental data in which the mass, volume, and end diastolic wall stress was measured in rats after coronary ligation and myocardial infarction (25). In these animals, there was a progressive increase in both the volume and mass of the left ventricle over time following infarction, and the end-diastolic wall stress was elevated at all times. Importantly, the ratio of mass to volume decreased progressively throughout the experimental period (from 2 to 100 days), indicating that the left ventricular volume was increasing out of proportion to the mass and suggesting that overload hypertrophy was occurring, perhaps in response to a persistently elevated end-diastolic wall stress.

Patency of Infarct-Related Artery

Other factors may contribute to the process of ventricular remodeling, besides the homeostatic and adaptive forces that have been discussed (Table 1). Patency of an infarct-related artery appears to provide some protection against late left ventricular enlargement. This relationship was first described by Jeremy and colleagues (26), who reported that late ventricular enlargement was more likely to occur in patients with a persistently occluded infarct-related artery than in patients with recanalized arteries or arteries that filled by collaterals. This relationship was confirmed by a prospective study of patients following a first acute anterior wall myocardial infarction. In this study (27), the presence of antegrade blood flow through an infarct-related artery, either by collaterals or by reperfusion therapy, protected against the development of left ventricular aneurysm formation. In our own studies, we observed that total occlusion of the infarct-related artery at 3 weeks following anterior myocardial infarction was a powerful predictor of further left ventricular enlargement at 1 year (28). Taken together, these data support the potential importance of a patent infarct-related artery, and one could speculate that its patency may serve to protect

Table 1 Factors that Contribute to Left Ventricular Remodeling

Homeostatic forces
Frank-Starling mechanism
Compensatory hypertrophy
Neurohumoral activation (?)
Increased wall stress
Patency of infarct-related artery
Severity of left ventricular systolic wall motion abnormalities
Hypertension
Vascular permeability (?)
Infarct location/depth

the vulnerable myocardium at the border zone of an infarct, an area that contributes greatly to late-phase ventricular enlargement (23).

Neurohumoral Activation

Another factor that may contribute to the regional hypertrophy that predicates left ventricular enlargement is neurohumoral activation. The potential deleterious role of neurohumoral activation in patients with congestive heart failure has been reviewed extensively in Chapters 3 and 4. One would anticipate the presence of elevated catecholamine levels in patients in the setting of an acute infarction, and a compensatory activation of the renin-angiotensin-aldosterone system in patients who develop congestive heart failure. An association between neurohumoral activation and left ventricular function, both in animals and in humans, has recently been described (29,30). Evidence is beginning to accumulate that neurohumoral activation can also occur in asymptomatic patients with left ventricular dysfunction. Neurohumoral profiles were obtained in 39 such patients within 1 month of acute anterior myocardial infarction in an effort to identify pathophysiological correlates of neurohumoral activity in the *absence* of overt congestive heart failure (31). In these patients, all of whom had a left ventricular ejection fraction of ≤45%, signs of activation of the renin-angiotensin-aldosterone system were identified. The administration of loop diuretics was the most powerful predictor of neurohumoral activation in these patients, and diuretics are known to activate the renin-angiotensin-system in normal individuals as well as in patients with mild congestive heart failure (32,33). However, in the subgroup of asymptomatic patients not on diuretics, the extent of the left ventricular wall motion abnormality correlated with increased levels of renin, angiotensin, and aldosterone (Fig. 4). Recently, Francis and colleagues (34) also identified evidence of neuroendocrine activation in 151 patients who had left ventricular dysfunction but were free of heart failure. These patients, all of whom were participants in Studies of Left Ventricular Dysfunction (SOLVD), a multicenter trial of enalapril in patients with left ventricular dysfunction (ejection fraction ≤35%), were found to have significantly higher plasma levels of norepinephrine, atrial natriuretic factor, arginine vasopressin, and renin activity than those of normal control subjects. Elevated levels of neurohormones, particularly angiotensin II, may play a role in the pathological sequence of ventricular hypertrophy and dilation (35,36) following myocardial infarction. These findings raise the suspicion that neurohumoral activation may participate in and promote the transition of asymptomatic left ventricular dysfunction to overt congestive heart failure.

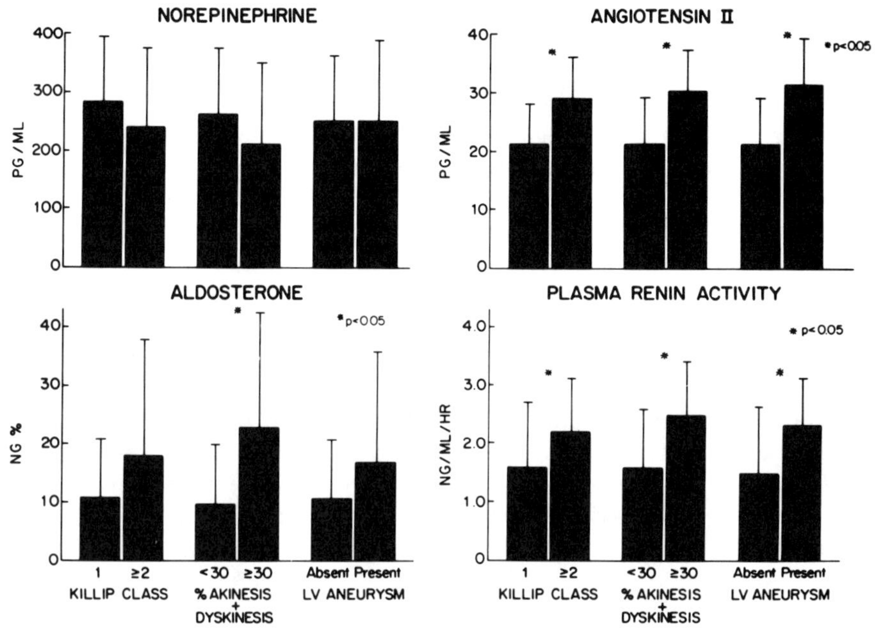

Figure 4 Plasma neurohumoral levels in 36 study patients not taking diuretics. Comparisons were made for each of the neurohormones shown in relation to the dichotomized clinical or angiographic variable listed on the horizontal axis. Statistically significant differences are indicated by the asterisk. Mean values ± standard deviation. Reprinted with permission (31).

Other Contributing Mechanisms

Weber and colleagues (37) recently described a potential relationship between altered permeability of intramyocardial arteries and left ventricular remodeling in a canine model of heart failure induced by rapid ventricular pacing. In the dilated ventricle secondary to rapid pacing, these investigators found that interstitial edema developed within 6 hours of onset of pacing coincident with medial swelling, proliferative changes, and perivascular and medial fibrosis in intramyocardial coronary arteries. If similar pathogenetic mechanisms contribute to left ventricular remodeling irrespective of the underlying disease, then it seems possible that this newly described mechanism (i.e., altered permeability) may also play a role in left ventricular remodeling following a myocardial infarction.

Since the classic description of Tennant and Wiggers (38) that the interruption of coronary blood flow leads to a local enfeeblement of contraction and systolic bulging, it has been apparent that mechanical forces play an important role in deforming the hypoperfused, noncontracting region. Dyskinesis is an important manifestation of this mechanical force that distends the noncontracting myocardium. The elongation and further thinning of the infarcted region that is observed with infarct expansion is an exaggeration of the response to the intracavitary distending forces. Modification of the distending or deforming forces acting on both the necrotic and viable myocardium can be expected to result in both acute and long-term changes in the extent of expansion of the infarct on the overall cavity size of the left ventricle and ultimately on the accompanying hypertrophy.

Elevations in systemic blood pressure can potentially increase the distending forces in the left ventricle. Experimentally, even transient modest pressure elevation by methoxamine infusion 1–5 h after coronary artery ligation exacerbated infarct expansion and thinning assessed 1 week after infarction (39). This study suggests that even relatively brief alterations in the loading conditions during the period of scar formation might have long-term implications on ventricular shape and size. Long-term augmentation in afterload produced by aortic banding 3 weeks before coronary artery ligation in rats increased the extent of left ventricular enlargement and infarct thinning (40). In a clinical study, Pierard et al. (41) demonstrated that infarct expansion was more likely to occur in patients with higher arterial pressure and systemic vascular resistance. The aggressive treatment of hypertension during the acute infarct period—to diminish afterload, myocardial oxygen demand, and possibly infarct size—may also help limit (short-term) left ventricular shape deformation.

Exercise represents a nonpharmacological mechanism for temporarily augmenting wall stress. The imposition of the hemodynamic stress of swimming to rats has been shown to cause greater scar thinning (42,43). In another study in the rat infarct model (44), a more moderate exercise program using daily treadmill activity during the first week of experimental infarction did not result in further distortion of the infarct region. Jugdutt et al. (45) studied the effects of an exercise program on left ventricular shape and function. The exercise program was instituted 15 days after infarction and continued for 3 months. In patients with extensive infarctions (defined as individuals with >18% akinesis or dyskinesis of the left ventricular contour), the group that exercised had echocardiographic evidence of deterioration in ventricular function and further distortion of infarct region topography with an increase in the expansion index and thinning ratio that was not observed in a matched control group. This important study illustrates that the hemodynamic stress of a graded exercise program can lead to a further distortion of left ventricular contour in patients with large Q-wave anterior infarctions and extensive wall motion abnormalities. This study raises a cautionary note that, although exercise after infarction is generally tolerated, the potential to adversely alter ventricular topography exists in highly selected patients.

PREVENTION OF LEFT VENTRICULAR REMODELING AND ENLARGEMENT

Animal Studies

Data are now available that support the concept that it is indeed possible to influence favorably the process of left ventricular remodeling after myocardial infarction. In an animal model of long-term infarction, the hypothesis was tested that the angiotensin converting enzyme (ACE) inhibitor captopril would favorably alter the loading conditions on the left ventricle and reduce the progressive enlargement regularly observed (46,47). Long-term therapy was begun long after any reduction of infarct size was possible and was associated with maintenance of cardiac output from a less-dilated ventricular cavity. The groups treated with ACE inhibitor had lower left ventricular volumes as a result of reduced distension (filling pressure) as well as an actual shift to the left (remodeling of left ventricular pressure-volume relation).

In this same experimental model of myocardial infarction and ventricular dysfunction, the risk of death during long-term follow-up was exponentially related to the extent of histological damage. Long-term therapy with captopril commencing 14 days after coronary ligation was associated with prolongation of survival (48). Analysis of subgroups using predefined criteria for histological damage demonstrated that the greatest improvement in survival was observed in the group with moderately sized infarcts (20–40% of the left ventricle), the same group in which earlier studies had demonstrated the greatest attenuation of ventricular enlargement with long-term therapy. These studies in the experimental infarct model emphasized that therapy to alter ventricular remodeling after myocardial infarction can, in fact, influence survival. Ventricular enlargement and dysfunction might favor the establishment of a positive feedback system whereby increases in systolic and diastolic wall stresses promote further ventricular enlargement that, according to Laplace's law, will further augment wall tension. Treatment with an ACE inhibitor was initiated to reduce the augmented "internal load" that the damaged ventricle sustains in an attempt to reduce wall stress and the resultant progressive enlargement. Captopril therapy was associated with a reduction in both arterial pressure and left ventricular end-diastolic pressure. In this same long-term infarct model in the rat, Raya and coworkers (49) demonstrated that long-term captopril therapy resulted in a lower mean circulatory filling pressure, in part attributed to both an augmentation in venous compliance and a reduction in blood volume. These effects on blood volume and venous capacitance produced by long-term captopril therapy were not observed in infarcted animals treated in the long term with equihypotensive doses of hydralazine that did not result in attenuation of ventricular enlargement. In contrast to arterial dilators such as hydralazine, ACE inhibition increases venous capacitance and has several additional actions that blunt the neurohumoral response to ventricular dysfunction, alter intrarenal hemodynamics, and promote sodium excretion resulting in reductions of both pre- and afterloads.

Human Studies

Flaherty and coworkers (50) compared the effects of a combination of intra-aortic balloon counterpulsation and intravenous nitroglycerin during the acute phase of infarction with conventional therapy without these interventions. This study was designed to examine the short-term effects of reducing wall stress on left ventricular geometry after infarction. Although the clinical outcomes were similar for both therapeutic groups, patients treated with the ventricular unloading regimen exhibited less echocardiographic evidence of lengthening of the noninfarct segment. Intravenous nitroglycerin—known to have profound dose-dependent acute effects on left ventricular filling pressure, arterial pressure, and regional myocardial blood flow—has been shown, in both experimental animals and patients, to be associated with a reduction in infarct size (51,52).

Jugdutt and Warnica (53) reported a randomized trial of placebo versus a carefully titrated regimen for nitroglycerin administration initiated within 12 hours of onset of pain in 310 patients. Creatinine kinase determinations of infarct size again confirmed the effectiveness of appropriately administered acute nitroglycerin in salvaging myocardium. An important aspect of this trial was the use of echocardiographic endpoints within the first 10 days of the infarction to evaluate short-term topographic changes of the left ventricle. The conventionally treated group showed echocardiographic evidence of infarct expansion that was not observed in the patients treated for approximately 2 days with titrated intravenous nitroglycerin. Although it is difficult to determine whether the beneficial effects of nitroglycerin resulted from limitation of infarct size, reduction in expansion of the infarcted region, or both, the active therapy group manifested a better-preserved left ventricular geometry and associated improved clinical outcome.

Two long-term studies in human subjects have been reported thus far that were prospectively designed to quantitate the effects of ACE inhibition (with captopril) on left ventricular size in patients after an acute myocardial infarction: Left ventricular volumes and function were measured approximately 3 weeks after infarction and reported 1 year later in survivors of first, transmural anterior infarcts (28). As would be expected, pronounced left ventricular enlargement and deformation were already present at baseline (Fig. 5). Patients were then randomized to placebo or captopril (50 t.i.d.) in addition to conventional therapy. Only placebo-treated patients showed further ventricular enlargement at 1 year; captopril-treated patients remained stable. These paired left ventriculograms after anterior infarction showed a pronounced heterogeneity in volume enlargement among patients. In the patients receiving placebo, the predictors of enlargement were the extent of wall motion abnormality (akinesis and dyskinesis) at the time of the baseline measurement and, as previously discussed, the patency of the vessel supplying the infarcted region high-risk group. These results confirmed the animal studies showing that ventricular enlargement can be a progressive process after anterior Q-wave infarction and that this process can be attenuated by long-term captopril therapy. In addition to the improvement in the primary ventriculographic endpoint, captopril treatment was associated with a prolonged exercise capacity.

Similar results have been reported by Sharpe et al. (54), who studied ventricular enlargement in 60 patients with inferior as well as anterior Q-wave infarctions with left-ventricular dysfunction. This study enrolled patients 1 week after infarction in three study groups (captopril 25 mg t.i.d., furosemide 40 mg daily, or placebo) and followed patients for 1 year. Using serial echocardiographic measurements of left ventricular volumes, they demonstrated that the placebo- and furosemide-treated groups had progressive ventricular enlargement that was not observed in patients treated with captopril therapy. The captopril-treated group also showed a significant improvement in the ejection fraction and stroke volume index over time.

The optimal timing for the initiation of ACE inhibition following acute myocardial infarction has not yet been determined. In a study performed by Pfeffer et al. (28), patients were randomized nearly 3 weeks after the acute event and by that time significant volume enlargement and remodeling had already occurred. Very recently, Nabel and colleagues (55) examined the effects of intravenous followed by oral captopril versus placebo therapy in a randomized trial of 38 patients treated with recombinant tissue-

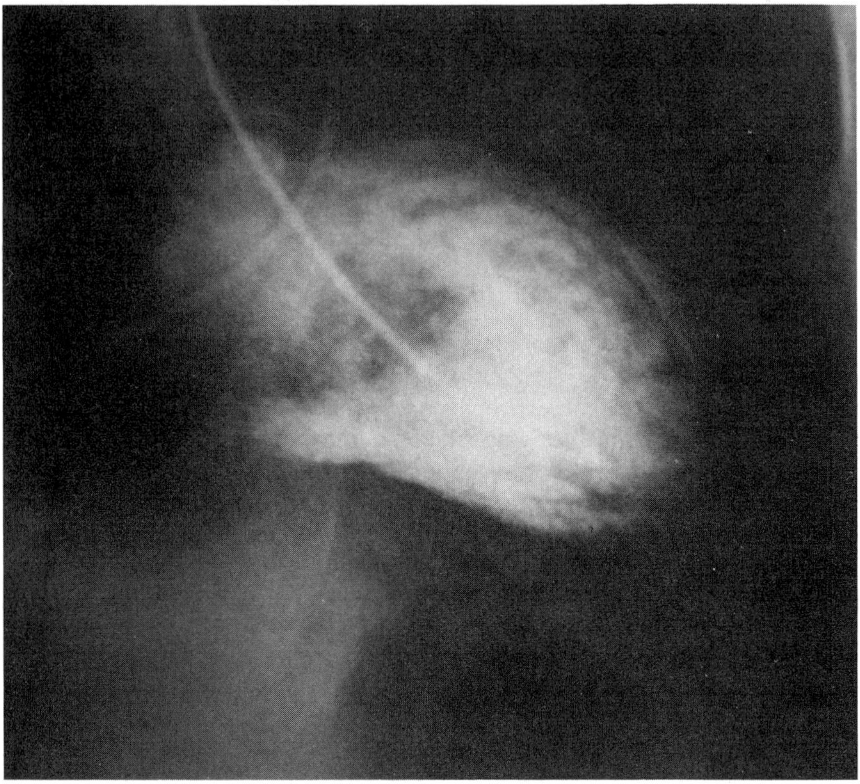

Figure 5 Angiogram of a remodeled left ventricle. A representative angiographic study (right anterior oblique view) obtained 3 weeks following an extensive anterior infarction. The diastolic contour is markedly deformed, as were the end-diastolic volume index (104; normal 70 ± 16 ml/m^2) and end-diastolic volume index (63; normal 24 ± 10 ml/m^2). This patient experienced further remodeling over the following year, with the end-diastolic volume index increasing to 160 ml/m^2 and the end-systolic volume index to 125 ml/m^2.

type plasminogen activator (rt-PA). In this study, the placebo-treated group showed a significant increase in the left ventricular end-diastolic volume when remeasured at day 7 while the end-diastolic volume decreased slightly in the captopril-treated group.

The beneficial effects of ACE inhibition therapy in preventing progressive ventricular enlargement after myocardial infarction in experimental animals and patients provided the rationale for the recently completed clinical trial of ACE inhibition following myocardial infarction, Survival and Ventricular Enlargement (SAVE) (56). This study of nearly 2300 patients in the United States and Canada, was designed to test the hypothesis that the long-term administration of captopril to survivors of infarction with left ventricular dysfunction (radionuclide ejection fraction ≤40%) but without clinical manifestations of heart failure will reduce mortality and prevent deterioration in left ventricular function over time. This study, completed in early 1992, demonstrated a 19% reduction in mortality in the captopril-treated group compared with the placebo group (Table 2). In addition, the incidence of both fatal and nonfatal major cardiovascular events was reduced in the captopril-treated group. The SAVE study enrolled patients within 3 to 16 days of an acute myocardial infarction, and patients were followed for an average of 42 months.

Another large multicenter trial designed to test the value of ACE inhibition in patients following acute MI was recently published (57). The Consensus II trial randomized 6090 patients within 24 h of an acute myocardial infarction, with 3046 patients assigned to the placebo group and 3044 patients assigned to treatment with enalapril. The follow-up period in this trial ranged from 41 to 180 days. In this study, which was terminated prematurely, enalapril failed to improve survival during the first 180 days after myocardial infarction.

Another large randomized trial (SOLVD) was recently completed that was designed to study the effect of an ACE inhibitor (enalapril) on the mortality and the development of CHF in patients with left ventricular dysfunction who were not receiving drug treatment for congestive heart failure (58). Patients enrolled in this study had left ventricular ejection fractions ≤35%.

Table 2 Effect of Captopril in Major Clinical Endpoints: Results from the SAVE Study

	Placebo (n = 1116)		Captopril (n = 1115)		Risk reduction
	No.	%	No.	%	%
Death (all causes)	275	24.6	228	20.4	19
Cardiovascular death and morbidity	448	40.1	359	32.2	24
Hospitalization for heart failure	192	17	154	13.8	22

In contrast with the SAVE and Consensus II trials, this was not specifically a post–myocardial infarction trial; it included patients with left ventricular dysfunction from a variety of causes. Over 4800 patients were randomized in this study, which demonstrated a 37% reduction in the development of heart failure ($p < 0.001$) and an 8% reduction in all causes of mortality, a result that failed to reach statistical significance.

SUMMARY

The acute and long-term changes in ventricular geometry (ventricular remodeling) after myocardial infarction are important processes affecting ventricular function and survival. Therapy to limit infarct size, enhance scar formation, reduce or prevent infarct expansion, and reduce ventricular wall stress can all favorably impact on the geometric metamorphosis that occurs following a myocardial infarction. Although a great deal of attention has been focused on the limitation of the initial damage during a myocardial infarction, the more insidious ventricular remodeling can also have an important impact on the ultimate outcome after infarction.

Although several factors appear to contribute to the process of left ventricular remodeling following a myocardial infarction, experimental and clinical data suggest that it is now possible to impact favorably on this process. Important questions that remain to be answered include the following: (1) What is the best therapy or combination of therapies to limit left ventricular remodeling after myocardial infarction? (2) Is left ventricular remodeling a consequence of left ventricular dysfunction irrespective of etiology? (3) Does prevention of left ventricular modeling improve patient survival? and (4) What is the optimal timing of therapy to prevent left ventricular remodeling? At the present time, many ongoing studies are addressing these and other questions pertaining to the pathogenesis and treatment of left ventricular remodeling, and it seems likely that further research on this topic will contribute to the management and outcome of patients with left ventricular dysfunction following myocardial infarction and in other settings as well.

REFERENCES

1. Kostuk WJ, Kazamias TM, Gander MP, Simon AL, Ross J. Left ventricular size after acute myocardial infarction: Serial changes and their prognostic significance. Circulation 1973; 47:1174–1179.
2. Hammermeister KE, DeRouen TA, Dodge HT. Variables predictive of survival in patients with coronary disease: Selection by univariate and multivar-

iate analyses from the clinical electrocardiographic, exercise, anteriographic, and quantitative angiographic evaluations. Circulation 1979; 59:421–430.
3. White HD, Norris RM, Brown MA, Brandt PWT, Whitlock RML, Wild CJ. Left ventricular end-systolic volume as the major determinant of survival after recovery from myocardial infarction. Circulation 1987; 76:44–51.
4. Lamas GA, Vaughan DE, Parisi AF, Pfeffer MA. Effects of left ventricular shape and captopril therapy on exercise capacity after anterior wall acute myocardial infarction. Am J Cardiol 1989; 63:1167–1173.
5. Pfeffer MA, Pfeffer JM, Fishbein MC, Fletcher PJ, Spadaro J, Kloner RA, Braunwald E. Myocardial infarct size and ventricular function in rats. Circ Res 1979; 44:503–512.
6. Hori M, Inoue M, Mishima M, Shimazu T, Abe H, Fukui S. Infarct size and left ventricular ejection fraction in acute myocardial infarction. Jap Circ J 1977; 41:1299–1309.
7. Klein MD, Herman MV, Gorlin R. A hemodynamic study of left ventricular aneurysm. Circulation 1967; 35:614–630.
8. Hutchins GM, Bulkley BH. Infarct expansion versus extension: Two different complications of acute myocardial infarction. Am J Cardiol 1978; 41:1127–1132.
9. Pirolo JS, Hutchins GM, Moore GW. Infarct expansion: Pathologic analysis of 204 patients with a single myocardial infarct. J Am Coll Cardiol 1986; 7:349–354.
10. Weisman HF, Bush DE, Mannisi JA, Weisfeldt ML, Healy B. Cellular mechanisms of myocardial infarct expansion. Circulation 1988; 78:186–201.
11. Eaton LW, Weiss JL, Bulkley BH, Garrison JB, Weisfeldt MD. Regional cardiac dilatation after acute myocardial infarction. N Engl J Med 1979; 300:57–62.
12. Burton AC. The importance of the shape and size of the heart. Am Heart J 1957; 54:801–810.
13. Schuster EH, Bulkley BH. Expansion of transmural myocardial infarction: A pathophysiologic factor in cardiac rupture. Circulation 1979; 60:1532–1538.
14. Jugdutt BI, Michorowski BL. Role of infarct expansion in rupture of the ventricular septum after acute myocardium infarction: A two-dimensional echocardiographic study. Clin Cardiol 1987; 10:641–652.
15. Theroux P, Ross Jr J, Franklin D, Covell JW, Bloor CM, Sasayama S. Regional myocardial infarction and dimensions early and late after myocardial infarction in the unanesthetized dog. Circ Res 1977; 40:158–165.
16. Erlebacher JA, Weiss JL, Eaton LW, Kallman C, Weisfeldt ML, Bulkley BH. Late effects of acute infarct dilation on heart size: A two-dimensional echocardiographic study. Am J Cardiol 1982; 49:1120–1126.
17. McKay RG, Pfeffer JM, Pasternak RC, Markis JE, Come PC, Nakao S, Alderman JD, Ferguson JJ, Safian RD, Grossman W. Left ventricular remodeling following myocardial infarction: A corollary to infarct expansion. Circulation 1986; 74:693–702.
18. Lamas GA, Pfeffer MA. Increased left ventricular volume following myocardial infarction in man. Am Heart J 1986; 111:30–35.

19. Pfeffer MA, Pfeffer JM, Fishbein MC, Fletcher PJ, Spandaro J, Kloner RA, Braunwald E. Myocardial infarct size and ventricular function in rats. Circ Res 1979; 44:503–512.
20. Pfeffer JM, Pfeffer MA, Fletcher PJ, Braunwald E. Progressive ventricular remodeling in rat with myocardial infarction. Am J Physiol 1991. In press.
21. Anversa P, Loud AV, Levicky V, Guideri G. Left ventricular failure induced by myocardial infarction. I. Myocyte hypertrophy. Am J Med 1985; 248:H876–H882.
22. Bogen DK, Rabinowitz SA, Needleman A, McMahon TA, Abelmann WH. An analysis of the mechanical disadvantage of myocardial infarction in the canine left ventricle. Circ Res 1980; 47:728–741.
23. Mitchell GF, Lamas GA, Vaughan DE, Pfeffer MA. Infarct expansion does not contribute to late left ventricular enlargement (abstr). Circulation 1989; 80(suppl II):II-589.
24. Weber KT, Janicki JS. The heart as a muscle-pump system and the concept of heart failure. Am Heart J 1979; 98:371–384.
25. Pfeffer JM, Pfeffer MA, Mirsky I, Steinberg CR, Braunwald E. Progressive ventricular dilatation and diastolic wall stress with myocardial infarction and failure (abstr.) Circulation 1982; 66(suppl II):II-66.
26. Jeremy RW, Allman KC, Bautovitch G, Harris PJ. Patterns of left ventricular dilation during the six months after myocardial infarction. J Am Coll Cardiol 1989; 13:304–310.
27. Hirai T, Fujita M, Nakajima H, Asanoi H, Yamanishi K, Ohno A, Sasayama S. Importance collateral circulation for prevention of left ventricular aneurysm formation in acute myocardial infarction. Circulation 1989; 79:791–796.
28. Pfeffer MA, Lamas GA, Vaughan DE, Parisi AF, Braunwald E. Effect of captopril on progressive ventricular dilatation after anterior myocardial infarction. N Engl J Med 1988; 319:80–86.
29. Mendez RE, Pfeffer JM, Ortola FV, Bloch KD, Anderson S, Seidman JG, Brenner BM. Atrial natriuretic peptide transcription, storage, and release in rats with myocardial infarction. Am J Physiol 1987; 253:H1449–H1455.
30. Phillips, PA, Sasadens, J, Hodsman GP, Horowitz J, Sattups A, Johnston CI. Plasma atrial natriuretic peptide in patients with acute myocardial infarction: Effects of streptokinase. Br Heart J 1989; 61:139–143.
31. Vaughan DE, Lamas GA, Pfeffer MA. Role of left ventricular dysfunction in selective neurohumoral activation in the recovery phase of acute myocardial infarction. Am J Cardiol 1990; 66:529–532.
32. Kudo SH, Clark M, Laragh J, Boru JS, Cody RJ. Identification of normal neurohumoral activity in mild congestive heart failure and stimulating effect on upright posture and diuretics. Am J Cardiol 1987; 60:1322–1328.
33. Bayliss J, Norell M, Canepa-Anson R, Sutton G, Poole-Wilson P. Untreated heart failure: clinical and neuroendocrine effects of introducing diuretics. Br Heart J 1987; 57:17–22.
34. Francis GS, Benedict C, Johnstone DE, Kirlin PC, et al. Comparison of neuroendocrine activation in patients with left ventricular dysfunction with and without congestive heart failure. Circulation 1990; 82:1724–1729.

35. Dzau VJ. Circulating versus local renin-angiotensin system in cardiovascular homeostasis. Circulation 1988; 77(suppl 1):4–13.
36. Pfeffer MA, Pfeffer JA, Braunwald E. Influence of chronic captopril therapy on the infarcted left ventricle of the rat. Circ Res 1985; 57:94–95.
37. Weber KT, Pick R, Silver MA, Moc GW, Janiki JS, Zucker IH, Armstrong PW. Fibrillar collagen and remodeling of dilated canine left ventricle. Circulation 1990; 82:1387–1401.
38. Tennant R, Wiggers CJ. The effect of coronary occlusion on myocardial contraction. Am J Physiol 1935; 112:351–361.
39. Hammerman H, Kloner RA, Alker KJ, Schoen FJ, Braunwald E. Effects of transient increased afterload during experimentally induced acute myocardial infarction in dogs. Am J Cardiol 1985; 55:566–570.
40. Nolan SE, Mannisi JA, Bush DE, Healy B, Weisman HF. Increased afterload aggravates infarct expansion after acute myocardial infarction. J Am Coll Cardiol 1988; 12:1318–1325.
41. Pierard LA, Albert A, Gillis F, Sprynger M, Carlier J, Kulbertus HE. Hemodynamic profile of patients with acute infarction at risk of infarct expansion. Am J Cardiol 1987; 60:5–9.
42. Kloner RA, Kloner JA. Short-term exercise has a prolonged effect on scar formation after experimental acute myocardial infarction. J Am Coll Cardiol 1983; 2:979–982.
43. Hammerman H, Schoen FJ, Kloner RA. Short-term exercise has a prolonged effect on scar formation after experimental acute myocardial infarction. J Am Coll Cardiol 1983; 2:979–982.
44. Hochman JS, Healy B. Effect of exercise on acute myocardial infarction in rats. J Am Coll Cardiol 1986; 7:126–132.
45. Jugdutt BI, Michorowski BL, Kappagoda CT. Exercise training after Q wave myocardial infarction: Importance of regional left ventricular function and topography. J Am Coll Cardiol 1988; 12:362–372.
46. Fletcher PJ, Pfeffer MA, Mirsky I, Steinberg CR, Braunwald E. Left ventricular diastolic pressure-volume relations in rats with healed myocardial infarction. Circ Res 1981; 49:618–626.
47. Pfeffer MJ, Pfeffer MA, Braunwald E. Influence of chronic captopril therapy on the infarcted left ventricle of the rat. Circ Res 1985; 57:84–95.
48. Pfeffer MA, Pfeffer JM, Steinberg C, Finn P. Survival after an experimental myocardial infarction: Beneficial effects of long-term therapy with captopril. Circulation 1985; 72:406–412.
49. Raya TE, Gay RG, Aguirre M, Goldman S. Importance of venodilation in prevention of left ventricular dilatation after chronic large myocardial infarction in rats: A comparison of captopril and hydralazine. Circ Res 1989; 64:330–337.
50. Flaherty JT, Becker LC, Bulkley BH, Weiss JL, Gersteinblith G, Kallman CH, Silverman KJ, Wei JY, Pitt B, Weisfeldt ML. A randomized prospective trial of intravenous nitroglycerine in patients with acute myocardial infarction. Circulation 1983; 68:576–578.

51. Borer JS, Redwood DR, Levitt B, Cagin N, Bianchi C, Vallin H, Epstein SE. Reduction in myocardial ischemia with nitroglycerin or nitroglycerin plus phenylephrine administered during acute myocardial infarction. N Engl J Med 1975; 293:1008–1012.
52. Jaffe AS, Geltman EM, Tiefenbrunn AJ, Ambos HD, Strauss HD, Sobel BE, Roberts R. Reduction of infarct size in patients with inferior infarction with intravenous glyceryl trinitrate: A randomized study. Br Heart J 1983; 49:452–460.
53. Jugdutt BI, Warnica JW. Intravenous nitroglycerin therapy to limit myocardial infarct size, expansion, and complications. Effects of timing, dosage, and infarct location. Circulation 1988; 78:906–919.
54. Sharpe N, Smith H, Murphy J, Hannan S. Treatment of patients with symptomless left ventricular dysfunction after myocardial infarction. Lancet 1988; i:255–259.
55. Nabel EG, Topol EJ, Galeana A, Ellis SG, et al. Randomized placebo-controlled trial of combined early intravenous captopril and recombinant tissue-type plasminogen activator therapy in acute myocardial infarction. J Am Coll Cardiol 1991; 17:467–473.
56. Pfeffer MA, Braunwald E, Moy LA, et al. Effect of captopril on mortality and morbidity in patients with left ventricular dysfunction after myocardial infarction. N Engl J Med 1992; 327:669–677.
57. Swedberg K, Held P, Kjekshus J, et al. Effects of early administration of enalapril on mortality in patients with acute myocardial infarction. N Engl J Med 1992; 327:678–684.
58. The SOLVD Investigators. Effect of enalapril on mortality and the development of heart failure in asymptomatic patients with reduced left ventricular ejection fractions. N Engl J Med 1992; 327:685–691.

TREATMENT

6

Assessment of Therapeutic Efficacy in Patients with Chronic Heart Failure

Thomas S. Rector and Jay N. Cohn
University of Minnesota Medical School, Minneapolis, Minnesota

The goals of medical therapy for chronic heart failure are to reduce disease-related disability and to prolong life. In dealing with a complex chronic syndrome such as heart failure, these therapeutic goals are difficult to assess. Furthermore, there is no assurance that an agent that improves quality of life will necessarily prolong life or that an agent effective in prolonging life will necessarily improve quality of life. Therefore, potential noncongruence of efficacy end point creates an additional clinical dilemma.

A number of surrogate measures have been utilized for disease-related disability, including hemodynamic effects of the therapy, measured changes in exercise tolerance, and improvement in physician-defined cardiac status. No surrogate end point has been shown to adequately predict a favorable effect on life expectancy. Since no medication can be expected to have a favorable effect on all patients to whom it is administered, even the results of carefully controlled trials cannot be extrapolated to individual patient response with certainty. The problem for the physician, therefore, is to seek sensitive and specific measures of efficacy that will allow differentiation between responders and nonresponders to the medical therapy. If a surrogate for a favorable effect on disability or survival could be identified, benefits of the treatment could theoretically be predicted by an intermediate end point.

The therapeutic goals in heart failure can be divided into three distinct phases. Hemodynamic benefit with an improvement in left ventricular dysfunction may be the primary goal in the acute management of patients with severe left ventricular failure being monitored in an intensive care unit. In this clinical situation an improvement in cardiac output and reduction of the elevated pulmonary capillary wedge pressure may be an adequate end point for clinical improvement that will allow the patient to become ambulatory. An intermediate goal in the management of heart failure is relief of symptoms and physical limitations, and an improvement in the quality of life. This therapeutic end point generally is sought over a 3- to 6-month period of therapy. The long-term therapeutic goal in heart failure is to prevent progression of the syndrome as indicated by delays in the onset of symptoms, hospitalization, and death. These preventive effects can be assessed only in long-term trials that provide the clinician with probabilities that an individual will benefit.

PHYSIOLOGICAL EFFECTS OF THERAPY

Most of the drugs in use for the treatment of heart failure have been identified on the basis of their favorable hemodynamic effects. The hemodynamic hallmarks of heart failure, a low cardiac output and an increased cardiac filling pressure, can be favorably influenced by diuretics, vasodilators, and inotropic agents. Monitoring of these variables by right heart catheterization in the intensive care environment can provide objective measures of the favorable effects of therapy. Long-term hemodynamic improvements may correspond with clinical improvement (1,2). However, acute changes in pulmonary artery pressures do not correspond with dyspnea (3). In addition, favorable acute hemodynamic effects may not translate into a long-term clinical benefit to the patient (4,5). Furthermore, the hemodynamically most effective dose may not be the most effective dose in terms of long-term disability or survival (6,7). Therefore, hemodynamic end points have only a limited role in the assessment of clinical efficacy of therapy.

Surrogates for cardiac filling pressure—including signs or symptoms of pulmonary congestion, radiologic evidence of cephalization of the pulmonary vasculature, bedside measurement of central venous pressure, changes in weight, and the appearance of peripheral edema—are commonly used in practice to monitor therapy. Jugular-venous pressure is perhaps the best noninvasive assessment of cardiac filling pressure available, and therefore it becomes an important end point for assessing the response to diuretic therapy. However, as many as 40% of patients with pulmonary capillary wedge pressures $\geq$22 mm Hg do not have an elevated jugular-venous pressure (8). The abdominojugular reflux test is a more sensitive indicator of an elevated pulmonary capillary wedge pressure (9).

The adequacy of cardiac output and its response to therapy is difficult to quantitate noninvasively. A small pulse volume as indicated by the pulse pressure, cutaneous vasoconstriction, renal sodium retention, and fatigue may be a manifestation of inadequate cardiac output or regional blood flow. Assessment of the effect of therapy on cardiac output can only crudely be made by measurement of these indirect indexes.

Measures of ventricular function can be made noninvasively by the use of echocardiography or radionuclide angiography. The calculation of left ventricular ejection fraction provides a fairly sensitive guide to the systolic performance of the left ventricle and may be useful to assess therapeutic responses. However, changes in measures of left ventricular systolic performance at rest do not always correspond with changes in functional capacity (10). The left ventricular ejection fraction is one of the best prognosticators of time to death (11). Unfortunately, how treatment-induced changes in the ejection fraction or other prognostic variables relate to changes in the probability of survival remains to be determined. More studies are needed to determine the sensitivity and specificity of long-term changes in physiologic measurements as indicators of therapeutic efficacy in chronic heart failure. However, reliable and comprehensive measures of disability due to heart failure are needed for these types of investigation.

EXERCISE TOLERANCE TESTS

Exercise tests seem to be logical, somewhat objective methods of measuring the symptoms of fatigue and dyspnea, particularly during physical activities. Many variables such as duration of exercise, peak oxygen consumption, and anaerobic threshold can differentiate patients with heart failure from healthy individuals. Cross-sectional studies have found these exercise variables to differ on average between patients grouped by functional class, but the degree of overlap is substantial. In addition, these findings based on between-patient variability do not directly address the longitudinal assessment of therapeutic efficacy, which focuses on within-patient variability.

Are changes in exercise measures congruent with changes in the symptoms and the secondary limitations patients experience? Although measures both of symptoms and of exercise capacity are commonly used in controlled trials, few have reported the relationship between these end points. Many reports seem to imply that symptomatic improvement and increases in exercise time correspond closely, since the means of measures of both trended in the same direction or were statistically significant. These oversimplifications may be challenged during scrutiny of the data in greater depth. Changes in the duration of a symptom-limited treadmill test were only weakly correlated with changes in ratings of breathlessness and tiredness during a 3-month study of xamoterol, digoxin, and placebo (12). All three treatment groups had a substantial proportion of subjects whose symptoms improved, did not change, or worsened, and this variability was not closely associated with the variability in exercise duration. Others have observed a similar association with changes in exercise duration and peak oxygen consumption (13,14). These findings suggest that one cannot use changes in the duration of symptom-limited exercise as an accurate indicator of changes in symptoms unless the magnitude of the change is substantial, such as an improvement in exercise duration of more than 2.5 min on a modified Naughton protocol (14).

One reason changes in maximal exercise tests do not correlate well with changes in the symptoms of fatigue and shortness of breath during daily activities may be that these end points involve different levels of cardiovascular stress. Submaximal exercise tests such as the 6-min walk and the self-powered treadmill might be more closely related to the physical limitations experienced by individuals with heart failure (15–17). Limb movement sensors may also be useful indicators of therapeutic effects, but validation studies are needed (18).

If serial exercise tests are used to assess therapeutic efficacy, efforts to eliminate placebo and training effects as well as methodologic inconsistencies are necessary. These demands restrict the practicality of exercise tests in many clinics. Furthermore, if a treatment improves an individual's cardiovascular function as determined by exercise tests, one still must determine if the magnitude of the increased ability makes a valuable difference in the patient's life before a therapeutic effect can be claimed.

DIRECT ASSESSMENT OF PATIENT OUTCOMES

In the absence of an adequate understanding of the complex causes of fatigue, dyspnea, and other symptoms that occur with heart failure, one must assess therapeutic efficacy by measuring the symptoms and their impact on an individual's life as well as possible. Patient reports are essentially unverifiable even with congruent physiologic observations and are difficult to quantitate, although a qualitative measure is sufficient to assess therapeutic efficacy. In addition, the influence of other comorbidities and psychosocial factors that vary independently of the fluctuations in heart failure and the effects of treatment create uncertainty. Nevertheless, the patient's self-assessment, ascertained in a systematic and unbiased manner, is very important for judging if a treatment benefits the recipient.

Consideration must be given to how one inquires about symptoms and the effects of a treatment. To reduce the caregiver's influence, the patient's viewpoints should be solicited before any other assessments or related comments. Many patients will be reluctant to disagree with a physician's opinion. Often the professional's functional classification is based on information other than direct patient inquiry or on a limited amount of patient feedback. Occurrences of discrepant patient and physician perceptions of the effect of a treatment are not surprising if they are based on different sets of data (19,20). Instructions to respondents should emphasize the importance of their opinions. Ample time should be allowed for the patient to think about the questions without interruptions. These simple procedures are often neglected in practice and during investigations.

A self-administered questionnaire will reduce bias in responses that is due to the method of asking questions and will decrease the time health care providers must spend in collecting good data. Like other methods of assessing symptoms, a questionnaire needs to be fairly comprehensive. Asking about different facets of fatigue and dyspnea can stimulate the respondent to think about how these symptoms have affected his or her life and increase the reliability of a questionnaire. One of the shortcomings of the New York Heart Association classification is its unstructured inquiry about a few nonspecific aspects of fatigue and dyspnea. Single items concerning tiredness or shortness of breath also do not encourage the respondent to consider systematically the many ways these symptoms may have altered working to earn a living or at home, social and recreational activities, sleep, relationships, emotions, cognitive function, the need for health care services, and so forth. Furthermore, all bothersome symptoms and side effects must be considered to determine the net result of a treatment. This type of in-depth inquiry is often shortchanged in favor of physiologic assessments that are useful for diagnosing heart failure and determining its severity but have questionable utility for judging therapeutic benefit.

In contrast to pharmacologic efficacy, values are an integral part of assessing therapeutic efficacy. If a treatment given to reduce symptoms does not yield a benefit the patient perceives as important, the treatment was not therapeutically effective. Therefore, the numeric values assigned to responses must represent the patient's values. The Specific Activity Scale asks patients if some common daily activities provoke symptoms but weighs each item by its metabolic equivalent, not its value to the respondent (21). In addition, the small set of physical activities that are part of this assessment may not represent the individual's primary concerns. Other dyspnea-fatigue indexes, including the New York Heart Association classification, inappropriately deemphasize the patient's values by having the physician rate the level of activity that causes symptoms or the level of discomfort.

The Sickness Impact Profile incorporates consensus values that may be different from the individual patient's (22). For example, impaired work is the most important dimension of this measure yet may not be the primary concern of older patients with heart failure. Many measures of symptoms and secondary limitations are therefore contrary to the common clinical practice of being responsive to the patient's primary complaints. Questions asking the respondents to indicate whether there has been an improvement, worsening, or no change at least allow them to self-define therapeutic efficacy, although their point of reference can change with the passage of time and intervening events. Other questionnaires ask how much each item impairs the individual's ability to live as he or she desires (14). Since each item uses the same response format, one can determine which limitations are most important and assess therapies by determining if they result in less impairment.

To evaluate therapeutic efficacy one needs to attribute longitudinal differences to an intervention regardless of the measure one uses. Reliance on objective measures that may be less susceptible to extraneous fluctuations can be misleading if, as previously discussed, they do not directly correspond with the patient's problems. Questionnaires that are focused on the sequelae of heart failure that can be affected by a treatment will reduce the extraneous variability in comparison with general or less specific measures of health status. In addition, repeated assessments using self-administered measures to establish a patient's status during stable periods are feasible and make changes during follow-up more interpretable. Through systematic, comprehensive, and unbiased inquiry, one can make a worthwhile assessment of whether or not a patient's limitations secondary to heart failure have been reduced in a useful way.

MORTALITY

Shortened life expectancy is being increasingly recognized as an adverse event in patients with chronic heart failure. The therapeutic goal of increasing life expectancy is therefore commonly being used as an end point for intervention trials. Identification of a survival benefit of a therapy for heart failure in a controlled clinical trial is most appropriately used by physicians as a mandate for this therapy in a similar patient population. Since no intermediate therapeutic end point can as yet be identified as a predictor for a favorable effect of an intervention on survival, the only appropriate response to such trial results is to administer the effective agent in the doses found to be effective. The decision-making process for the physician, therefore, is to be certain that the patient under treatment is represented in the therapeutic trial and that no adverse events occur to counteract the theoretical benefits of the therapy on life expectancy.

One problem that has plagued clinical study of heart failure end points is the attempt to distinguish the mechanism of death in a given patient. Many controlled studies of heart failure have identified progressive pump failure as the cause of death in fewer than half of patients and sudden unexpected death suggestive of a ventricular arrhythmia as a common cause of death. These distinct mechanisms of the terminal event raise the possibility that the efficacy of treatments to prolong survival would be monitored differently. Attempts to identify useful prognostic variables have been hindered by the uncertain classification of death in individual patients, since death often occurs in the absence of direct observation and may have many contributing factors.

SUMMARY

Therapeutic efficacy should be defined as the extent of achievement of the goals of medical care for heart failure, which are to reduce disease-related disability and to prolong life. Our understanding of the complex pathophysiology of this heterogeneous condition continues to progress, but more studies are needed to apply this new knowledge to the assessment of therapeutic efficacy. Medications are designed to improve various physiologic abnormalities that are characteristic of the syndrome of heart failure. Monitoring of physical signs, hemodynamics, and exercise performance can help determine the physiologic effects of an intervention, but these end points have yet to be proven as sensitive and specific indicators of beneficial patient outcomes. More efforts are required to develop and systematically use reliable and valid patient self-assessments of the effects of treatments. Subsequently, physiologic end points need to be validated as indicators of therapeutic efficacy. Randomized, controlled trials can only determine if a treatment has a reasonable chance of providing treatment-related benefit to an individual with heart failure. If a patient tolerates a potentially effective medication, perhaps the treatment should be utilized. The task of identifying those who truly benefit remains in the realm of the art of medicine, with all its uncertainty.

REFERENCES

1. Packer M, Medina N, Yushak M, Meller J. Hemodynamic patterns of response during long-term captopril therapy for severe chronic heart failure. Circulation 1983; 68:803–812.

2. Sharpe DN, Murphy J, Coxon R, Hannan SF. Enalapril in patients with chronic heart failure: a placebo-controlled, randomized, double-blind study. Circulation 1984; 70:271–278.
3. Gibbs JSR, Keegan J, Wright C, Fox KM, Poole-Wilson PA. Pulmonary artery pressure changes during exercise and daily activities in chronic heart failure. J Am Coll Cardiol 1990; 15:52–61.
4. Leier CV, Binkley PF, Starling RC, Huss-Randolph P. Disparity between improvement in left ventricular function and changes in clinical status and exercise capacity during chronic enoximone therapy. Am Heart J 1989; 117:1029–1098.
5. Colucci WS, Alexander RW, Williams GH, Rude RE, Holman BL, Konstam MA, Wynne J, Mudge GH, Braunwald E. Decreased lymphocyte beta-adrenergic-receptor density in patients with heart failure and tolerance to the beta-adrenergic agonist pirbuterol. N Engl J Med 1981; 305:185–190.
6. Kubo SH, Gollub S, Bourge R, Rahko P, Cobb F, Jessup M, Brozena S, Brodsky M, Kirlin P, Shanes J, Konstam M, Gradman A, Morledge J, Cinquegrani M, Singh S, LeJemtel T, Nicklas J, Troha J, Cohn JN for the Pimobendan Multicenter Research Group. Beneficial effects of pimobendan on exercise tolerance and quality of life in patients with heart failure. Results of a multicenter trial. Circulation 1992; 85:942–949.
7. Packer M, Carver JR, Rodeheffer RJ, Ivanhoe RJ, DiBianco R, Zeldis SM, Hendrix GH, Bommer WJ, Elkayam U, Kukin ML, Mallis GI, Sollano JA, Shannon J, Tandon PK, DeMets DL for the PROMISE Study Research group. Effect of oral milrinone on mortality in severe chronic heart failure. N Engl J Med 1991; 325:1468–1475.
8. Stevenson LW, Perloff JK. The limited reliability of physical signs for estimating hemodynamics in chronic heart failure. JAMA 1989; 261:884–888.
9. Ewy GA. The abdominojugular test: technique and hemodynamic correlates. Ann Intern Med 1988; 109:456–460.
10. Engler R, Ray R, Higgins CB, McNally C, Buxton WH, Bhargava V, Shabetai R. Clinical assessment and follow-up of functional capacity in patients with chronic congestive cardiomyopathy. Am J Cardiol 1982; 49:1832–1837.
11. Cohn JN, Rector TS. Prognosis of congestive heart failure and predictors of mortality. Am J Cardiol 1988; 62:25A–30A.
12. Blackwood R, Mayou RA, Garnham JC, Armstrong C, Bryant B. Exercise capacity and quality of life in the treatment of heart failure. Clin Pharmacol Ther 1990; 48:325–332.
13. Feinstein AR, Fisher MB, Pigeon JG. Changes in dyspnea-fatigue ratings as indicators of quality of life in the treatment of congestive heart failure. Am J Cardiol 1989; 64:50–55.
14. Rector TS, Cohn JN with the Pimobendan Multicenter Research Group. Assessment of patient outcome with the Minnesota Living with Heart Failure Questionnaire: Reliability and validity during a randomized, double-blind, placebo controlled trial of pimobendan. Am Heart J 1992; 124:1017–1025.

15. Guyatt GH, Thompson PJ, Berman LB, Sullivan MJ, Townsend M, Jones NL, Pugsley SO. How should we measure function in patients with chronic heart and lung disease? J Chron Dis 1985; 38:517–524.
16. Lipkin DP, Scriven AJ, Crake T, Poole-Wilson PA. Six minute walking test for assessing exercise capacity in chronic heart failure. Br Med J 1986; 292:653–655.
17. Parameshwar J, Hedambrink J, Sparrow J, Wright C, Park A, Tweed J, Poole-Wilson PA. A new exercise test for the assessment of heart failure: use of a self powered treadmill. Br Heart J 1989; 61:421–425.
18. Davies SW, Jordan SL, Lipkin DP. Use of limb movement sensors as indicators of the level of everyday physical activity in chronic congestive heart failure. Am J Cardiol 1992; 69:1581–1586.
19. Conradson TB, Ryden L, Ahlmark G, Saetre H, Persson S, Nyquist O, Wernersson B. Clinical efficacy of hydralazine in chronic heart failure: one-year double-blind placebo-controlled study. Am Heart J 1984; 108:1001–1006.
20. Captopril Multicenter Research Group. A placebo-controlled trial of captopril in refractory chronic congestive heart failure. J Am Coll Cardiol 1983; 2:755–763.
21. Goldman L, Cook EF, Mitchell N, Flatley M, Sherman H, Cohn PF. Pitfalls in the serial assessment of cardiac functional status. How a reduction in "ordinary" activity may reduce the apparent degree of cardiac compromise and give a misleading impression of improvement. J Chron Dis 1982; 35:763–771.
22. Bergner M, Bobbitt RA, Carter WB, Gilson BS. The sickness impact profile: development and final revision of a health status measure. Medical Care 1981; 15:787–805.

7

Diuretics for the Treatment of Heart Failure

Philip Alexander Poole-Wilson
National Heart & Lung Institute, London, United Kingdom

INTRODUCTION

Diuretics are much the most commonly used group of drugs in the treatment of heart failure. Diuretics are used not only to treat the syndrome of acute heart failure, but also as an essential part of the treatment of chronic heart failure, with the exception of one or two rare conditions, such as chronic pericarditis (1) or some forms of pulmonary hypertension. Few carefully designed studies are available to demonstrate their efficacy. This is partly because the drugs were introduced into clinical practice at a time when the methodology for drug trials in chronic heart failure was not well developed, and partly because the efficacy of diuretics in congestive heart failure is readily apparent to the clinician; a placebo-controlled clinical trial would be an inappropriate method for assessing efficacy.

The standard treatment for chronic heart failure a decade ago was the combination of diuretics and digoxin. The availability of the angiotensin converting enzyme (ACE) inhibitors and the demonstration that these drugs further improve both morbidity (2,3) and mortality (4–6) has changed that recommendation, so that today the standard treatment for chronic heart failure is a diuretic with an ACE inhibitor. In selected patients digoxin may be added (Table 1).

HEART FAILURE WITH SALT AND WATER RETENTION

A discussion of the use of diuretics in heart failure is dependent on a consensus concerning the definition of heart failure. "Heart failure" is a generic term used by doctors to convey information regarding a syndrome. Many attempts have been made to define heart failure, but most of these definitions have depended on particular biochemical or physiological entities (7). A pragmatic definition is that heart failure is a clinical syndrome caused by an abnormality of the heart and recognized by a characteristic pattern of hemodynamic, renal, neural, and endocrine responses (8). Whenever the heart is damaged, by whatever mechanism, compensatory mechanisms within the heart itself and within the whole body are activated (7,9). The commonest response in chronic heart failure is the retention of salt and water. This is caused by an inability of the kidney to secrete sodium, attributable to the altered hemodynamics within the kidney—a consequence of both a reduction of perfusion pressure (9) and, to a lesser extent, of an increase in the venous pressure (10).

For practical purposes, heart failure can be considered as three syndromes: acute heart failure (sometimes referred to as acute pulmonary edema), circulatory collapse (sometimes referred to as shock, characterized by low cardiac output, reduced blood pressure, and oliguria), and chronic heart failure (7). A further distinction should be made between ventricular dysfunction, in which there is damage to the ventricle but only a minimal

Table 1 Treatment of Chronic Heart Failure

General	No added salt	Treat hypertension
	Maintain optimal weight	Detect alcohol abuse
	Stop smoking	Prevent coronary disease
	Encourage exercise	
Mild	Thiazide/loop diuretic	?? potassium therapy
	ACE inhibitor	
	Digoxin if atrial fibrillation	
Moderate	Loop diuretic	?? potassium therapy
	ACE inhibitor	
	Combine diuretics	
Severe	Increase loop diuretic	Transplant
	Combine diuretics	? inotropic drug
	Metolazone	? digoxin
	ACE inhibitor	? spironolactone
	Nitrates	

compensatory response, and chronic or overt heart failure. Left ventricular dysfunction is particularly common after a small myocardial infarct when the ventricle has unquestionably been damaged but there is no evidence of sodium and water retention. By contrast, chronic heart failure is characterized by left ventricular dysfunction with evidence of sodium and water retention. This is the terminology used in this chapter.

HISTORY

Diuretics were introduced into medical therapy for heart failure sometime after 1920. At that time the diuretic action of mercury was observed when the substance was used for the treatment of syphilis (11). Similar observations with the sulfonylureas led to the discovery of the carbonic anhydrase inhibitors. Modification of these molecules resulted in the discovery of the thiazide diuretics, introduced into clinical practice in 1957 (12,13). The loop diuretics followed. Before this era the treatment of heart failure was difficult and the prognosis poor or even desperate. Fluid retention could be treated only by blood letting, leeches, the insertion of Southey's tubes into the edematous limbs, prolonged bed rest, or digitalis glycosides. Withering (14) believed that at least part of the benefit obtained from the use of digitalis was the consequence of a diuretic effect. Nitrates were another group of drugs to be used for heart failure as early as the 19th century, although it is possible that some of their benefit was due to the relief of angina pectoris mimicking chronic heart failure.

The recent demonstration of the benefit that accrues from the use of ACE inhibitors in the management of heart failure (3–5,15) has led to the recommendation that the combination of a diuretic and an ACE inhibitor, rather than digoxin with diuretics, should now be first-line treatment for patients with overt heart failure. The value of digoxin for patients with heart failure in sinus rhythm is controversial (16,17).

CLASSIFICATION OF DIURETICS

There are now a large number of diuretics available for the treatment of patients with heart failure. Several excellent reviews have been published that describe their pharmacology (18–23). The different sites of action in the kidney of some of the commoner diuretics are shown in Table 2. Some agents can cause diuresis by an action on the hemodynamics in the kidney; these are not traditionally referred to as diuretics, although they certainly have a diuretic effect. The ACE inhibitors have many actions, which not only cause diuresis when the ACE inhibitor is given alone (24) but also can increase the diuretic action of conventional diuretics (25,26). Although

Table 2 Sites of Action of Diuretics in the Kidney

Tubular function
1. Proximal convoluted tubule
Carbonic anhydrase inhibitors
Osmotic agents
Metolazone
Mercurial diuretics
2. Ascending limb of the loop of Henle (thick)
Furosemide
Bumetanide
Ethacrynic acid
Mercurial diuretics
3. Early distal convoluted tubule
Bendrofluazide
Chlorothiazide
Hydrochlorothiazide
Indapamide
Metolazone
4. Late distal convoluted tubule and collecting ducts
Amiloride
Triamterene
Spironolactone
Renal hemodynamics
Xanthines
Calcium antagonists
Angiotensin converting enzyme inhibitors

a classification based on the site of action is conventional, a more clinically relevant classification is into thiazide diuretics, loop diuretics (sometimes called high-ceiling diuretics), and potassium-sparing diuretics. The loop diuretics are by far the most powerful, and potassium-sparing diuretics are used almost exclusively to prevent the potassium loss associated with a loop or thiazide diuretic.

SIDE EFFECTS OF DIURETICS

The major side effects of the diuretics are shown in Table 3. Although this may appear a formidable list, in general side effects are rare and do not represent a major therapeutic problem. Gout can cause a distressing episode for the patient. The insidious onset of diabetes mellitus following the use of thiazides or loop diuretics may be missed unless repeated blood glucose measurements and urine tests are made. Thiazide diuretics are

Table 3 Common Adverse Effects of Diuretics

Electrolyte abnormalities	**Metabolic abnormalities**
Hypokalemia*	Glucose intolerance (diabetes)*
Hyponatremia	Lipid changes (raised LDL and VLDL, unchanged HDL)
Hypomagnesemia	Hyperuricemia (gout)*
Variable calcium excretion	Thrombocytopenic purpura
Hyperkalemia with K^+-retaining diuretics	Increased platelet aggregation
Metabolic alkalosis	Activation of the renin-angiotensin system*
	Increased blood viscosity
General effects particularly common in the elderly	
Hypovolemia with fatigue and even dizziness*	
Azotemia*	
Urinary incontinence*	
Cardiac effects	
Arrhythmias*	
?? effect on contractility	

*Important side effects.

known to cause a small increase in total cholesterol, in low-density lipoprotein cholesterol, and in very low-density lipoprotein cholesterol, with little if any effect on high-density lipoprotein cholesterol. These effects might be of importance in patients being treated with thiazide diuretics for hypertension (27), when treatment with the diuretic may be continued over many years, but in patients with heart failure the effect is likely to be trivial. That is because the mortality rate from heart failure is 50% in approximately 4 years even if a population with mild heart failure is considered (5,28,29). In patients with heart failure due to severe and extensive coronary heart disease, such minor changes are unlikely to have sufficient effect on the regression of atheromatous plaque to alter ventricular function and prognosis.

Harmful drug interactions with diuretics are few. The most important is the reduction of diuretic effect when loop diuretics are given in combination with nonsteroidal anti-inflammatory drugs. This effect is probably caused by interference with the vasodilator action of prostaglandins within the kidney. Ototoxicity can be exacerbated when loop diuretics are used in combination with aminoglycoside antibiotics, as can nephrotoxicity with cephalothin.

Much the most serious complication of the use of diuretics is hypokalemia. This effect occurs with thiazide and loop diuretics and is dose-related (30,31). The evidence linking hypokalemia with cardiac arrhythmias comes from animal experiments, studies of myocardial infarction and sudden death, large epidemiological studies, exercise testing, and studies of hospitalized patients (32,33). Hypokalemia is uncommon in patients on low-dose thiazide diuretics (31) for the treatment of hypertension and is less common in patients with heart failure (34). Patients with heart failure have a complex hormonal response, and total body potassium is often reduced, especially in patients with severe heart failure. This may be accounted for partly by a net loss of potassium and partly by the accompanying muscle atrophy and cachexia.

A loss of intracellular potassium is of less importance than a fall of extracellular potassium, because the concentration within the cell is high (approximately 150 mm/L) and the extracellular concentration is low (Table 4). The electrical potential across cell membranes, including that of heart muscle, is more critically dependent on the extracellular than on the intracellular potassium concentration. A low plasma potassium level lowers the resting membrane potential, increases conduction velocity, increases the duration of the action potential, increases the rate of spontaneous depolarization, alters the refractory period, and reduces the threshold potential. Many symptoms are caused by hypokalemia, including muscle weakness and tiredness, but much the most important consequence is the increased propensity for arrhythmias, particularly if the patient is receiving digoxin (32,33,35,36). Several causes other than diuretics need to be considered in the differential diagnosis of hypokalemia (Table 4). Inadequate diet is relatively common in the elderly (37).

Cardiac arrhythmias are common in heart failure because of damage to the heart muscle. Sudden death may occur in as many as 50% of patients. Controversy exists as to whether such a sudden death is attributable to an

Table 4 Causes of Hypokalemia

Gastrointestinal loss	Inadequate intake
	Vomiting
	Diarrhea
Renal loss	Diuretics
	Steroids
	Liquorice
	Endocrine disease
	Renal-tubular acidosis
	Ureterosigmoidostomy
Cellular shifts	Alkalosis
	Glucose and insulin
	Periodic paralysis

opportunistic arrhythmia or whether an arrhythmia is merely the common pathway for eventual demise in patients with inadequate cardiac function. In any event, arrhythmias of almost any cause are exacerbated by hypokalemia. Normal practice is to take measures to avoid or treat hypokalemia.

AVOIDANCE OF HYPOKALEMIA

Simple dietary advice may increase the intake of potassium (Table 5). Potassium supplements in general do not contain sufficient potassium to restore the plasma potassium level to normal on a permanent basis. Potassium tablets are large and both unpleasant and difficult to swallow. There are complications, such as gastrointestinal erosions and erosions in the esophagus that can result in the formation of a stricture. This has been reported in patients with a large left atrium, which may press on the esophagus and cause a large potassium tablet to lodge repeatedly at a particular site.

Special consideration should be given to the use of diuretics in elderly patients. The major problems in such patients are hypovolemia, azotemia,

Table 5 Clinical Approach to Diuretic-Induced Hypokalemia

Prevention of hypokalemia	
1. Diet	
2. Low dose of thiazides	
3. Early detection of hypokalemia by frequent measurements	
4. Potassium supplements (marginally effective)	
5. Combined diuretic and angiotensin converting enzyme inhibitor	
6. Potassium-sparing diuretics	
Potassium supplements	
One tablet 'Slow-K'	8 mmol
One tablet 'Sandoz-K', effervescent K	12 mmol
One banana (112 g)	11 mmol
Fresh orange juice (1 cup, 250 ml)	13 mmol
One raw but ripe tomato (100 g)	6 mmol
Carlsberg lager	4 mmol/L
Milk	35 mmol/L
Body content of potassium	
Total potassium	3500 mmol
Intracellular potassium	3430 mmol
Extracellular potassium	70 mmol
Plasma potassium content	16 mmol
Plasma potassium concentration	3.5–4.5 mmol/L
Intake and excretion	90 mmol/day

and urinary incontinence. Heart failure is difficult to diagnose in the elderly. Often patients with small but fibrosed and hypertrophied hearts have symptoms of shortness of breath and fatigue. These patients can be improved by diuretics, but side effects are common if the dose is increased too high in the face of continuing symptoms.

TREATMENT OF ACUTE HEART FAILURE

The treatment of acute heart failure employs an intravenous dose of a loop diuretic combined with morphine. This combination is known to be effective, and the clinical situation is not one in which it is possible to undertake carefully designed, placebo-controlled clinical trials. The mechanism of action of the diuretic is not clear. Some data suggest that the benefit of thiazide diuretics occurs before the onset of diuresis and is attributable to vasodilatation (38). On the other hand, other work has indicated that the use of loop diuretics intravenously results in reflex activation of hormonal systems, including the renin-angiotensin system, such that vasoconstriction occurs over the initial 20 min (39). The left ventricular end-diastolic pressure may fall modestly, but the cardiac output is also reduced (40,41). If such an effect were to occur in clinical practice, it might not be observed in patients with acute pulmonary edema in intensive care who have been partly sedated with morphine at the same time. Recent work has indicated that the effectiveness of intravenous nitrates may equal or surpass that of the conventional treatment for acute heart failure, in that not only is the left ventricular end-diastolic pressure reduced but cardiac output is increased (40).

An important consideration in the treatment of acute heart failure is that the pulmonary edema and shortness of breath are a consequence of and directly related to the left ventricular end-diastolic pressure (7,42). Almost any therapy that reduces this pressure is effective. Often in acute heart failure there is not retention of sodium and water because the event follows acute damage to the myocardium, such as a myocardial infarction. Under these circumstances small shifts occur in the fluid volumes between the systemic and pulmonary circulation, causing an increase in the pressure in the left atrium and pulmonary veins that leads directly to the symptom of shortness of breath. This situation should be contrasted with that of chronic heart failure, where there is almost no relationship between the left atrial pressure and the symptom that limits exercise, be it shortness of breath or fatigue (42). In chronic heart failure the origin of symptoms is considerably more complex. Symptoms may be related in part to altered ventilatory and hemodynamic physiology in the lungs but very largely to the metabolic and neurohumoral consequences of poor peripheral flow and of atrophy and metabolic changes in skeletal muscle (43).

TREATMENT OF CHRONIC HEART FAILURE WITH DIURETICS

The purpose of treatment in chronic heart failure is to alleviate symptoms and improve prognosis. Diuretics are the key component of therapy (Table 1), since they are the most powerful clinical agents that eliminate and prevent edema either in the lungs or in the peripheral circulation. The efficacy of diuretics in chronic heart failure has never been established formally. This is partly because diuretics became available before the era when it was thought possible to undertake clinical trials in severe heart failure and partly because the benefit accruing from the use of these drugs is blindingly obvious. The early observational studies with diuretics reported dramatic improvements. More recently, further evidence has been obtained with regard to the efficacy of diuretics. Bayliss et al. (44) made careful measurements, including an exercise test, in patients with untreated heart failure. The patients had never received any form of treatment. They subsequently were treated with a loop diuretic and a potassium-sparing diuretic for a period of 1 month. There was a mean loss of weight of 4 kg, and the exercise time doubled. Although the number of patients was small, there was no control group, and the study was not blind, the size of the benefit was so great that it is more than unlikely, indeed unreasonable to believe, that such an effect was not attributable to the drugs. Similar studies have been undertaken in patients with more severe heart failure (45). Richardson et al. (46) undertook a double-blind study comparing the effect of a diuretic alone or an ACE inhibitor alone in a group of patients who had heart failure and previously documented evidence of sodium and water retention. The purpose of the study was to determine whether an ACE inhibitor alone was sufficient therapy for these patients. In the event, 4 of the 14 patients developed increasing shortness of breath, and the study was terminated. Although this study did not have a control group, the outcome would suggest not only that ACE inhibitors alone are insufficient treatment for patients with left ventricular dysfunction and previously diagnosed sodium and water retention (overt heart failure), but also that the diuretic itself confers substantial benefit on the patient.

The dose of diuretic can be difficult to determine. Usually patients with heart failure and sodium retention need a diuretic indefinitely. There is a subgroup of patients who have been treated with a diuretic for an acute exacerbation of heart failure—for example, during myocardial infarction—and who are never reassessed as to the continuing need for the drug.

Patients can be instructed in how to alter the dose of diuretics within a predetermined range by daily measurements of body weight at home. On the basis of clinical examination, a chest x-ray, and biochemical investigations, physicians are able to assess patients accurately enough to return the volumes of the body fluid compartments to normal (47).

There is no evidence from clinical trials that diuretics improve prognosis in patients with heart failure, but, again, that conclusion is so strongly supported by clinical observation that any trial would be unlikely to gain ethical approval. In the past, congestive heart failure has been treated by bed rest on the grounds that this will lead to improved ventricular function and bring about diuresis. Alternative methods have included bloodletting, drainage of edema directly from the leg, and the use of leeches. This era of what now seems almost primitive medicine was ended with the introduction of diuretics into modern treatment. It is unlikely that diuretics will ever be tested with regard to prognosis.

Until recently, diuretics were given alone to patients with heart failure. There is much to be gained by the judicious use of drug combinations. Although formal studies are few, clinical experience suggests that drug combinations increase diuresis without the side effects of high-dose loop diuretics (48,49). The dose of a loop diuretic can often be reduced after the introduction of a thiazide and/or a potassium-sparing diuretic. In patients with gross edema and fluid retention, hemofiltration can be avoided by using a loop diuretic with a thiazide diuretic, a potassium-sparing diuretic, and metolazone, all at the same time (50). Care is needed to avoid hypovolemia and severe electrolyte disturbance.

DIURETICS AND THE NEUROHUMORAL SYSTEM

Five studies (44,51–54) have now shown that in left ventricular dysfunction or early heart failure with sodium and water retention the plasma renin activity is not increased. This is in contrast to the plasma concentration of atrial natriuretic peptide or noradrenaline. These two systems are activated and may be markers of early heart failure. The normal plasma renin seems to be the result of two conflicting control mechanisms for the renin-angiotensin system. A fall in blood pressure activates the system (9), but expansion of fluid volumes suppresses it. In very severe untreated heart failure, plasma renin is increased despite substantial sodium and water retention (55).

The major stimulant to activation of the renin-angiotensin system in heart failure is the use of diuretics (44,56). Thus it is possible to consider activation of the renin-angiotensin system by diuretics as a major side effect of diuretics, and the logical conclusion would be the use of a diuretic with an ACE inhibitor. The combination of a diuretic with an ACE inhibitor has additional advantages, such as avoidance of hypokalemia and improvement of hyponatremia.

Recent trials have shown that the introduction of an ACE inhibitor for patients treated with a diuretic improves exercise capacity, reduces hospital admissions for heart failure, and prolongs life (3–6). In patients with left ventricular dysfunction alone, the ACE inhibitors have also been shown to prevent hospital admissions, delay the onset of heart failure, and reduce the number of ischemic episodes, namely, unstable angina and myocardial infarction. The reason for the latter is entirely unclear and may be an effect of ACE inhibitors on the vessel wall and those processes leading to atheroma and an unstable plaque. If plasma renin activity is not elevated in left ventricular dysfunction, the ACE inhibitors would not be expected to have a great effect. However, it is possible that ACE inhibitors have a direct effect on the myocardium such as to alter the function and components of the renin-angiotensin system, which are within the myocardium (an autocrine or paracrine effect). Further evidence for such an effect has been obtained from experiments in which ACE inhibitors appear to remodel the myocardium following myocardial infarction. There are, however, alternative explanations for the reduced onset of heart failure in patients on an ACE inhibitor. Therapy with ACE inhibitors alone is of some benefit in chronic congestive heart failure (24), although substantially less so than diuretic therapy. If a patient were on an ACE inhibitor at the time of progression from left ventricular dysfunction to overt heart failure, it may be that some benefit would accrue. Thus, it is not yet clear whether a patient with left ventricular dysfunction needs to be on an ACE inhibitor indefinitely in order to prevent progression to heart failure, or whether the ACE inhibitor could be introduced with a diuretic at the time that sodium and water retention develops, with a similar benefit. That, of course, would require close medical observation of the patient.

CONCLUSION

Diuretics are the mainstay of therapy for patients with congestive heart failure and are likely to remain so. Although side effects are well described, in general these are not of great importance. The drugs are well tolerated. The combination of a diuretic with an ACE inhibitor is entirely logical. Indeed, a patient receiving a diuretic for the treatment of heart failure should also be given an ACE inhibitor unless there is a contraindication. Diuretics are the most powerful of the drugs known to bring benefit to patients with heart failure. The proper use of diuretics requires careful assessment of fluid volumes, attention to electrolyte imbalance, and the prudent use of diuretic combinations.

REFERENCES

1. Anand I, Ferrari R, Kalra GS, Wahi PL, Poole-Wilson PA, Harris PC. Pathogenesis of edema in constrictive pericarditis: studies of body water and sodium, renal function, hemodynamics, and plasma hormones before and after pericardiectomy. Circulation 1991; 83:1880–1887.
2. Poole-Wilson PA, Lindsay D. Advances in the treatment of chronic heart failure. Two steps forward, one step back. Br Med J 1992; 304:1069–1070.
3. Lindsay DC, Poole-Wilson PA. Angiotensin-converting enzyme inhibitors or vasodilators as therapy in chronic heart failure: a review of the trials. J Cardiovasc Pharmacol 1992; 19(suppl 4):S45–S55.
4. Cohn JN, Johnson G, Ziesche S, Cobb F, Francis GS, Tristani F, Smith R, Dunkman WB, Loeb H, Wong M, Bhat G, Goldman S, Fletcher RD, Doherty J, Hughes CV, Carson P, Cintron G, Shabetai R, Haakenson C. A comparison of enalapril with hydralazine-isosorbide dinitrate in the treatment of chronic congestive heart failure. N Engl J Med 1991; 325:302–310.
5. The SOLVD Investigators. Effect of enalapril on survival in patients with reduced left ventricular ejection fractions and congestive heart failure. N Engl J Med 1991; 325:293–302.
6. Kleber FX, Niemoller L, Doering W. Impact of converting enzyme inhibition on progression of chronic heart failure: results of the Munich Mild Heart Failure Trial. Br Heart J 1992; 67:289–296.
7. Poole-Wilson PA. In: Julian DG, Camm AJ, Fox KF, Hall RJC, Poole-Wilson PA, eds. Diseases of the Heart. Vol. 1. London: Balliere-Tindall, 1989:24–36.
8. Poole-Wilson PA. Heart failure. Med Int 1985; 2:866–871.
9. Harris P. Congestive cardiac failure: central role of the arterial blood pressure. Br Heart J 1987; 58:190–203.
10. Firth JD, Raine AE, Ledingham JG. Raised venous pressure: a direct cause of renal sodium retention in oedema? Lancet 1988; 1:1033–1035.
11. Pugh LGC, Wyndham CL. The circulatory effects of mercurial diuretics in congestive heart failure. Clin Sci 1949; 8:11–19.
12. Novello FC, Sprague JM. Benzothiadiazine dioxides as novel diuretics. J Am Chem Soc 1957; 79:2028–2029.
13. Slater JDH, Nabarro JDN. Clinical experience with chlorothiazide. Lancet 1958; 1:124–126.
14. Withering W. An Account of the Foxglove, and Some of Its Medical Uses: With Practical Remarks on Dropsy, and Other Diseases. London: GJJ and J Robinson, 1785.
15. The CONSENSUS Trial Study Group. Effects of enalapril on mortality in severe congestive heart failure. Results of the Cooperative North Scandina-

vian Enalapril Survival Study (CONSENSUS). N Engl J Med 1987; 316:1429–1435.
16. Poole-Wilson PA, Robinson K. Digoxin—a redundant drug in the treatment of congestive heart failure. Cardiovasc Drugs Ther 1989; 2:733–741.
17. Gibbs JSR, MacLachlan D, Poole-Wilson PA, Fox KM. Ambulatory pulmonary artery pressure: development of a new system for measurement, recording and data analysis (abstr). Eur Heart J 1991; 12(suppl):79.
18. Lant A. Diuretics. Clinical pharmacology and therapeutic use (Part II). Drugs 1985; 29:162–188.
19. Lant A. Diuretics. Clinical pharmacology and therapeutic use (Part I). Drugs 1985; 29:57–87.
20. Puschett JB. Clinical pharmacologic implications in diuretic selection. Am J Cardiol 1986; 57:6A–13A.
21. Diuretics in Heart failure. Trends and Developments. London: Royal Society of Medicine Services, 1987.
22. Progress in Pharmacology. Clinical Pharmacology and Therapeutic Uses of Diuretics. Vol. 6. No. 3 Stuttgart: Gustav Fischer Verlag, 1988.
23. Chatterjee K, Gersh BJ, Kaplan NM, et al. Drugs for the Heart. Philadelphia: W. B. Saunders, 1991.
24. Anand IS, Kalra GS, Ferrari R, Wahi PL, Harris PC, Poole-Wilson PA. Enalapril as initial and sole treatment in severe chronic heart failure with sodium retention. Int J Cardiol 1990; 28:341–346.
25. Cleland JG, Gillen G, Dargie HJ. The effects of furosemide and angiotensin-converting enzyme inhibitors and their combination on cardiac and renal haemodynamics in heart failure. Eur Heart J 1988; 9:132–141.
26. Odemuyiwa O, Gilmartin J, Kenny D, Hall RJ. Captopril and the diuretic requirements in moderate and severe chronic heart failure. Eur Heart J 1989; 10:586–590.
27. Swales JD. Antihypertensive drugs and plasma lipids. Br Heart J 1991; 66:409–410.
28. Kannel WB, Savage D, Castelli WP. In: Braunwald E, Mock MB, Watson JT, eds. Congestive Heart Failure. Current Research and Clinical Applications. New York: Grune and Stratton, 1982:15–30.
29. Smith WM. Epidemiology of congestive heart failure. Am J Cardiol 1985; 55:3A–8A.
30. Cranston WI, Juel-Jenson BE, Semmence AM, Jones RPCH, Forbes JA, Mutch LM. Effects of oral diuretics on raised arterial pressure. Lancet 1963; 2:966–970.
31. Carlsen JE, Kober L, Torp-Pedersen C, and Johansen P. Relation between dose of bendrofluazide, antihypertensive effect, and adverse biochemical effects. Br Med J 1990; 300:975–978.
32. Poole-Wilson PA. Hypokalemia induced by thiazide diuretics in the treatment of hypertension: a cause for concern, not nihilism. Postgrad Med J 1983; 59(suppl 3):137–139.

33. Singh BN, Hollenberg NK, Poole-Wilson PA, Robertson JIS. Diuretic-induced potassium and magnesium deficiency in relation to drug-induced QT prolongation, cardiac arrhythmias, and sudden death. J Hypertension 1992; 10:301–316.
34. Morgan DB, Davidson C. Hypokalemia and diuretics: an analysis of publications. Br Med J 1980; 280:905–908.
35. Kassirer JP, Harrington JT. Diuretics and potassium metabolism: a reassessment of the need, effectiveness and safety of potassium therapy. Kidney Int 1977; 11:505–515.
36. DiBianco R, Shabetai R, Kostuk W, Moran J, Schlant RC, Wright R. A comparison of oral milrinone, digoxin, and their combination in the treatment of patients with chronic heart failure. N Engl J Med 1989; 320:677–683.
37. Maclennan WJ. Diuretics in the elderly: how safe? Br Med J 1988; 296:1551–1552.
38. Dikshit K, Vyden JK, Forrester JS, Chatterjee K, Prakash R, Swan HJ. Renal and extrarenal hemodynamic effects of furosemide in congestive heart failure after acute myocardial infarction. N Engl J Med 1973; 288:1087–1090.
39. Francis GS, Siegel RM, Goldsmith SR, Olivari MT, Levine TB, Cohn JN. Acute vasoconstrictor response to intravenous furosemide in patients with chronic congestive heart failure. Ann Intern Med 1985; 103:1–6.
40. Nelson GI, Silke B, Ahuja RC, Hussain M, Taylor SH. Haemodynamic advantages of isosorbide dinitrate over frusemide in acute heart-failure following myocardial infarction. Lancet 1983; 1:730–733.
41. Taylor SH, Silke B, Nelson GI. Principles of treatment of left ventricular failure. Eur Heart J 1982; 3(suppl D):19–43.
42. Lipkin DP, Poole-Wilson PA. Symptoms limiting exercise in chronic heart failure (editorial). Br Med J 1986; 292:1030–1031.
43. Poole-Wilson PA. The origin of symptoms in patients with chronic heart failure. Eur Heart J 1988; 9(suppl H):49–53.
44. Bayliss J, Norell M, Canepa-Anson R, Sutton G, Poole-Wilson P. Untreated heart failure: clinical and neuroendocrine effects of introducing diuretics. Br Heart J 1987; 57:17–22.
45. Anand IS, Kalra GS, Harris P, Poole-Wilson PA, Panzali A, De Giuli F, Ferrari R. Diuretics as initial and sole treatment in chronic cardiac failure. Cardioscience. 1991; 2:273–278.
46. Richardson A, Bayliss J, Scriven AJ, Parameshwar J, Poole-Wilson PA, Sutton GC. Double-blind comparison of captopril alone against frusemide plus amiloride in mild heart failure. Lancet 1987; 2:709–711.
47. Anand IS, Veall N, Kalra GS, Ferrari R, Sutton G, Lipkin D, Harris P, Poole-Wilson PA. Treatment of heart failure with diuretics: body compartments, renal function and plasma hormones. Eur Heart J 1989; 10:445–450.
48. Channer KS, Richardson M, Crook R, Jones JV. Thiazides with loop diuretics for congestive heart failure. Lancet 1990; 1:922–923.
49. Allman S, Norris RJ. An open, parallel group study comparing a frusemide/amiloride diuretic and a diuretic containing cyclopenthiazide with sustained

release potassium in the treatment of congestive cardiac failure—a multicentre general practice study. J Int Med Res 1990; 18:17B–23B.
50. Kiyingi A, Field MJ, Pawsey CC, Yiannikas J, Lawrence JR, Arter WJ. Metolazone in treatment of severe refractory congestive cardiac failure. Lancet 1990; 335:29–31.
51. Brown JJ, Davies DL, Johnson VW, Lever AF, Robertson JI. Renin relationships in congestive cardiac failure, treated and untreated. Am Heart J 1970; 80:329–342.
52. Remes J, Tikkanen I, Fyhrquist F, Pyorala K. Neuroendocrine activity in untreated heart failure. Br Heart J 1991; 65:249–255.
53. Francis GS, Benedict C, Johnstone DE, Kirlin PC, Nicklas J, Liang C, Kubo SH, Rudin-Toretsky E, Yusuf S. Comparison of neuroendocrine activation in patients with left ventricular dysfunction with and without congestive heart failure. Circulation 1990; 82:1724–1729.
54. Kubo SH, Clark M, Laragh JH, Borer JS, Cody RJ. Identification of normal neurohormonal activity in mild congestive heart failure and stimulating effect of upright posture and diuretics. Am J Cardiol 1987; 60:1322–1328.
55. Anand IS, Ferrari R, Kalra GS, Wahi PL, Poole-Wilson PA, Harris PC. Edema of cardiac origin. Studies of body water and sodium, renal function, hemodynamic indexes, and plasma hormones in untreated congestive cardiac failure. Circulation 1989; 80:299–305.
56. Ikram H, Chan W, Espiner EA, Nicholls MG. Haemodynamic and hormone responses to acute and chronic frusemide therapy in congestive heart failure.Clin Sci 1980; 59:443–449.

8

Cardiac Glycosides in the Treatment of Heart Failure

Marc D. Tischler
University of Vermont College of Medicine, Burlington, Vermont

Elliott M. Antman
Brigham and Women's Hospital and Harvard Medical School, Boston, Massachusetts

INTRODUCTION

Two centuries have passed since the publication of a classic treatise on the foxglove by William Withering (1). It was not until the late 1920s, however, that digitalis was demonstrated to have a positive inotropic effect, when it was shown to enhance the contractile state of intact heart preparations (2). Since that time, despite considerable debate regarding its basic mechanism of action and risk:benefit ratio when used clinically (3), digitalis has remained a primary agent in the pharmacologic management of congestive heart failure. While most physicians acknowledge the utility of digitalis preparations in patients with congestive heart failure complicated by supraventricular tachyarrhythmias, controversy has surrounded the efficacy of digitalis preparations in patients with heart failure and normal sinus rhythm. As early as 1920, Sir James Mackenzie stated that clinical benefits of digitalis were found mainly to "occur in one condition, auricular fibrillation, or its allied condition, auricular flutter" (4). But Henry Christian and followers argued that digitalis had a "striking effect on those changes in the patient which are brought about by cardiac insufficiency, and this effect appears irrespective of whether or not the pulses are regular" (5). A variety of different patterns of digitalis use can be found clinically, and

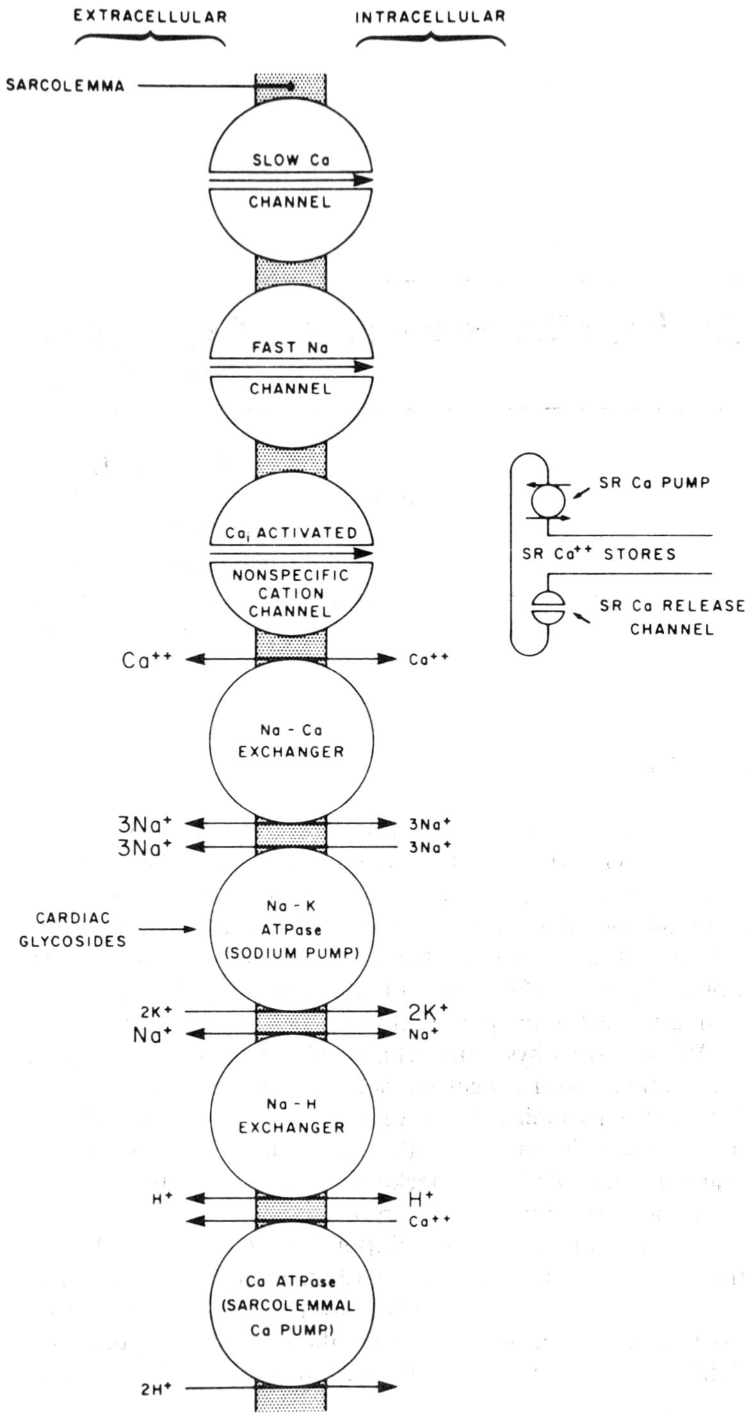
EXTRACELLULAR
INTRACELLULAR
SARCOLEMMA
SLOW Ca CHANNEL
FAST Na CHANNEL
Ca$_i$ ACTIVATED NONSPECIFIC CATION CHANNEL
SR Ca PUMP
SR Ca^{++} STORES
SR Ca RELEASE CHANNEL
Ca^{++}
Ca^{++}
Na - Ca EXCHANGER
3Na$^+$
3Na$^+$
3Na$^+$
3Na$^+$
CARDIAC GLYCOSIDES
Na - K ATPase (SODIUM PUMP)
2K$^+$
Na$^+$
2K$^+$
Na$^+$
Na - H EXCHANGER
H$^+$
H$^+$
Ca^{++}
Ca ATPase (SARCOLEMMAL Ca PUMP)
2H$^+$

concerns over the safety and efficacy of digoxin in heart failure continue to be discussed in the literature (6,7).

The current widespread prescription of new vasodilator drugs and increasing realization that the clinical syndrome of heart failure is composed of a heterogeneous group of conditions, including those in which systolic performance is unimpaired but relaxation or diastolic compliance is dis-

---

Figure 1 Selected components regulating cellular calcium homeostasis in myocardial membrane systems. (1) The slow calcium channel, a voltage-sensitive protein complex that carries the slow inward calcium current during phase 2 of the cardiac action potential, provides the pulse of intracellular calcium $[CA^+]_i$ that triggers calcium-induced release of a much larger amount of activator calcium from stores in the sarcoplasmic reticulum (SR). The arrow indicates the principal direction of ion movement when the channel is activated. (2) The fast sodium channel, another voltage-sensitive structure, mediates the upstroke of the cardiac action potential; this depolarization event results in activation of the slow calcium channel. (3) A putative intracellular calcium-activated nonspecific cation channel, less well characterized than the preceding components (1 and 2), is thought to account for the transient depolarizing (and hence arrhythmogenic) inward current that occurs in response to toxic doses of cardiac glycosides. (4) The sodium-calcium exchanger is a membrane component that mediates the facilitated, bi-directional exchange of sodium for calcium across the sarcolemmal membrane. This process is sensitive to membrane potential because of the asymmetry of charge movement inherent in the stoichiometry of the process (three sodium ions for every calcium ion). (See text for explanation of the role of this exchanger in the inotropic mechanism of digitalis.) (5) The NaK-ATPase, or sodium pump—the cardiac glycoside–binding site—is located on the outward-facing surface of the alpha subunit of this enzyme, which mediates the active transport of sodium and potassium ions against their respective concentration gradients. (6) The sodium–hydrogen exchanger, an amiloride-sensitive protein, mediates the electroneutral exchange of sodium for hydrogen ions and helps to facilitate the accumulation of intracellular sodium (and hence intracellular calcium) in response to cardiac glycosides (see text and Fig. 2). (7) The sarcolemmal calcium pump has a relatively low-capacity but high affinity ATP-dependent ion-transport protein that extrudes calcium from cardiac cells against a large electrochemical gradient and helps to maintain the low levels of intracellular calcium ions that prevail during diastole. To the right of the sarcolemmal membrane are represented (8) the sarcoplasmic-reticulum ATP-dependent calcium pump that is responsible for diastolic relaxation by rapid sequestration of calcium at end systole, and (9) the ryanodine-sensitive sarcoplasmic-reticulum calcium-release channel that accounts for calcium-induced release of most of the calcium that activates contractile proteins in mammalian myocardium. (From Ref. 3.)

turbed, have added to the complexity of clinical decision making in caring for patients with heart failure. Recently, a few rigorous attempts have been made to assess prospectively the efficacy of digitalis in a randomized, double-blinded fashion (8–12). These studies, however, are in many cases flawed and require critical review.

MECHANISM OF ACTION

It is now generally agreed that the inotropic effects of cardiac glycosides result from the binding to and inhibition of NaK-ATPase (13). Cardiac glycosides bind with high affinity and specificity to an inhibitory site on the alpha subunit of NaK-ATPase, producing complete inhibition of sodium and potassium transport by that enzyme unit. As a result of inhibition of NaK-ATPase, intracellular sodium accumulates, leading to activation of the sodium-calcium exchanger, a membrane component that facilitates bidirectional exchange of sodium for calcium across the sarcolemmal mem-

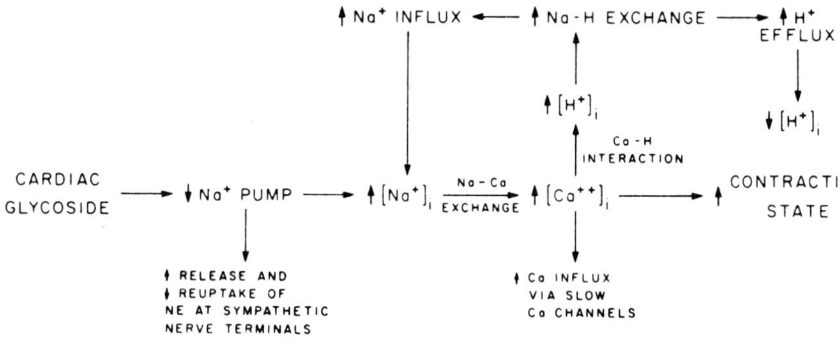

Figure 2 Mechanisms of modulation of myocardial function by cardiac glycosides. In addition to the horizontal sequence leading from cardiac glycoside–induced inhibition of the sodium-ion pump to enhanced myocardial contractile state, three ancillary processes are shown: enhanced norepinephrine (NE) release and reduced reuptake at cardiac sympathetic-nerve terminals, which may occur in experimental circumstances but has doubtful clinical relevance; an enhanced slow inward calcium current with increased calcium influx through slow calcium channels in response to an increased concentration of intracellular calcium ions over a limited range of values for these ions; and decreased intracellular pH (increased $[H^+]_i$) in response to increased intracellular calcium, leading to enhanced sodium–hydrogen exchange and hence augmentation of the rise in intracellular sodium ($[Na^+]_i$) caused by sodium-pump inhibition. (From Ref. 3.)

brane (Fig. 1) (14,15). The process tends toward an equilibrium in which any increase in the intracellular concentration of sodium favors increased calcium entry and reduced calcium extrusion. The increase in intracellular calcium concentration has, in turn, been shown to augment myocardial contractile function (16). Additional cellular mechanisms participate in the inotropic effect of cardiac glycosides. These include increased calcium entry through slow calcium channels (17), stimulation of release and blockade of reuptake of norepinephrine from adrenergic nerve terminals (18), and alterations of the sodium-hydrogen exchange process (19) (Fig. 2).

PHARMACOKINETICS AND BIOAVAILABILITY

Digoxin is the most commonly prescribed digitalis preparation by virtue of its flexibility of routes of administration and intermediate duration of action, and the ready availability of assays of its serum concentration (20). To circumvent problems with digoxin bioavailability, the FDA developed requirements whereby all digoxin tablets marketed in the United States must have an in vitro dissolution rate no greater than 90% in 15 min and no less than 65% in 1 h (21.)

Digoxin is predominantly excreted via the renal route, and in young normal subjects the elimination half-life is approximately 36 h, irrespective of the route of administration (22). Approximately 37% of total body stores of digoxin is removed daily. In older patients with cardiovascular disease but normal blood urea nitrogen and creatinine levels, an excretory half-life of 48 h is probably a more accurate estimate of the rate of clearance of digoxin. It is imperative that maintenance doses of digoxin be adjusted to compensate for altered renal function. It is noteworthy that approximately 10% of the population carry gut flora that are capable of metabolizing digoxin into inactive reduction products (23). Antibiotic therapy in these patients might cause important alterations in the state of digitalization.

Other Cardiac Glycosides

Digitoxin is the least polar of the cardiac glycosides and is 97% bound to serum albumin (24). As opposed to digoxin, the elimination half-life is in the range of 4 to 6 days, irrespective of renal function, and renal clearance of unchanged digitoxin is minor (25). Elimination of digitoxin occurs predominantly through metabolic change.

Ouabain, a parenterally available cardiac glycoside, has a half-life of approximately 21 h. Deslanoside is a digoxin analogue with a terminal glucose moiety that renders it poorly absorbed from the gastrointestinal tract and therefore suitable for parenteral use only (26). Acetylstrophanthidin is a semisynthetic acetyl ester of the aglycone strophanthidin and has the advantage of a short half-life (2.3 h) and a short duration of clinical effect.

DRUG INTERACTIONS WITH CARDIAC GLYCOSIDES

Drugs Affecting Absorption of Cardiac Glycosides

Cholestyramine (27), colestipol (28), pectin (20), and neomycin (30) have all been shown to decrease the absorption of cardiac glycosides from the gut, thereby necessitating higher loading and maintenance doses than usual. Alternatively, discontinuation of one of these agents can lead to digitalis toxicity if the digoxin dosage is not reduced.

Interactions with Cardioactive Drugs

Quinidine (31,32), verapamil (33,34), and amiodarone (35,36) have all been shown to decrease the total body clearance of digoxin by both renal and nonrenal mechanisms. Quinidine also appears to decrease the volume of distribution of digoxin (37). Therefore, careful monitoring of serum digoxin levels is indicated whenever one of these agents is administered to a patient receiving maintenance digoxin therapy. In general, the maintenance digoxin dose should be halved to avoid an increase in steady-state serum digoxin concentrations once a new equilibrium is established.

SERUM AND PLASMA LEVELS

Most currently available tests of serum and plasma levels of cardiac glycosides rely on radioimmunoassay methodologies. Because of the narrow margin between toxic and therapeutic doses, these determinations should not be relied on as the sole basis for diagnosing digitalis toxicity. Rather, they should be interpreted in the context of all the available clinical information.

Serum level data are useful in situations characterized by unexpected responses to digitalis, such as underdigitalization on standard doses or unexpected toxicity.

DIGITALIS TOXICITY

In a survey of over 4300 digitalis-treated patients in Boston hospitals between 1966 and 1975, adverse reactions attributed to digitalis were reported in 12% but were believed to have contributed to death in only two individuals, both of whom had severe coexisting illnesses (38). These observations were made before the development of assays for serum digoxin levels or the ready availability of digoxin-specific Fab fragments.

The first clinical report of the use of purified digoxin-specific Fab fragments for the treatment of advanced digitalis toxicity was in 1976 (39). Subsequently, a multicenter clinical trial was undertaken and was recently completed. A total of 150 patients with potentially life-threatening digitalis toxicity were treated with Fab fragments; 80% had complete resolution of all symptoms and signs of digitalis toxicity, and 10% were improved (40). In the subset of patients with digitalis-induced cardiac arrest, 54% survived to hospital discharge. This compares favorably with the 100% mortality for a similar cohort reported by Gaultier and Bismuth (41).

DIGITALIS THERAPY AFTER ACUTE MYOCARDIAL INFARCTION

The question of whether digoxin increases mortality in patients recovering from acute myocardial infarction has sparked considerable controversy (42,43). Seven nonrandomized trials have been performed examining survival after acute myocardial infarction in patients treated and not treated with digitalis preparations (44). Significant differences in recruitment criteria and definition of congestive heart failure severely limit the generalizability of these reports. Even so, in six of these studies, there was no significant difference in mortality in treated and untreated groups (Table 1). In the one trial demonstrating an increased mortality in the cohort of patients treated with digoxin (45), the overall mortality in the control group was only 1.8%, suggesting the possibility of selection bias leading to incorporation of less ill patients in the control group. Additionally, the definition of congestive heart failure (presence of rales, leg edema, or both) was somewhat unusual. In our view, when one accounts for baseline characteristics predictive of mortality, the added risk of digoxin therapy, if present at all, appears to be sufficiently small that only an extremely large prospective, randomized trial would have the power to detect any adverse effect on survival (46,47).

CLINICAL USE OF DIGOXIN IN CONGESTIVE HEART FAILURE

Hemodynamic Effects: Evidence for Positive Inotropic Effects

Augmentation of myocardial contractility by digitalis has been demonstrated by virtually every study investigating the hemodynamic effects of

Table 1 Comparison of Seven Nonrandomized Studies of the Effect of Digitalis on Survival After Myocardial Infarction

Parameter	U. Rochester Heart Attack Follow-up Program 1981	Coronary Artery Study Group 1983	U. California Myocardial Infarction Study 1984	Presbyterian Hospital Myocardial Infarction Study 1985	Beta-Blocker Heart Attack Trial 1985	Multicenter Investigation on the Limitation of Infarct Size 1986	Multicenter Post-Infarction Program 1987
Enrollment period	1973–1976	1974–1979	1969–1982	1974–1980	1978–1980	1978–1983	1979–1980
Inclusion criteria	Definite or probable AMI	Definite AMI; chest pain syndrome	Definite AMI	Definite AMI	Definite AMI	Definite AMI	Definite AMI
Time of enrollment	Within 3 wk of AMI	Within 2 mo of AMI	Within 3 wk of AMI	Within 3 wk of AMI	Within 3 wk of AMI	Within 18 h of onset of chest pain	Within 3 wk of AMI
Number of patients analyzed	812	892/1592	1300	504	1921/3837	903	728
Duration of follow-up	4 mo	55 mo (av.)	12 mo	23 mo	25 mo	25 mo	22 mo
Mortality end point	All causes	All causes	All causes	All causes	All causes	All causes	All causes
% on digitalis	19	21	37	45	13	31	31
1-yr survival	—	90	86	86	95	91	91
Statistically significant independent predictors of survival	Female sex, smoking, diabetes, previous infarction, NYHA functional class	Age, rales, edema, number of diseased vessels, LV wall motion score	Age, MI, angina, CHF, maximum HR in hospital	LV failure in CCU, AF in CCU, cardio-megaly on CXR, VPC frequence	16 variables	LVEF, age, ST elevation, beta-blockers, diuretics, complex VPC	LVEF, NYHA class, VPC frequency, BUN, rales, age, edema, diabetes
Statistical methods used	Modified logistic regression	Cox survival analysis	Cox survival analysis	Cox survival analysis	Logistic regression	Cox survival analysis	Cox survival analysis
p value	≤0.01	≤0.10	≤0.10	≤0.10	≥0.05	≥0.30	≤0.001

AF = atrial fibrillation; AMI = acute myocardial infarction; BUN = blood urea nitrogen; CHF = congestive heart failure; CCU = coronary care unit; CXR = chest X-ray; EF = ejection fraction; HR = heart rate; LV = left ventricle; VPC = ventricular premature contraction.

Source: Ref. 44.

Table 2 Hemodynamic Responses to Digoxin

Response	Reference
Increased LVEF	8,11,66
Reduced PCW	48
Shortened QS_2I	47
Increased % LV fractional shortening	9
Increased LV stroke work index	48

EF = ejection fraction; LV = left ventricle; PCW = pulmonary capillary wedge pressure; STI = systolic time intervals.

digitalis (Table 2). Unfortunately, the end points in these studies have been extremely heterogeneous. Carliner et al., using oral digoxin in eight patients in normal sinus rhythm, documented a dose-related positive inotropic effect as assessed by reduction in the duration of systole (QS_2I) following 2 weeks of therapy (48). The efficacy of digoxin in patients with moderately severe to severe congestive heart failure and left ventricular dilation due to coronary artery disease or idiopathic dilated cardiomyopathy was evaluated by Arnold et al. in 1980 (49). In a small cohort of nine patients with well-quantitated systolic ventricular dysfunction, invasive hemodynamic measurements were carried out during long-term digoxin therapy and again after digoxin was discontinued for 6 to 7 weeks (or sooner in four patients who experienced clinical deterioration 12 to 31 days after withdrawal of digoxin). Hemodynamic deterioration with digoxin withdrawal as indicated by a decrease in left ventricular stroke work index and increase in pulmonary capillary wedge pressure occurred in all nine patients; this deterioration was reversed with resumption of digitalis therapy.

In a particularly well designed trial, Guyatt et al. conducted a double-blinded, placebo-controlled crossover study of 20 patients in normal sinus rhythm with congestive heart failure and echocardiographic evidence of left ventricular dysfunction (fractional shortening $< 28\%$; left ventricular end-diastolic diameter > 3.2 cm/m^2) (9). They demonstrated a statistically significant improvement in fractional shortening and a trend toward reduced left ventricular end-diastolic dimension following 7 weeks of digoxin therapy when compared with 7 weeks of matched placebo.

Clinical Benefits

Following their review of 16 studies published between 1960 and 1982 designed to evaluate the efficacy of digitalis in patients with congestive heart failure and normal sinus rhythm, Mulrow et al. concluded that only two trials were both double-blinded and placebo-controlled and, hence, could provide unbiased information (50). Ambiguous entry criteria and nonrandomized design limited the generalizability of many other trials.

The first placebo-controlled, double-blinded trial of digitalis in congestive heart failure was published by Dobbs et al. in 1977 (51). Using a crossover design, they found that 16 of 46 patients with stable heart failure exhibited clinical deterioration when placebo was substituted for digoxin. Unfortunately, 13 patients had atrial arrhythmias, and the authors failed to specify how many of the 16 patients who required digitalis were in atrial fibrillation on entry into the trial. The study is also flawed in that no data were provided on other therapeutic interventions (e.g., diuretics) employed during the crossover period.

Lee et al. reported a placebo-controlled, double-blinded crossover study of 25 patients in normal sinus rhythm with chronic heart failure (12). Fourteen patients had improvement in a clinical heart failure score following therapy with digoxin. Six of the 11 patients who failed to improve had no symptoms of heart failure at baseline (heart failure score = 0) and hence were incapable of demonstrating any improvement with therapy, two suffered from ischemic disease but had normal ejection fractions, and another four had hypertrophic cardiomyopathy with well-preserved systolic function. Clinically significant systolic ventricular dysfunction was not evident in these latter six patients, and digoxin would therefore not be expected to result in symptomatic improvement. It seems more plausible that the pathophysiological mechanism of dyspnea in these patients was the now more widely appreciated problem of diastolic dysfunction and elevated left ventricular end-diastolic pressure (52–54). The study is also limited by the nonstandardized heart failure scoring system, although Gheorghiade et al. did use a similar scoring system in their evaluation of the combined use of digoxin, vasodilators, and diuretics (55).

Guyatt et al. conducted one of the more rigorous placebo-controlled, double-blinded crossover studies of digoxin versus placebo in 20 patients with clinically symptomatic heart failure and well-documented functional disability and quantitated systolic ventricular dysfunction (9). Clinical deterioration manifested by subjective dyspnea occurred in seven patients during placebo therapy, while none deteriorated after crossing over from placebo to digoxin ($p < 0.02$). Small differences in a 6-min walking test (411 m vs. 392 m; $p = 0.055$) and left ventricular fractional shortening (21% vs. 17%; $p = 0.004$) favored the digoxin group.

More recently, Sullivan et al. performed maximal treadmill testing in conjunction with respiratory gas exchange analysis on 11 patients with chronic congestive heart failure (New York Heart Association [NYHA] class II–III) under conditions where digoxin was and was not part of the therapeutic regimen (56). All 11 patients were in normal sinus rhythm and were confirmed to have systolic ventricular dysfunction. The mean ejection fraction of the group was 24% ± 10%. Patients on digoxin were studied at a time when stable serum digoxin levels were obtained and again following a 2- to 4-week period of drug washout. Significant improvements in oxygen uptake were observed with digoxin during submaximal exercise (3.0 mph, 0% grade), at the gas exchange anaerobic threshold, and at maximal exercise (mean increase of 2.6 ml/kg/min; $p < 0.02$). Resting heart rate was significantly higher (91 ± 16 vs. 102 ± 16 beats/min; $p < 0.05$) and resting systolic blood pressure was significantly reduced (130 ± 23 vs. 121 ± 15; $p < 0.05$) in the absence of digoxin. Thus, in this cohort of patients with moderate chronic congestive heart failure, digoxin was associated with important improvements in exercise capacity.

DiBianco and colleagues recently reported a compelling large-scale clinical trial designed to examine the effects of digitalis on exercise tolerance in patients with heart failure and normal sinus rhythm (8). They randomly allocated 230 patients with moderately severe heart failure (71% NYHA class III or IV) despite chronic therapy with digitalis and diuretics to one of four groups: therapy with digoxin, milrinone, both drugs, or placebo. The effects of each regimen were compared during a 12 week double-blind trial. Treatment with milrinone increased exercise capacity modestly, but neither monotherapy with milrinone (82 s or 19% improvement) nor combination with digoxin (48 s or 10% improvement) offered any advantage over digoxin alone (64 s or 14% improvement); when given with diuretics but not digoxin, milrinone was associated with a markedly increased frequency of clinical deterioration at 2 weeks and 3 months (Table 3). Digoxin significantly improved exercise tolerance ($p < 0.03$) and produced a small but statistically significant increase in mean left ventricular ejection fraction when compared with placebo (+1.7%; $p < 0.01$). Milrinone alone or milrinone plus digoxin was associated with increased asymptomatic ventricular arrhythmia and an increased incidence of nonsustained ventricular tachycardia when compared with placebo or digoxin alone. The study had insufficient numbers of patients and duration of follow-up to achieve the power needed to evaluate an effect on mortality.

Digitalis and Vasodilators

While there is a general consensus that digitalis improves cardiac performance in patients with chronic heart failure due to systolic dysfunction (Table 4), present-day therapeutic decisions often rest on evidence regarding the relative safety and efficacy of alternative therapeutic modalities as well as the benefits of combined therapy. The Captopril-Digoxin Multicenter Re-

Table 3 Comparison of Oral Milrinone and Digoxin

	Placebo	Digoxin	Milrinone	D + M
ETT	—	+14% ($p < 0.03$)	+19% ($p < 0.006$)	+10%
LVEF	−2.0%	+1.7% ($p < 0.01$)	+0.2% (NS)	+2.1% ($p < 0.005$)
Clinical deterioration (2 wk)	—	3.0%	20.0% ($p < 0.05$)	—
Increased vea	11.0%	0%	22.0%	15.0%

D + M = digoxin plus milrinone; ETT = exercise tolerance test; LVEF = left ventricular ejection fraction; VEA = ventricular ectopic activity.
Source: Ref. 8.

Table 4 Hemodynamic Effects of Digoxin and Vasodilators

	↑ EF	↓ PCW	↓ SVR	↑ Exercise duration	Reference
Digitalis	+ +	+ +	+	+	8,9,10,11,29
Vasodilators	+	+	+ +	+ +	10,11,40,41
Combined	+ + +	+ + +	+ + +	+ + +	35,42,43

EF = ejection fraction; PCW = pulmonary capillary wedge pressure; SVR = systemic vascular resistance.

search Group Study (11) represents the first direct comparison of sustained treatment with digitalis versus vasodilators. Using pretrial end points of left ventricular ejection fraction and exercise duration, 300 patients with left ventricular ejection fraction less than or equal to 40% and mild to moderate congestive heart failure on diuretic therapy were randomly assigned to captopril, digoxin, or placebo after a period of withdrawal from therapy with digoxin and/or vasodilators and stabilization of the diuretic regimen. Notably, *patients who did not tolerate digoxin withdrawal were not included in the study group*. After 6 months of treatment, digoxin and captopril reduced to a similar extent (45%) the need for hospitalizations and emergency room visits for exacerbations of heart failure. Exercise duration significantly increased with captopril (mean increase 82 s vs. 35 s on placebo; $p < 0.05$) while the improvement on digoxin (54 s vs. 35 s on placebo) was not statistically significant. Mean exercise capacity was not statistically different in the digoxin and captopril groups. Overall, left ventricular ejection fraction increased from 26.0% to 30.4% in the digoxin group compared with an increase from 26.0% to 27.8% in the captopril group ($p < 0.05$) and from 26.3% to 27.2% in the placebo group ($p < 0.01$). There is a "built-in" recruitment bias in the design of this study in that those patients who could not tolerate withdrawal of digoxin therapy were not randomized. This bias may have diluted the possible favorable effect of digoxin.

In the Enalapril Versus Digoxin French Multicenter Study, 142 patients with NYHA class II to IV congestive heart failure (43% class II; 40% class III; 12% class IV) were treated for 2 to 4 weeks with digoxin and diuretics and were then randomized to receive either enalapril plus diuretics or digoxin plus diuretics for the subsequent 8 weeks (10). After 8 weeks of therapy, a significant improvement in NYHA classification was observed in 22 of 63 patients in the enalapril group (35%) and in 17 of 61 (28%) in the digoxin group (difference not significant). Similarly, the duration of exercise was significantly improved in both treatment groups ($p < 0.005$) compared with placebo but did not differ significantly between treatment groups. As with previous trials, the sample size and length of follow-up (2 months) were insufficient to permit any meaningful conclusions regarding mortality.

The German and Austrian Xamoterol Study Group Trial compared digoxin to xamoterol, a partial β_1-agonist. In this trial, 433 patients with mild to moderate heart failure (24% NYHA class I; 63% NYHA class II) were randomized to treatment with digoxin, xamoterol, or placebo for a 3-month treatment period (57). This study has several major limitations. The entry criteria were designed to focus on less severely ill patients (the majority of patients were NYHA class I or II and only 25% were on maintenance therapy with diuretics). There is also ascertainment bias, as evidenced by the high incidence of withdrawal after randomization (over 16% of randomized patients withdrew from treatment before completing the protocol). Patients treated with xamoterol achieved statistically significant increases in exercise duration (299 s vs. 263 s, $p < 0.001$), work performed (19.3 kJ vs. 15.5 kJ, $p < 0.001$), and subjective improvements in breathlessness (Likert scale, $p < 0.001$) and tiredness (Likert scale, $p < 0.001$) when compared with placebo. Digoxin improved subjective symptoms of breathlessness (Likert scale, $p < 0.05$) and tiredness (Likert scale, $p < 0.05$) when compared with placebo. Digoxin also increased exercise duration (279 s vs. 263 s) and work performance (17.1 kJ vs. 15.5 kJ). These differences, however, were insufficient to achieve statistical significance. In view of the fact that the trial appeared to select digoxin nonresponders, many of whom were relatively asymptomatic and may not have had systolic left ventricular dysfunction, it is difficult to make any definitive statements based on the observations of this trial.

Combined Therapy

Early studies demonstrated increases in cardiac index and reductions in systemic vascular resistance in patients on stable doses of vasodilators upon acute administration of digoxin (58,59). Valuable clinical data were obtained from the VHeFT-I and CONSENSUS studies that showed improved survival in patients receiving baseline diuretics and maintenance therapy with digoxin who were further randomized to the addition of vasodilators compared with placebo (60,61). Despite these observations, there have been few systematic investigations of the combined hemodynamic and clinical effects of digitalis and vasodilators.

Cantelli et al. published an early study on the combined hemodynamic effects of a cardiac glycoside and an angiotensin converting enzyme (ACE) inhibitor. In a small sample of eight patients with chronic congestive heart failure treated acutely with digoxin or captopril alone and then in combination, they demonstrated additive effects on the reduction in left ventricular filling pressures and increase in stroke volume index (62).

Gheorghiade et al. studied 11 patients with NYHA class IV heart failure after therapy with diuretics and vasodilators but without cardiac glycosides (55). After an initial period averaging 4.7 days during which doses of diuretics and vasodilators were optimized, substantial improvement in signs and symptoms of heart failure was reported. The addition of intravenous digoxin at this point increased the cardiac index by 30% (from 2.6 $\pm$ 0.7 to 3.3 $\pm$ 0.6 L/min/m^2), left ventricular stroke work index by 62% (from 27 $\pm$ 16 to 43 $\pm$ 23 g$*$m/m^2), and left ventricular ejection fraction by 38% (from 0.21 to 0.29) and decreased mean pulmonary capillary wedge pressure by 29% (from 24 $\pm$ 7 to 17 $\pm$ 4 mm Hg). In a subset analysis, the greatest response to digoxin was noted to occur in those patients with persistent hemodynamic evidence of left ventricular dysfunction after aggressive therapy with diuretics plus vasodilators.

Using more clinically oriented end points, Gheorghiade and colleagues (63) extended their original observations and reported additive beneficial effects of digoxin and captopril at rest and during exercise in patients with severe chronic congestive heart failure and sinus rhythm (Table 5). Trends toward improvement in maximum exercise time were observed in response to monotherapy with digoxin or captopril. However, the increase reached statistical significance (+40%; $p < 0.01$) only with the combined administration of digoxin and captopril. It is worth noting that digoxin alone and

Table 5 Captopril and Digoxin in Advanced CHF

		Control	IV captopril	IV digoxin	C + D
CI	(Rest)	—	NS	+23% ($p < 0.03$)	+43%
	(Exercise)	—	+33% ($p < 0.02$)	+24% ($p < 0.09$)	+61%
PCWP	(Rest)	—	−24% ($p < 0.003$)	−34% ($p < 0.004$)	−35%
	(Exercise)	—	NS	−11% ($p < 0.04$)	−24%
SWI	(Rest)	—	NS	+52% ($p < 0.01$)	+75%
	(Exercise)	—	NS	+44% ($p < 0.01$)	+87%
MAX EX TIME		—	NS	NS	+40% ($p < 0.01$)
LVEF		19%	—	—	24% ($p < 0.001$)
(NE)	(pg/ml)	795	NS	604 ($p < 0.03$)	639 ($p < 0.04$)

Table 2. *Adapted from Gheorghiade et al. (63). CHF = congestive heart failure; IV = intravenous; C + D = captopril plus digoxin; CI = cardiac index; PCWP = pulmonary capillary wedge pressure; SWI = stroke work index; MAX EX TIME = maximal exercise time; LVEF = left ventricular ejection fraction; (NE) = plasma concentration of norepinephrine; NS = not significant.
Source: Ref. 63.

in combination with captopril reduced plasma norepinephrine (NE) concentration while captopril alone did not. This finding is of particular interest in light of the known adverse prognostic significance of plasma NE levels in patients with heart failure (64). Possible explanations for the observed reduction in NE concentration after intravenous digoxin include withdrawal of tonically elevated sympathetic tone in response to acute improvement in cardiac function versus the known ability of digitalis to sensitize the baroreceptor reflex and augment hypotensive and bradycardic effects of baroreceptor stimulation (65,66).

IMPLICATIONS FOR TREATMENT

Diagnostic Subsets

Taken collectively, the available data seem to indicate a positive treatment effect from the use of digitalis in appropriately selected subsets of patients with congestive heart failure. The work of Guyatt et al. (9) and DiBianco et al. (8) confirms the prior investigation of Lee et al. demonstrating a benefit of digitalis in the management of patients in normal sinus rhythm with heart failure due to systolic ventricular dysfunction (12). In the subset of patients with supraventricular arrhythmias and systolic left ventricular failure, digoxin also remains a useful drug. Similarly, in patients at risk for either symptomatic hypotension or renal dysfunction with vasodilator therapy, digoxin is a more attractive initial therapeutic intervention than ACE inhibitors.

In patients with minimal left ventricular systolic dysfunction, the relative benefits of digoxin are less well established. The heterogeneity of diagnostic criteria used in most trials attempting to compare therapeutic options in the management of heart failure precludes comparison between trial cohorts (Table 6) (16). Because of disparate enrollment criteria, conflicting results of these trials may simply be due to baseline differences in the patient populations under study. For example, it is unlikely that digoxin will improve the patient with elevated left heart filling pressures and dyspnea on the basis of hypertrophic cardiomyopathy with a well-preserved left ventricular ejection fraction. The xamoterol study (36) is another example; in that study the proportion of patients who had heart failure on the basis of diastolic dysfunction was not specified. It is clear, however, that a significant number of study patients had evidence of active ischemic heart disease. It is not surprising that xamoterol, a drug with appreciable β_1-adrenergic antagonist action, might prove more beneficial than digoxin in patients with active ischemia.

In the absence of uniform entry criteria, it is difficult to generalize from many of these earlier studies. What is required is the establishment of explicit standardized diagnostic criteria so that well-defined patient populations can be studied (16). For instance, rather than relying on nonspecific clinical indices of congestive heart failure such as rales and peripheral edema, more uniform pathophysiologic references such as degree of systolic dysfunction should be employed. In this fashion, it would be possible to define specific patient cohorts that would, in turn, allow for generalization to an individual patient.

Table 6 Flaws in Existing Clinical Trials of Cardiac Glycosides

1. Unspecified enrollment criteria.
2. Nonuniform clinical diagnostic criteria for congestive heart failure.
3. Poor documentation of systolic left ventricular dysfunction.
4. Heterogeneous treatment end points.
5. Inadequate sample sizes to detect differences in mortality.
6. Selection biases.
   a. low even rates in control groups
   b. randomization only of patients intolerant of digoxin withdrawal

Mortality

The only trials to demonstrate a significant reduction in mortality in heart failure patients are the CONSENSUS and V-HeFT-I trials (Table 7). In CONSENSUS, a 40% reduction in mortality at 6 months was observed in 253 NYHA Class IV patients randomized to either enalapril or placebo. Notably, virtually every patient in the trial was also receiving maintenance digoxin therapy (60). The V-HeFT-I trial randomized 642 patients with chronic congestive heart failure with reduced exercise tolerance despite maintenance treatment with digoxin and diuretics to receive additional double-blinded treatment with placebo, prazosin, or the combination of hydralazine plus isosorbide dinitrate. Mortality was significantly reduced in the hydralazine/isosorbide dinitrate group (risk reduction 34%, $p < 0.03$ when compared with placebo) at 2-year follow-up. Beyond 3 years of

Table 7 Comparison of the CONSENSUS and V-HeFT Trials

	CONSENSUS			VHeFT		
Parameter	Rx*		Placebo	Rx†		Placebo
Number of patients	127		126	186		273
Mean age	71		70	58		58
% Male	70		71	100		0
% CAD	72		74	44		44
% HTN	24		19	40		43
% DM	24		21	17		25
Duration of						
CHF <6 mo	4		9	10		20
6mo–1.5 yr	24		16	23		27
1.5–4.0 yr	23		21	25		22
>4 yr	47		52	32		31
LVEF	—		—	30		30
MORTALITY						
n (%)						
6 mo	36(26%)	$p < 0.002$	55(44%)	—		—
1 yr	46(36%)	$p < 0.001$	66(52%)	23(12%)	—	53(20%)
2 yr	—		—	47(26%)	$p < 0.03$	94(34%)

CAD = coronary artery disease; CHF = congestive heart failure; DM = diabetes mellitus; HTN = hypertension; LVEF = left ventricular ejection fraction.
* Enalapril.
† Hydralazine-nitrates.
Source: Refs. 60, 61.

Table 8 Unresolved Questions

1. Does digoxin improve clinical symptoms in patients with mild left ventricular systolic dysfunction?
2. Does monotherapy with digoxin prolong life in patients with various degrees of left ventricular systolic dysfunction? Which subgroups derive maximum benefit?
3. Does the combination of digoxin and vasodilators offer *incremental improvement* in subjective symptoms, exercise performance, hemodynamic parameters, or mortality reduction when compared with either agent alone? In which subsets of patients?

follow-up, the treatment effect was no longer statistically significant, although the trend persisted (61). Three large, ongoing multicenter randomized clinical trials comparing various vasodilators with placebo in patients with left ventricular dysfunction, using mortality as a primary trial endpoint, are V-HeFT-II, SAVE, and SOLVD.

As is evident from the preceding discussion, the only way to answer definitively the important unresolved questions (Table 8) regarding the effects of digitalis on quality of life *and* mortality in patients with heart failure would be to conduct a large-scale multicenter trial randomizing several thousand patients with well-defined ventricular systolic dysfunction of varying severity to therapy with digoxin versus placebo. An ideal study would need to take into account the fact that modest differences in overall mortality (e.g., 20%) would necessitate extremely large sample sizes. Table 9 illustrates simplified examples of the results of sample size calculations based on various event rates and desired levels of significance. To detect a 20% reduction in mortality, one would need to enroll 2860 patients to

Table 9 Sample Size Calculations

Mortality in placebo group	Mortality in intervention group	Total number of patients required to be randomized*
50%	25%	150
50%	40%	1056
25%	12.5%	365
25%	20%	2860
12.5%	10%	6460

* $\alpha = 0.05$, 2-tailed power = 90%.

Table 10 Multivariate Analysis

1. Age
2. Sex
3. History of angina
4. History of myocardial infarction
5. History of ventricular ectopy
6. Diabetes
7. Hypertension
8. Renal dysfunction
9. Chronic lung disease
10. Goldman index (68)
11. Concurrent medications
12. Left ventricular ejection fraction

achieve a power of 90% at a 95% level of significance. No previous study has approached these numbers. The statistical analysis of such a study would first involve univariate testing for correlations between clinical characteristics, therapeutic interventions, and events. Variables with univariate correlations with the outcome of interest and variables with an expected a priori association would then be considered in a multivariate analysis aimed at developing an expression for the risk of cardiac death. An example of variables likely to be included in such a model is presented in Table 10.

CONCLUSIONS

The National Institutes of Health is currently designing a large-scale multicenter trial addressing many of these issues. Pending the outcome of this and other such trials, the available evidence supports the use of digoxin in certain subsets of patients with congestive heart failure. In symptomatic patients with congestive heart failure complicated by supraventricular tachyarrhythmias, there is general consensus that digoxin remains a first-line therapeutic agent. Similarly, in symptomatic patients with systolic left ventricular dysfunction who are at risk for developing either hypotension or renal dysfunction on vasodilator therapy, digoxin remains a valuable therapeutic option. As illustrated in Table 5, the combination of digoxin plus vasodilator therapy offers a potent hemodynamic combination that may be of considerable benefit to certain patients, in particular those with reduced systolic function and elevated systemic vascular resistance. Until the aforementioned large prospective trials have been completed, clinical decisions will continue to be based on the limited available data tempered by clinical judgment as to the risk:benefit ratio in a given patient, especially one with only mildly reduced left ventricular systolic function.

REFERENCES

1. Withering W. An Account of the Foxglove, and Some of Its Medical Uses: With Practical Remarks on Dropsy, and Other Diseases. London: GGJ and J Robinson, 1785.
2. Wiggers CJ, Stimson B. Studies on cardiodynamic actions of drugs. III. The mechanism of cardiac stimulation by digitalis and g-strophanthin. J Pharmacol Exp Ther 1927; 30:251–269.
3. Smith TW. Digitalis. Mechanisms of action and clinical use. N Engl J Med 1988; 318:358–365.
4. Mackenzie J, Christian H, eds. Chronic diseases of the heart. In: The Oxford Medicine, Vol. 2. Oxford: Oxford University Press:1920; 387–492.
5. Christian HA. Digitalis effects in chronic cardiac cases with regular rhythm in contrast to auricular fibrillation. Med Clin North Am 1922; 5:1173–1190.
6. Smith TW. Should digoxin be the drug of first choice after diuretics in chronic congestive heart failure: protagonist's viewpoint. J Am Coll Cardiol 1988; 12:267–271.
7. Pitt B. Should digoxin be the drug of first choice after diuretics in chronic congestive heart failure: antagonist's viewpoint. J Am Coll Cardiol 1988; 12:271–273.
8. DiBianco R, Shabetai R, Kostuk W, Moran J, Schlant RC, Wright R. A comparison of oral milrinone, digoxin, and their combination in the treatment of patients with chronic heart failure. N Engl J Med 1989; 320:677–683.
9. Guyatt GH, Sullivan MJJ, Fallen EL, Tihal H, Rideout E, Halcrow S, Nogradi S, Townsend M, Taylor DW. A controlled trial of digoxin in congestive heart failure. Am J Cardiol 1988; 61:371–375.
10. Beaunes J. Comparison of enalapril versus digoxin for congestive heart failure. Am J Cardiol 1989; 63:22D–25D.
11. The Captopril-Digoxin Multicenter Research Group. Comparative effects of therapy with captopril and digoxin in patients with mild to moderate heart failure. JAMA 1988; 259:539–544.
12. Lee DC, Johnson RA, Bingham JB, Leahy M, Dinsmore RE, Goroll AH, Newell JB, Strauss HW, Haber E. Heart failure in outpatients: a randomized trial of digoxin versus placebo. N Engl J Med 1982; 306:699–705.
13. Marban E, Smith TW. Digitalis. In: Fozzard HA, Haber E, Jennings RB, Katz AM, Morgan HE, eds. The Heart and Cardiovascular System. New York: Raven Press, 1986:1573–1596.
14. Eisner DA, Lederer WJ. Na-Ca exchange: stoichiometry and electrogenicity. Am J Physiol 1985; 248:C189–C202.
15. Barry WH, Hasin Y, Smith TW. Sodium pump inhibition, enhanced calcium influx via sodium-calcium exchange, and positive inotropic response in cultured heart cells. Circ Res 1985; 56:231–241.

16. Wier WG, Hess P. Excitation-contraction coupling in cardiac Purkinje fibers: effects of cardiotonic steroids on the intracellular [Ca] transient, membrane potential and contraction. J Gen Physiol 1984; 83:395–415.
17. Eisner DA, Lederer WJ, Vaughn-Jones RD. The quantitative relationship between twitch tension and intracellular sodium activity in sheep cardiac Purkinje fibers. J Physiol (Lond) 1984; 355:251–266.
18. Hougen TJ, Spicer N, Smith TW. Stimulation of monovalent cation active transport by low concentration of cardiac glycosides: role of catecholamines. J Clin Invest 1981; 68:1207–1214.
19. Kim D, Cragoe EJ Jr, Smith TW. Relations among sodium pump inhibition, Na-Ca and Na-H exchange activities, and Ca-H interaction in cultured chick heart cells. Circ Res 1987; 60:185–193.
20. Smith TW, Braunwald E, Kelley RA. The management of heart failure. In: Braunwald E, ed. Heart Disease: A Textbook of Cardiovascular Medicine. 3d ed. Philadelphia: WB Saunders, 1988:485–543.
21. Harter JG, Skelley JP, Steers AW. Digoxin: the regulatory viewpoint. Circulation 1974; 49:395–398.
22. Antman EM, Smith TW. Pharmacokinetics of digitalis glycosides. In Smith TW, ed. Digitalis Glycosides. New York: Grune and Stratton, 1986:45–60.
23. Lindenbaum J, Rund DG, Butler VP, Tse-End D, Saha JR. Inactivation of digoxin by the gut flora: reversal by antibiotic therapy. N Engl J Med 1981; 305:789–791.
24. Doherty JE, deSoyza N, Kane JJ, et al. Clinical pharmacokinetics of digitalis glycosides. Prog Cardiovasc Dis 1978; 21:141–158.
25. Solomon HM, Reich S, Spirt N, Abrams WB. Interactions between digitoxin and other drugs in vitro and in vivo. Ann NY Acad Sci 1971; 179:362–369.
26. Berman B. On the fate of orally administered 3H-lanatoside C in man. Eur J Clin Pharm 1972; 5:11–18.
27. Hall WH, Shappell SD, Doherty JE. Effect of cholestyramine on digoxin absorption and excretion in man. Am J Cardiol 1977; 39:213–216.
28. Bazzano G, Bazzano GS. Digitalis intoxication. Treatment with a new steroid-binding resin. JAMA 1972; 220:828–830.
29. Brown DD, John PR, Warner SL. Decreased bioavailability of digoxin due to hypercholesterolemic interventions. Circulation 1978; 58:164–172.
30. Lindenbaum RA, Maulitz RM, Butler VP. Inhibition of digoxin absorption by neomycin. Gastroenterology 1976; 71:399–404.
31. Doering W, Konig E. Ansteig der digoxinkonzentration im serum unter chinidinmedikation. Med Klin 1978; 73:1085–1088.
32. Ejvensson G. Effect of quinidine on plasma concentrations of digoxin. Br Med J 1978; 1:278–280.
33. Klein HO, Lang R, Weiss E. The influence of verapamil on serum digoxin concentration. Circulation 1982; 65:998–1003.
34. Pedersen KE, Dorph-Pedersen A, Hvidt S, Klitgaard NA, Kudsn FN. Digoxin-verapamil interaction. Clin Pharm Ther 1981; 30:311.
35. Moysey JO, Jaggaro NSV, Grundy EN, Chamberlain DA. Amiodarone increases plasma digoxin concentrations. Br Med J 1981; 282:272–273.

36. Nademanee K, Kannan R, Hendrickson J, Ookhtens M, Kay I, Singh B. Amiodarone–digoxin interaction: Clinical significance, time course of development, potential pharmacokinetic mechanisms and therapeutic implications. J Am Coll Cardiol 1984; 4:111–116.
37. Hager WD, Fenster P, Mayersohn M, Perrier D, Graves P, Marcus F, Goldman S. Digoxin-quinidine interaction. Pharmacokinetic evaluation. N Engl J Med 1979; 300:1238–1241.
38. Greenblatt DR. Digitalis glycosides. In: Miller, Greenblatt DR. Drug Effects in Hospitalized Patients: Experiences of the Boston Collaborative Drug Surveillance Program 1966–1975. New York: John Wiley & Sons, 1976:38–40.
39. Smith TW, Haber E, Yeatman L, Butler VP Jr. Reversal of advanced digoxin intoxication with Fab fragments of digoxin-specific antibodies. N Engl J Med 1976; 294:797–800.
40. Antman EA, Wenger T, Butler VP Jr, Haber E, Smith TW. Treatment of life-threatening digitalis intoxication with digoxin-specific antibody fragments: final report of a multicenter study. Circulation 1990; 81:1744–1752.
41. Gaultier M, Bismuth C. L'intoxication digitalique aigüe. La Revue du Practicien 1978; 28:4565–4579.
42. Moss AJ, DeCamilla J, Davis H. Cardiac death in the first 6 months after myocardial infarction: Potential for mortality reduction in the early posthospital period. Am J Cardiol 1977; 39:816–820.
43. Ryan TJ, Bailey KR, McCabe CH, Luk S, Fisher LD, Mock MB, Killip T. The effect of digitalis on survival in high-risk patients with coronary artery disease. Circulation 1983; 67:735–742.
44. Bigger JT, Rolnitzky LM, Fless JL. Possible adverse effects of digitalis therapy after myocardial infarction. In: Francis GS, Alpert JS, eds. Modern Coronary Care. Boston: Little, Brown: 1990:557–571.
45. Moss AJ, Davis HT, Conard DL, DeCamilla J, Odoroff CL. Digitalis associated cardiac mortality after myocardial infarction. Circulation 1983; 64:1150–1156.
46. Muller JE, Turi ZG, Stone PH, Rude RE, Raabe DS, Jaffe AS, Gold HK, Gustafson N, Poole WK, Passamani E, Smith TW, Braunwald E, and the MILIS Study Group. Digoxin therapy and mortality after myocardial infarction. N Engl J Med 1986; 314:265–271.
47. Yusuf S, Wittes J, Bailey K, Furberg C. Digitalis—a new controversy regarding an old drug: the pitfalls of inappropriate methods. Circulation 1986; 73:14–18.
48. Carliner NH, Gilbert SA, Pruitt AW, Goldberg LI. Effects of maintenance digoxin therapy on systolic time intervals and serum digoxin concentrations. Circulation 1974; 50:94–98.
49. Arnold SB, Byrd RC, Meister W, Melmon K, Cheitlin MD, Bristow JD, Parmley WW, Chatterjee K. Long-term digitalis therapy improves left ventricular failure in heart failure. N Engl J Med 1980; 303:1443–1448.

50. Mulrow C, Feussner JR, Velez R. Reevaluation of digitalis efficacy: new light on an old leaf. Ann Intern Med 1984; 101:113–117.
51. Dobbs SM, Kenyon WL, Dobbs RJ. Maintenance of digoxin after an episode of heart failure: placebo-controlled trial in outpatients. Br Med J 1977; 1:749–752.
52. Grossman W, McLaurin LP. Diastolic properties of the left ventricle. Ann Intern Med 1976; 84:316–326.
53. DeMaria AN, Wisenbaugh T. Identification and treatment of diastolic dysfunction: role of transmital Doppler recordings. J Am Coll Cardiol 1987; 9:1106–1107.
54. Labowitz AJ, Pearson AC. Evaluation of left ventricular diastolic function: clinical relevance and recent Doppler echocardiographic insights. Am Heart J 1987; 114:836–851.
55. Gheorghiade M, St. Clair J, St. Clair C, Beller GA. Hemodynamic effects of intravenous digoxin in patients with severe heart failure initially treated with diuretics and vasodilators. J Am Coll Cardiol 1987; 9:849–847.
56. Sullivan M, Atwood E, Myers J, Feuer J, Hall P, Kellerman B, Forbes S, Froelicher V. Increased exercise capacity after digoxin administration in patients with heart failure. J Am Coll Cardiol 1989; 13:1138–1143.
57. The German and Austrian Xamoterol Study Group. Double-blind placebo-controlled comparison of digoxin and xamoterol in chronic heart failure. Lancet 1988; i:489–493.
58. Raabe DS. Combined therapy with digoxin and nitroprusside in heart failure complicating acute myocardial infarction. Am J Cardiol 1979; 43:990–994.
59. Cantelli I, Pavesi PC, Parchi C, Naccarella F, Brachetti D. Acute hemodynamic effects of combined therapy with digoxin and nifedipine in patients with chronic heart failure. Am Heart J 1983; 106:308–315.
60. CONSENSUS Trial Study Group. Effects of enalapril on mortality in severe congestive heart failure; results of the Cooperative North Scandinavian Enalapril Survival Study. N Engl J Med 1987; 316:1429–1435.
61. Cohn JN, Archibald DG, Ziesche S, Franciosa JA, Harston WE, Tristani FE, Dunkman WB, Jacobs W, Francis GS, Flahr KH. Effect of vasodilator therapy on mortality in chronic congestive heart failure: Results of a Veterans Administration Cooperative Study. N Engl J Med 1986; 314:1547–1552.
62. Cantelli I, Vitolo A, Lombardi G, Bomba E, Brachetti D. Combined hemodynamic effects of digoxin and captopril in patients with congestive heart failure. Curr Ther Res 1984; 36:323–331.
63. Gheorghiade M, Hall V, Lakier JB, Goldstein S. Comparative hemodynamic and neurohumoral effects of intravenous captopril and digoxin, and their combination in patients with severe heart failure. J Am Coll Cardiol 1989; 13:134–142.
64. Cohn JN, Rector TS. Prognosis of congestive heart failure and predictors of mortality. Am J Cardiol 1988; 62:25A–30A.

65. Ferrari A, Gregorini L, Ferrari ML, Preti L, Mancia G. Digitalis and baroreceptor reflexes in man. Circulation 1981; 63:279–285.
66. Imamura T, Takeshita A, Ashihara T, Yamamoto K, Hoka S, Nakamura M. Digitalis-induced augmentation of cardiopulmonary baroreflex control of forearm vascular resistance. Circulation 1985; 71:11–16.
67. Goldman L, Caldera DL, Nussbaum SR, Southwick F, Kragstad D, Murray B, Burke D, O'Malley T, Gorolli A, Kaplan C, Nolan J, Carabello B, Slater E. Multifactorial index of cardiac risk in noncardiac surgical procedures. N Engl J Med 1977; 297:845–850.

9

Vasodilators in the Therapeutics of Heart Failure

B. Silke
The Queen's University of Belfast, Belfast, Northern Ireland

INTRODUCTION

The increasing incidence of heart failure over the past two decades can in part be attributed to an aging population as well as increased survival following myocardial infarction. More precise diagnostic methods have led to the early recognition of the syndrome even in the presymptomatic phase. Heart failure occurs in approximately 1% of the population by the age of 60; its prevalence doubles in each successive decade, and it occurs in 8% of those aged 80 to 89. It is estimated that in the United States alone 400,000 new cases of congestive heart failure are diagnosed each year and between 3 and 4 million people are affected (1,2). The 1-year survival rate varies, depending on selection, between 35% and 70%, but 5-year survival is uniformly poor (3).

It is increasingly recognized that heart failure following myocardial infarction is a time-dependent process; disturbance in cardiac geometry results in (asymptomatic) cardiac dilatation, which may precede symptomatic cardiac failure by months or even years. The development of heart failure after myocardial infarction is not inevitable; however, echocardiographic studies suggest that clinical methods underestimate the risk; moreover progressive deterioration of cardiac function in the presymptomatic phase may occur without symptoms.

The immediate goals of therapy remain relief of symptoms, improvement in the quality of life, and possibly prolongation of survival. However, the emphasis on survival as a primary end point may be misguided; many individuals might prefer an improved, productive, and enjoyable life at unaltered longevity rather than mere extension in unproductive life. The mortality benefits accrue to only a few of those treated; the widely acclaimed CONSENSUS trial with enalapril in severe heart failure demonstrated improved survival comparing the actively treated group with the placebo group. However, survival was on average extended by only 2 weeks following enalapril compared with the placebo control (4). Clearly this cannot be hailed as a major advance—symptomatic improvement and augmented exercise capacity need to be considered. The normally slowly progressive process may be interrupted at any stage by rapid deterioration or by sudden death.

The acute symptomatic relief of heart failure depends on appropriate therapy, usually with loop diuretics; these agents relieve disabling dyspnea. Short-term studies suggest they improve hemodynamic function and exercise capacity (5). With the evidence that both angiotensin converting enzyme (ACE) inhibitor therapy and vasodilators improve survival, diuretic therapy alone is rarely contemplated. Current evidence suggests that ACE inhibitors (possibly because of their effects on central sympathetic outflow) may be more effective in improving survival than direct-acting vasodilators. Practicing physicians might therefore consider it inappropriate or unethical not to include an ACE inhibitor, as the first-line vasodilator agent, in a heart failure treatment regimen. The crucial question then becomes not whether but at which stage to introduce an ACE inhibitor; other vasodilators may be considered in patients in whom ACE inhibitors are contraindicated or poorly tolerated. A subsidiary role may be for direct-acting vasodilators in combination therapy with ACE-inhibiting drugs.

The mechanisms and theoretical basis for the application of vasodilators in heart failure have been previously reviewed (6,7) but will be briefly summarized. The clinical evidence favoring the use of these agents to alter the symptomatic progress of the disease, including impact on quality of life, needs to be determined, and finally their effects in relation to survival data need to be considered.

HEMODYNAMIC PROFILE AND SYMPATHETIC ACTIVATION IN CHRONIC HEART FAILURE

Optimization of therapy with any drug depends on a detailed appreciation of its spectrum of pharmacodynamic activity when applied in a given pathophysiological circumstance. This is particularly true when considering the clinical application of vasodilator drugs in heart failure. Vasodilator therapy, in general terms, attempts to reduce the abnormally high peripheral vascular resistance produced by the deranged hemodynamic mechanisms; the falling contractile response and diminished stroke volume become a self-sustaining loop with progressive cardiac dilatation and pumping insufficiency. The primary abnormality of heart failure is inability to maintain contractile activity and cardiac stroke output appropriate to the metabolic needs of the various regional vascular territories. The hemodynamic abnormality is illustrated in Table 1; with the absolute fall in cardiac stroke output, blood flow to vital organs, including cerebral and coronary circulation, is maintained, and indeed flow to skeletal musculature is preserved, at least at rest. Flow to other territories, including skin, splanchnic, and renal regional flow, is reduced to between 10% and 53% of normal.

As a consequence, immediate and longer-term circulatory adjustments are initiated. Hypotension due to diminished cardiac pumping function results in activation of arterial baroreceptors, and failure to maintain cardiac stroke output results in dilatation of the left ventricle. The increased left ventricular filling pressure and volume results in further stimulation of stretch receptors in the left atrium and pulmonary veins. The combination of such output from baroreceptors and stretch receptors comprises the afferent limb of a circulatory reflex involving the vasomotor center in the brain; the final common efferent output being mediation through the sympathetic nervous system. Sympathetic fibers to the heart terminate near β-adrenoceptors in the atrial sinus and atrial node; their activation results in an increased heart rate and facilitation of a conduction of atrial impulses to the ventricle. Sympathetic stimulation of β-adrenoceptors increases car-

Table 1 Regional Blood Flow Distribution (L/min) in Congestive Heart Failure

	Normal	Mildly impaired	Severely impaired
Cardiac output	5.8	4.4	3.4
Cerebral	0.75	0.6 (80%)	0.5 (67%)
Renal	1.1	0.65 (59%)	0.35 (32%)
Coronary	0.25	0.3 (120%)	0.3 (120%)
Skeletal muscle	1.2	1.2 (100%)	1.2 (100%)
Skin	0.5	0.15 (30%)	0.05 (10%)
Splanchnic	1.4	1.2 (80%)	0.8 (53%)
Other organs	0.6	0.3 (75%)	0.2 (50%)

diac contractility and reduces ventricular compliance, increasing the sensitivity of the intrinsic mechanism (Frank-Starling). The overall result is therefore to increase contractile activity in an attempt to maintain left ventricle pumping activity.

In addition, there is a second efferent system involving sympathetic pathways to the peripheral vasculature; stimulation of α-adrenoceptors increases the arterial resistance and redistributes blood from the peripheral to the central circulation. Arterial compliance diminishes, and such reflexes, by facilitating an expansion of the central volume, support hemodynamics despite a diminished cardiac stroke volume. The maintenance of systemic arterial blood pressure is facilitated by the increase in venous return.

The vasodilator therapies aim to modulate this disordered impedance; provided the left ventricular filling pressure does not fall below a critical level (probably 15–20 mm Hg), a reduced impedance usually augments cardiac function, improving cardiac stroke volume (Fig. 1). This is a direct consequence of the sensitivity of the stressed and dilated heart to loading conditions.

It is fashionable to characterize vasodilator agents as being predominantly active on veins or arteries and to describe their effects in terms of actions on preload (i.e., changing end-diastolic volume and pressure) or afterload (i.e., resistance vessels). Of course, this is oversimplistic; the end-diastolic volume is an important component of left ventricular afterload, and drugs that act on capacitance vessels must reduce afterload as a

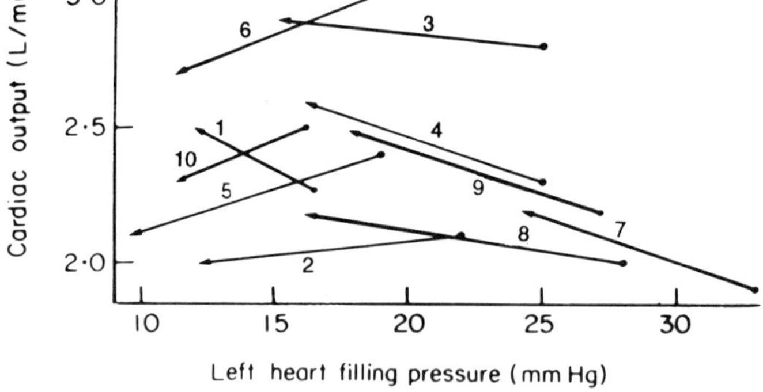

Figure 1 Actions of nitrates on cardiac output in relationship to filling pressures achieved in acute heart failure. (From Ref. 7.)

consequence. Nonetheless, the distinction is useful because there are distinct hemodynamic differences between drugs related to their predominant target vasculature; drugs that venodilate usually are effective in reducing pulmonary artery wedge pressure (left ventricular end-diastolic pressure equivalent) at unchanged cardiac output (Fig. 2). They may be expected

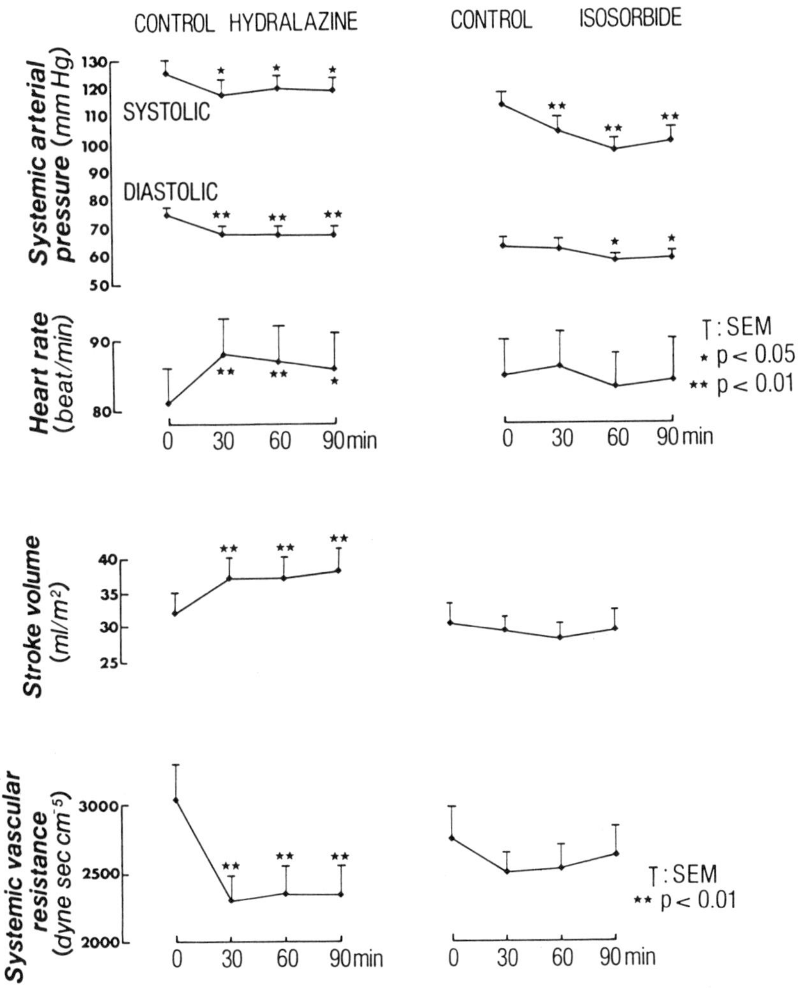

Figure 2 Comparison of actions of predominantly arteriolar (hydralazine) or venodilation (isosorbide dinitrate) in acute heart failure following myocardial infarction. (From Ref. 11.)

to alleviate symptoms of dyspnea due to stimulation of pulmonary stretch receptors. Therapeutic agents acting on resistance vessels improve cardiac stroke output at unchanged left ventricular filling pressure and might be expected to improve symptoms such as fatigue, usually associated with low flow states to skeletal muscle.

The impact of different and potentially usefully vasodilators in chronic heart failure will be considered; ACE inhibitors, slow-calcium channel blocking agents, and compounds with combined inotropic and vasodilator actions are the subject of other chapters and will not be considered.

PRAZOSIN

The selective postsynaptic α_1-adrenoceptor antagonist prazosin is a quinazoline derivative that is relatively selective for the postjunctional α_1-adrenoceptor; little effect is seen on the presynaptic (α_2) adrenoceptor (8). Earlier nonselective alpha-blockers such as phentolamine resulted in generalized vasodilatation of all regional vascular territories; theoretically, the diversion of blood to nonessential tissues might limit the increase to exercising muscles, with a suboptimal improvement in exercise capacity. In addition, a selective postjunctional α_1-antagonist is less likely to increase heart rate and limit the myocardial oxygen-wasting effects that would accrue from the combined reduction in left ventricular afterload and preload. For these reasons, selective α_1-adrenoceptor antagonism would be expected to confer theoretical advantages over nonselective vasodilatation such as that mediated by the venodilator nitrates and the arteriolar dilator hydralazine (9). In contrast to the tachycardia following nonselective alpha-blockade with phentolamine (10) and nonspecific vasodilators such as hydralazine (11), prazosin appears to exert a negative chronotropic effect, which is of particular therapeutic advantage in the context of heart failure (12).

Prazosin is an orally effective balanced vasodilator with actions on both arterioles and veins, and its circulatory profile resembles that of intravenous nitroprusside. Following oral administration, peak actions can be demonstrated by 45 min and appear to persist for at least 6 h. The actions of oral prazosin on the hemodynamic profile of patients with chronic heart failure have been reported in detail (13). In the majority of studies the major influence of the first dose of prazosin was a substantial reduction in the left heart filling pressure with little change in the accompanying cardiac output. It has been demonstrated (14,15) that the reduction in left heart filling pressure at rest achieved by prazosin was also maintained during dynamic exercise and that the increment in cardiac output and stroke volume was similar to the pretreatment control. However, these studies and also those of others (16) demonstrated that the initial hemodynamic impact was attenuated during long-term therapy (Fig. 3). Comparison of prazosin and captopril demonstrated that the latter was superior in terms of clinical efficacy and long-term hemodynamics (17). Moreover, in the VHeFT-I trial (18) prazosin was not different from placebo in terms of overall patient outcome and survival. Therefore, despite the initial favorable hemodynamic profile induced by prazosin in acute and chronic heart failure, the development of tolerance would appear to limit much of its long-term potential in patients with heart failure.

The α_1-adrenoceptor antagonist terazosin (19) has also been shown to have beneficial hemodynamic effects in chronic heart failure, but again its long-term efficacy is uncertain. Thus, despite the attractive theoretical basis for selective blockade of α_1-adrenoceptors in chronic heart failure, clinical experience to date has been disappointing. In view of both the lack of sustained hemodynamic improvement and the apparent lack of impact on survival, the clinical case for the use of selective α_1-adrenoceptor agents in the long-term treatment of heart failure is not sustainable.

HYDRALAZINE

Hydralazine is an orally effective vasodilator whose actions predominantly influence left ventricular afterload (20). Studies in acute heart failure dem-

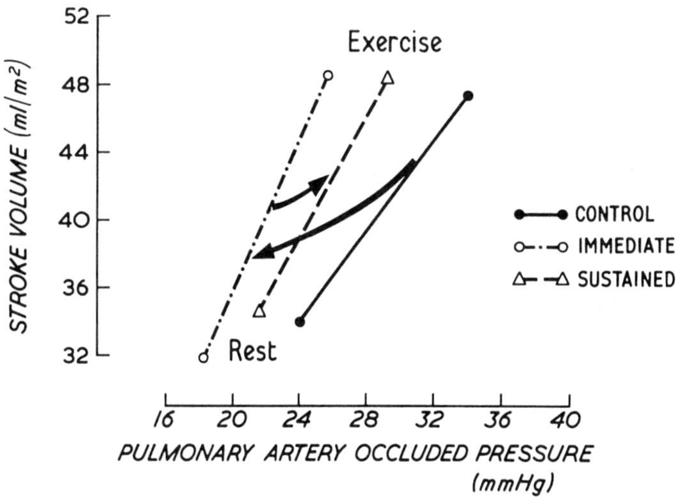

Figure 3 Immediate and sustained actions of prazosin, at rest and during treadmill walking, in chronic heart failure. (From Ref. 15.)

onstrated a predominant action in lowering systemic vascular resistance, with increased forward blood flow and minor secondary falls in left ventricular filling pressure (21). The actions of the drug are usually evident by 30 min and persist for up to 6 h.

The hemodynamic response to vasodilation in heart failure is variable and heavily influenced by the loading conditions (22). Patients with high levels of systemic vascular resistance appear to show the greatest hemodynamic response to hydralazine, and indeed the degree of left ventricular enlargement has been stated to be a good predictor of hemodynamic benefit (23). However, long-term hydralazine therapy has not been without its problems. There is uncertainty as to its sustained hemodynamic efficacy (24,25), and the reflex tachycardia frequently encountered may limit therapy. Notwithstanding these limitations, the VHeFT-I study (18) demonstrated that combined hydralazine/isosorbide dinitrate therapy reduced mortality in patients with mild to moderate heart failure who were already treated with digoxin and diuretic. The VHeFT-1 trial also demonstrated a statistically significant, albeit small, improvement in exercise capacity in patients randomly assigned to hydralazine/isosorbide treatment compared with either placebo or prazosin. Thus a case can be made for such balanced vasodilator treatment, particularly in those subjects in whom ACE inhibitors are poorly tolerated. However, VHeFT-II (26) suggested that the mortality reduction achieved with the hydralazine/isosorbide combination (18%) was less than that attained with enalapril (26% and 25%, VHeFT I and II respectively). Thus the place of hydralazine/isosorbide combination therapy in chronic congestive heart failure is uncertain, although it is possible that direct-acting vasodilators such as hydralazine may confer additional benefits in heart failure patients already receiving ACE inhibitor therapy.

Vascular side effects with hydralazine are frequent and include headache, flushing, and nausea and vomiting; however, these may be attenuated with continued treatment. Drug fever, skin rashes, and other idiosyncratic reactions may occasionally occur, and fluid retention/edema may be a problem. The potential for expansion of the intravascular fluid volume with consequent stimulus for left ventricular hypertrophy during hydralazine therapy is an unresolved issue. The lupus-like syndrome may occur in up to 15% of patients, particularly with high-dose therapy (> 400 mg of hydralazine daily). Antinuclear antibodies in the circulation occur in a higher percentage of individuals. Hydralazine is an example of a compound subject to genetic polymorphism, and individuals with slow acetylator status may be particularly at risk of developing both the lupus syndrome and peripheral neuropathy due to pyridoxine deficiency.

NITRATES

Nitrates are widely used in the treatment of acute and chronic heart failure (27). Their hemodynamic impact is the result of dilatation of both arteries and veins. At low therapeutic concentrations (< 0.2 ng/ml) they are relatively venoselective, with progressive actions on the systemic circulation with increasing doses (28). Venodilation results in peripheral pooling of blood in capacitance vessels. The reduction in venous return reduces cardiac preload (end-diastolic volume) and wall tension, and excessive reduction in central filling pressures may limit or result in a fall in cardiac output (29) (Fig. 4). In normal individuals the reduction in normal right heart filling pressures and consequent fall in cardiac output can precipitate nitrate syncope. However, in patients with chronic heart failure and elevated filling pressures, nitroglycerin reduces left ventricular filling pressure with either no change or improvement in cardiac output. The actions of nitroglycerin usually begin within a few minutes, are maximum by 10 to 15 min, and persist for at least half an hour. Reduction on the order of 10 mm Hg would on average be achieved in patients in whom left ventricular filling pressures are elevated (29).

Nitrates have been developed in a variety of different formulations and routes of administration that make them useful in varying clinical situations. Despite mild cardioacceleration, maximum oxygen consumption decreases, and this is a major aspect of the useful antianginal action of nitrates. Arteriolar dilation may reduce systemic blood pressure with reflex tachycardia. In ischemic heart disease this will offset some of the desirable aspects of nitrate therapy by reducing coronary perfusion and by oxygen-wasting effects of the augmented heart rate. In cardiac failure, with the marked sensitivity to loading conditions, augmented cardiac stroke output usually follows reduction of the pressure workload; however, with the down-regulation of cardiac β-adrenoceptors reflex tachycardia may be less problematic than in patients with more normal cardiac function (27).

In acute situations, continuous intravenous infusion of glyceryl trinitrate has been used to produce a titratable improvement in the hemodynamics of acute heart failure. Initial doses on the order of 10 μg/min would be used, increasing by increments of 10 μg/min every 5 min to a maximum dose of approximately 100 μg/min. Alternative choices for acute administration include the long-acting isosorbide dinitrate, available in either sublingual or oral formulations. Prolonged controlled-release systems have been developed that allow sustained nitrate effect to be maintained with once-daily or twice-daily dosing schedules. Methemoglobinemia may occur with long-term use of high-dose nitrate therapy.

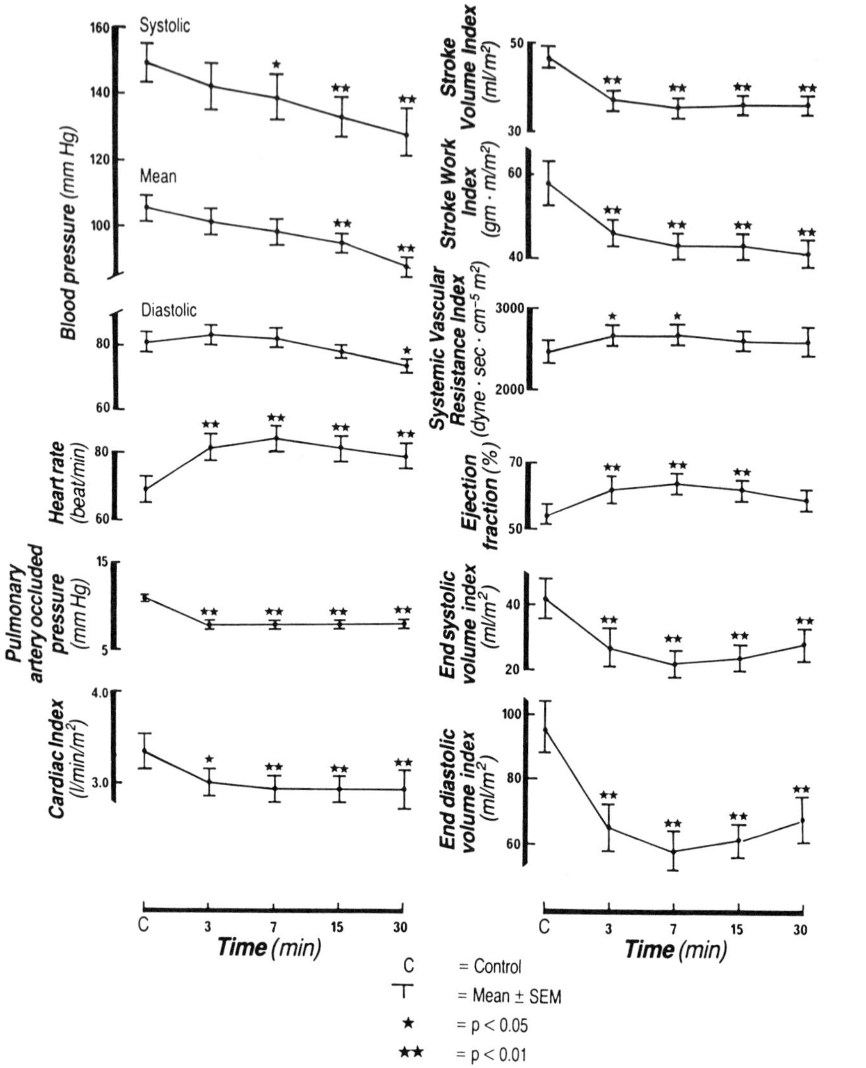

Figure 4 Actions of nitroglycerin (buccal route) on hemodynamic and radionuclide variables in ischemic heart disease.

Recent investigations have revealed some of the mechanisms by which nitrates achieve their hemodynamic actions. The nitrate molecule enters the vascular smooth muscle cell, where either nitric oxide or *S*-nitrosothiol is formed. These compounds then interact with the intracellular enzyme guanylate cyclase, leading to the formation of cyclic GMP, which results in vasodilatation (30). An important problem with all sustained use of nitrate preparations is the propensity to develop tolerance (31,32). This time-related decrease of initial hemodynamic impact occurs following constant-dose intravenous infusion and may be more rapid in the pulmonary than in the systemic circulation (33). Cross-tolerance between different nitrate compounds occurs. Intermittent therapy or therapeutic regimes that allow a low-dose or nitrate-free interval at some stage during the 24-h period may prevent tolerance or encourage "detolerance" by the next scheduled dose (Fig. 5).

The complex problem of tolerance to sustained nitrate therapy is incompletely understood (30). Reduced sulfhydryl groups are necessary in vascular smooth muscle to denitrate organic nitrates and form nitric oxide

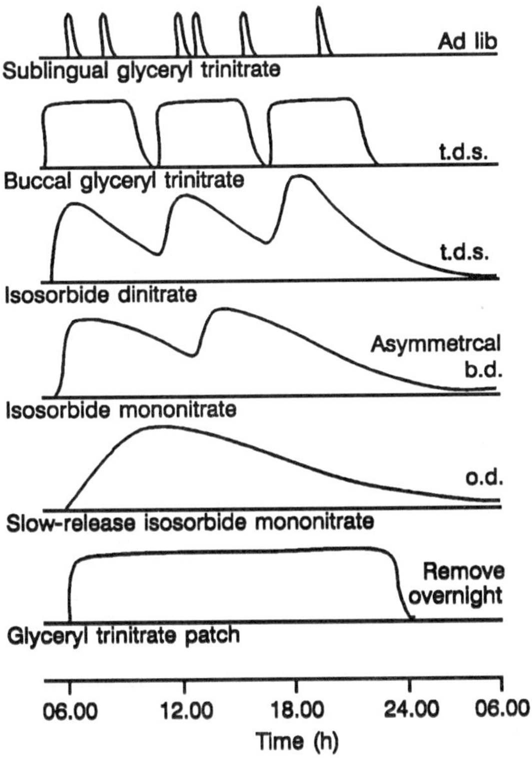

Figure 5 Suggested schema to administer nitrate to prevent tolerance development. (After Ref. 32.)

and nitrosothiols. Nitric oxide is thought to be endothelium-derived relaxing factor (EDRF)—the endogenous agent. Both nitric oxide and nitrosothiols result in production of cyclic guanosine monophosphate, which induces vasodilatation by reducing cytosolic calcium. Nitrate tolerance is thought to be due primarily to depletion of reduced sulfhydryl groups, which impairs nitric oxide production with resultant secondary insufficiency of cyclic GMP. Detolerance of vascular smooth muscle has been demonstrated in vitro and in vivo with the use of cysteine or alternative sulhydryl donors (28,31).

Thus, the objective of nitrate therapy is to alter the hemodynamic profile over the greatest duration of the day, balanced against the risk of developing tolerance. This may be achievable only by providing a nitrate-free interval or by using a formulation that allows relatively low nitrate exposure at some time during the 24 h. This may be achieved by intermittent transdermal (32,34) (Fig. 6), oral (31), or modified delivery systems (35). Tolerance may be related in part to neurohumoral activation, and the use of drugs such as captopril (36) or thiazide diuretics (37) to counter such neurohumoral activation may partially offset the tendency to induce tolerance.

The impact of nitrate therapy on cardiovascular mortality in postinfarction patients has been overviewed in a pooled meta-analysis (38). The risk reduction was 0.52 in seven studies of intravenous nitrate therapy, 0.88 in five studies of oral therapy, and 0.68 in all 12 studies (32% reduction in mortality; 95% confidence limits, 12% to 47%). Specific data on heart failure are more scanty. Short-term hemodynamics are improved, with a reduction in left ventricular filling pressure and a maintained or slightly reduced cardiac output. Exercise capacity is improved during submaximal supine bicycle work, but there is some time before this is maximized and before oxygen utilization improves at a given workload (39,40). The improved exercise capacity is maintained over at least 3 to 4 months. Mortality data on the combination of isosorbide and hydralazine in the VHeFT I study (18) demonstrated a 34% mortality reduction over 2 years in comparison with placebo. In VHeFT II (24), isosorbide/hydralazine induced greater improvement in hemodynamics (ejection fraction) and in objective exercise oxygen utilization compared with enalapril; however, mortality effects were significantly worse than with ACE inhibition. Planned studies of the impact of nitrates on heart failure mortality include the ISIS-4 study (nitrates vs. captopril plus magnesium) and the Italian GISSI-3 trial comparing nitrates and lisinopril. Current evidence indicates that nitrates may be useful in improving hemodynamics and exercise capacity in chronic heart failure; in this regard they may be more effective than ACE inhibition. Although the latter therapy has proven mortality advantages, the possible

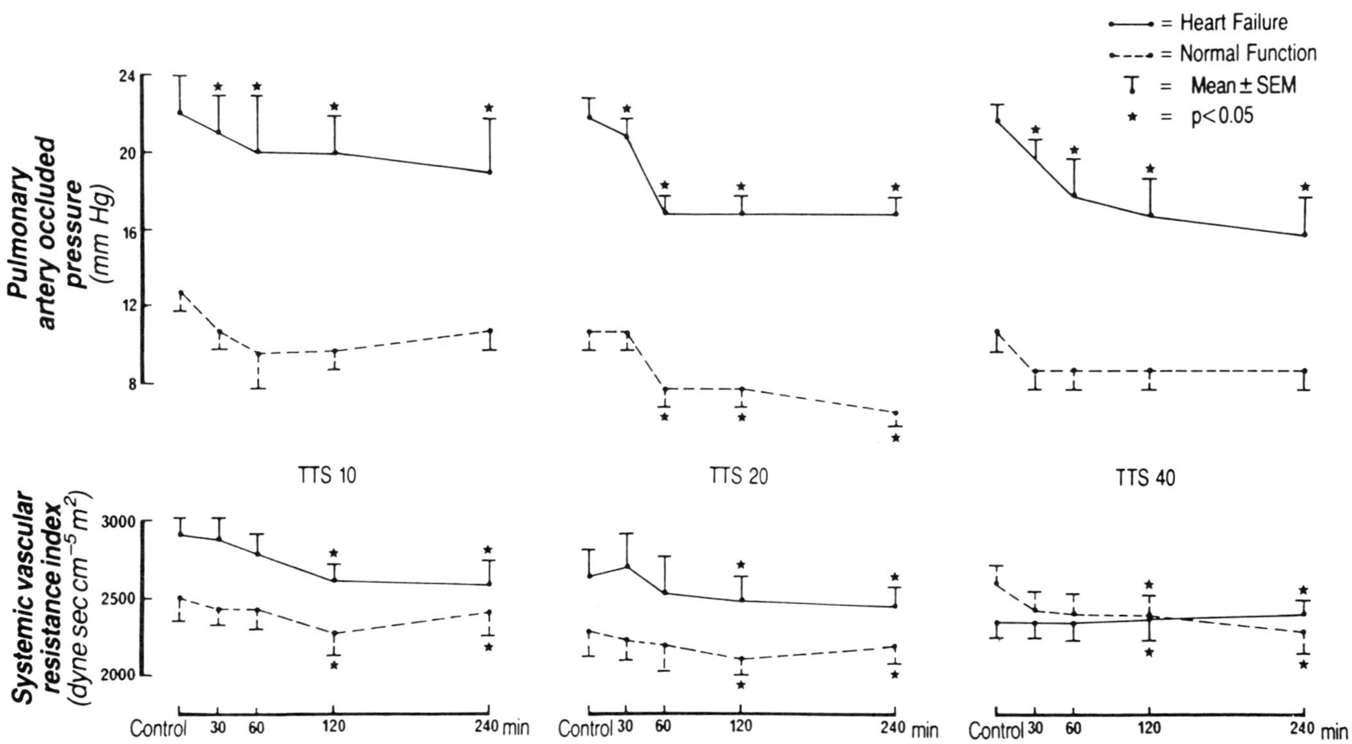

Figure 6 Hemodynamic dose-response actions of transdermal nitroglycerin in patients with or without left ventricular decompensation following acute myocardial infarction. Transdermal delivery at 10, 20, or 40 mg/24 h.

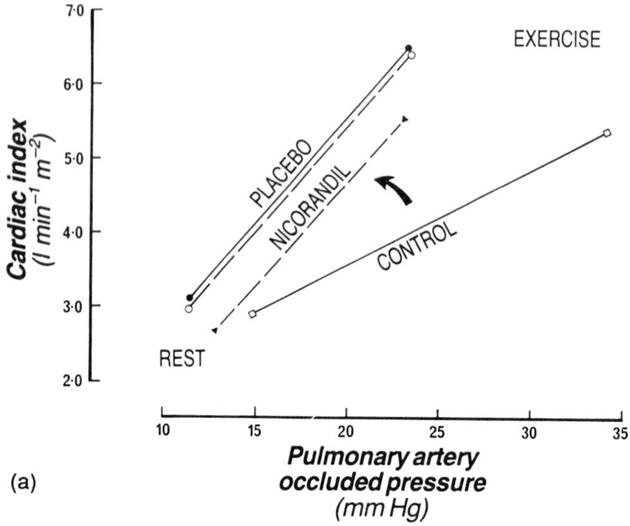

(a)

Figure 7 Effect of nicorandil on cardiac pumping indexes in angina pectoris with left ventricular decompensation. Patients assigned randomly to placebo or treatment; observations (a) at rest and (b) during 4-min supine bicycle exercise. (From Ref. 43.)

further impact on exercise capacity and mortality from the addition of nitrates to ACE inhibition remains to be established.

NICORANDIL

Nicorandil is a nicotinamide derivative that is also structurally a nitrate; thus, it possesses a hybrid structure (41). Experimentally, it has arteriolar dilator actions that might be expected to benefit heart failure patients. It preferentially dilates resistance vessels and induces hyperpolarization of cardiac and vascular smooth muscle cells, resulting in mild negative inotropic/chronotropic and vasodilator effects. In experimental animals at a dose level that resulted in doubling of coronary blood flow, no adverse effects on sinus rate, atrioventricular conduction time, or myocardial contractile force were described (42). The hemodynamic effects of 20 mg of nicorandil were evaluated at rest and during supine bicycle exercise in a placebo-controlled, double-blind study of patients with LV dysfunction (43). At rest, nicorandil reduced all components of systemic arterial pressure without change in cardiac or stroke volume indexes or heart rate. Resting pulmonary artery occluded pressure without change in left ven-

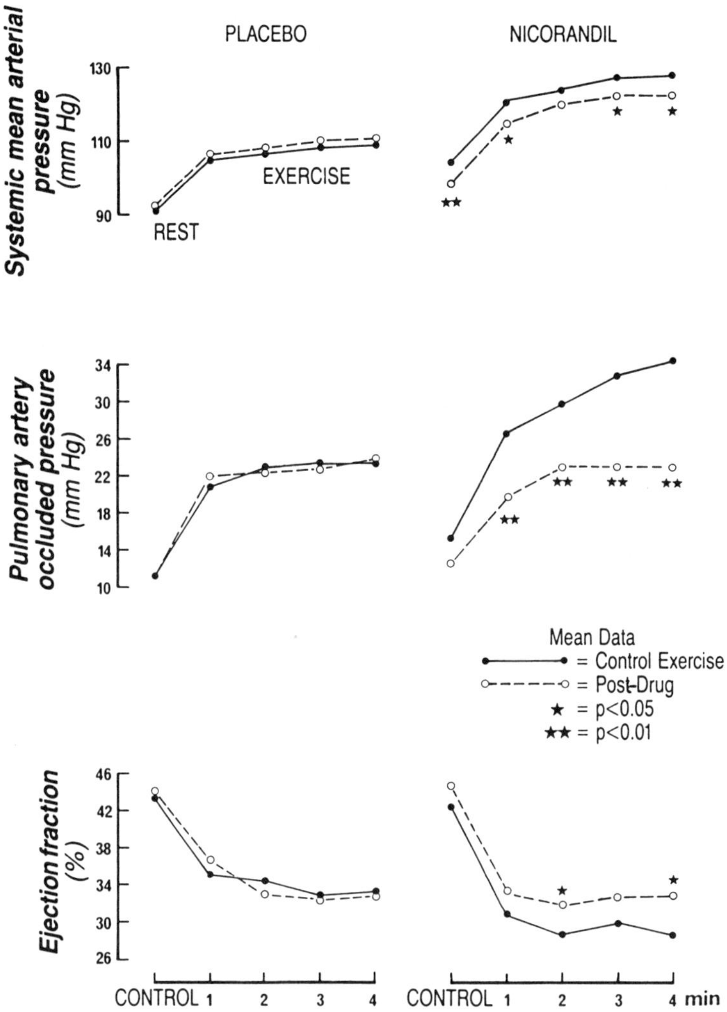

(b)

tricular ejection fraction or calculated systemic vascular resistance. The effects were evident by 7 min from oral dosing, reached their maximum at 30 min, and showed some attenuation by 60 min. Comparing exercise effects at 60 min with a control predrug period demonstrated falls in exercise systemic arterial pressure and left ventricular filling pressure, without change in cardiac pumping indexes, and a small increase in left ventricular ejection fraction (Fig. 7). These data suggested beneficial hemodynamic effects that were particularly evident during exercise-induced acute heart failure, as left heart filling pressures fell but cardiac pumping indexes were maintained.

These results were very similar to the hemodynamic impact of 15 mg of nicorandil in nine patients with severe coronary disease (44). Left ventricular filling pressure reductions were not associated with altered cardiac or stroke volume indexes, although this study demonstrated somewhat greater effects on systemic arterial pressure. The effects of nicorandil 5 mg sublingually during pacing-induced angina (45) were reductions in end-diastolic filling pressure with substantial falls in left ventricular systolic volumes and dramatic improvement in ejection fraction. The extent and degree of dyskinesia induced during angina was substantially offset by premedication with nicorandil (46). In a further study in ischemic patients, nicorandil significantly augmented resting coronary sinus flow and reduced coronary vascular resistance (47). Similarly, Suryapranata et al. (48) reported significant (9% to 15%) dilatation of normal and stenosed coronary arteries following 20 and 40 mg nicorandil.

These results suggest that nicorandil has useful coronary vasodilator and systemic circulatory activity resulting in balanced actions on the circulation. During the stress of angina these effects tend to maintain cardiac stroke volume indexes and improve left ventricular filling pressures, ejection fraction, and systolic volume indexes.

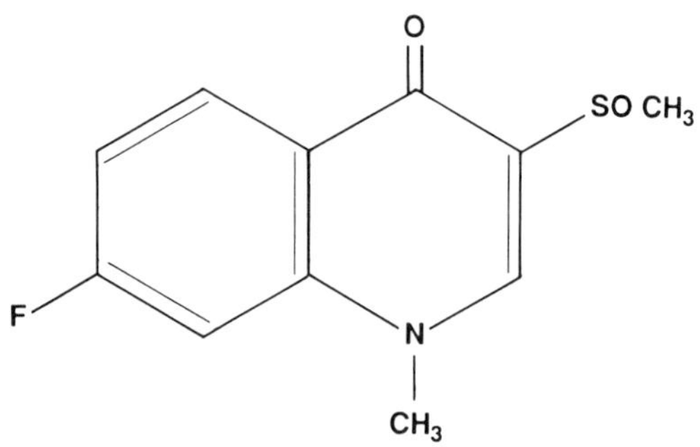

Figure 8 Flosequinan, a 7-fluorinated quinolone.

FLOSEQUINAN

Flosequinan (Fig. 8) is a novel 7-fluorinated quinolone with cardiovascular activity likely to prove useful in the therapeutics of heart failure. Animal pharmacology data indicate that its arterial and venous dilating activity is due both to the parent compound flosequinan and its major metabolite, flosequinoxan. The compound has vasodilator actions on both arteries and veins with little reflex tachycardia (49). The mechanism of the vasodilator action is incompletely understood; it does not appear to affect classical receptors or ion channels directly and it is not an ACE inhibitor. Flosequinan modulates the phosphatidylinositol pathway, attenuating inositol 1,4,5-triphosphate (IP_3) levels and protein kinase C activity (50). The decrease in calcium sensitivity associated with flosequinan-induced relaxation of human resistance vessels in vitro (51) may result from attenuation of protein kinase C activity. Flosequinan is rapidly and extensively absorbed but hepatic "first pass" results in bioavailability of the order of 72%; metabolism is by hepatic S-oxidation to form the sulphone metabolite flosequinoxan, which is then excreted in the urine. The plasma half-life of the parent compound in humans is 1.6 h and that of the major metabolite flosequinoxan 30–40 h, which may explain why a single dose is hemodynamically active for up to 24 h.

Animal studies have indicated some inotropic activity (52–55), but with marked interspecies variation (49). Clinical studies in heart failure patients have indicated little or no direct inotropic activity (56,57); the tissue levels required to inhibit phosphodiesterase are much higher than those achieved during effective clinical therapy, questioning the relevance of basic observations on PDE inhibition at high dosage to human studies (58). Volunteer studies have demonstrated a fall in vascular resistance and an increase in forearm blood flow (59); others demonstrated that the regional effects of flosequinan include an augmented forearm and hepatic blood flow and a reduced renal vascular resistance (60).

The hemodynamic activity of flosequinan has been assessed in 11 open studies of 165 patients, of whom 153 were in New York Heart Association Class 3 or 4 heart failure (57,61–63). Over the dose range between 75 and 150 mg beneficial effects in terms of reduction in right atrial and pulmonary artery occluded pressure, fall in vascular resistance, and increase in cardiac output occurred within a half hour of dosing, with peak action of about 1–2 h. Effects on systemic arterial blood pressure were minimal. Hemodynamic activity was sustained for 24 h when 40–44% of the peak effect remained following the 100-mg oral dose. The data over the dose range

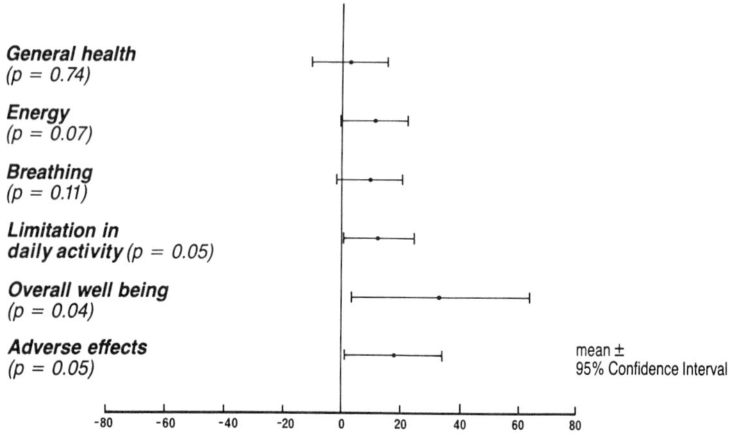

Figure 9 Effect of flosequinan versus placebo (difference) on quality of life. Score assessed by visual analogue questionnaire in 16 patients with New York Heart Association Class II/III heart failure in 2-month crossover study. (From Ref. 64.)

75–150 mg suggested a flat dose response effect; moreover, chronic dosing did not appear to be associated with tolerance or attenuation of the initial hemodynamic response. However, 150 mg resulted in a higher heart rate without additional hemodynamic benefit, thus the optimum hemodynamic dose appeared to be 100 or 125 mg. These effects may explain the symptomatic improvement (Fig. 9) during sustained therapy (64).

In severe chronic cardiac failure due to ischemic heart disease, 20 patients were treated with flosequinan 100 mg daily or placebo (double-blind) in addition to preexisting diuretic/digoxin (65). After 8 weeks of therapy, flosequinan significantly improved treadmill exercise time, increased peak achieved oxygen consumption, and improved the New York Heart Association symptom grade when compared with placebo. Flosequinan was well tolerated with few adverse effects. In a further study, Elborn et al. (66) investigated the resting minute ventilation and respiratory rate following flosequinan 100 mg. During submaximal exercise at approximately 50% of peak uptake, minute ventilation, carbon dioxide production, and venous lactate levels were reduced on flosequinan compared with placebo.

Further hemodynamic studies with flosequinan have been completed in chronic heart failure. Its actions on left ventricular performance and cardiac contractility were determined in 10 severe CHF patients during combined left and right heart catheterization. Sixty minutes following 100 mg flosequinan orally, peak left ventricular dp/dt increased (940 to 1050 mm Hg/s) with a fall in PWP (32 to 26 mm Hg); cardiac index increased (2.1 to 2.3 L/min/m^2). The authors inferred increased inotropism from the increase in contractility and fall in PWP at unchanged arterial pressure and sympathetic tone (56). The hemodynamic and neurohumoral actions of flosequinan were evaluated at 90 min and 8 days of therapy in ten patients with moderate chronic congestive heart failure. Acute administration of 100 mg orally resulted in a decrease of preload, with a reduction of left ventricular end-diastolic volume and pressure, pulmonary capillary wedge pressure, and right atrial pressure. Acutely, there were no changes in heart rate, cardiac index, stroke volume, peripheral vascular resistance, ejection fraction, and dp/dt. Chronic application for 8 days (100 mg/day) showed persistent effects on preload, with an augmented cardiac index (2.2 to 2.8 L/min/m^2) and stroke volume (57 to 74 ml). Peripheral vascular resistance decreased by 28%. Already by 8 days, bicycle exercise capacity increased significantly (383 to 422 s) with a concomitant decrease of dyspnea. Although plasma renin concentration was elevated at 90 min, by day 8 both atrial natriuretic peptide and 6-keto-prostaglandin F1-α decreased significantly (57).

A number of studies have determined the hemodynamic effects of flosequinan in acute heart failure. Extended monitoring of 100-mg flosequinan over 3 days demonstrated peak hemodynamic improvement between 1 and 2 h after oral administration. On day 1 pulmonary capillary wedge pressure (PCWP) was reduced from 27.8 to 13.0 mm Hg and cardiac output (CO) increased from 3.3 to 4.5 L/min. After 12–16 h the effect was slightly attenuated but remained significant at 24 h. A similar response was observed after the doses given on days 2 and 3. At 72 h, PCWP was 15.5 mm Hg and CO 3.8 L/min. Heart rate was slightly increased only at 2 h after the initial dose; the response to subsequent doses was similar to the response to the first dose (67,68). In ten patients with severe acute-onset heart failure complicating acute myocardial infarction (MI) resistant to high IV doses of diuretics, nitrates, and dobutamine, flosequinan (100 mg) was added to conventional therapy at 3–8 days after infarction. Hemodynamic measurements were performed every hour for 4 h after administration, without any other drug being added. The nitrate infusion rate was kept constant. Flosequinan improved hemodynamics, the effect peaked at 1 to 2 h, and remained at this level at 4 h. Pulmonary capillary wedge pressure decreased from 27.2 to 16.4 mm Hg, and cardiac output increased from 3.5 to 4.1 L/min. Cardiac index, stroke index, and left ventricular stroke work index were significantly increased at unaltered heart rate. Flosequinan administration was not associated with symptomatic hypotension (69).

Although the beneficial effects of flosequinan have been demonstrated in patients with severe heart failure, its efficacy has been less studied in patients with early heart failure (64). In 24 such patients (NYHA II), the effects of 4 weeks flosequinan (50 mg) versus placebo were determined on exercise capacity, cardiac function, and symptoms. No difference was found in measured variables except for left ventricular fractional shortening which increased by 2.9% in the flosequinan versus −1.3% in the placebo group. However, flosequinan increased exercise time 704 to 763 s and the oxygen uptake at the anaerobic threshold (13.8 to 16.7 mL/min kg), and improved symptoms (70).

Three pivotal placebo-controlled parallel group studies of flosequinan in patients with heart failure refractory to digoxin and diuretics, demonstrated significantly greater increases in exercise tolerance compared with placebo (71–73). Two other exercise studies compared flosequinan with either the angiotensin converting enzyme inhibitors captopril (74) or enalapril (75). Both demonstrated similar efficacy (increased exercise tolerance) for flosequinan and comparator over at least a 3-month period. The addition of flosequinan 75–125 mg to baseline diuretic/digoxin therapy, improved bicycle capacity and quality of life parameters equivalent to the ACE inhibitor enalapril (Fig. 10).

In a fourth major study, the flosequinan ACE Trial (FACET), flosequinan was given in addition to an ACE inhibitor plus diuretic and digoxin; a once-daily 100-mg dose produced significant additional improvements in exercise tolerance and quality of life compared with placebo, and the combination was well tolerated (76).

Flosequinan may be a promising vasodilator for the treatment of pulmonary hypertension. It appears to exert selective activity on the pulmonary vascular bed (77); in eight patients with cor pulmonale studied over a 24-h period, pulmonary hemodynamics were favorably altered relative to systemic values and resulted in improved oxygen delivery (78).

Thus flosequinan appears to be a balanced vasodilator with a proven efficacy in the treatment of chronic heart failure. The most common side effect is headache, which occurs in approximately 30% of all patients receiving flosequinan, although the incidence for heart failure patients alone appears somewhat lower (21%). Taste disturbance is also noted due to the drug's excretion in saliva. Interestingly, consistent reductions in blood urea and bilirubin have appeared in several studies with flosequinan compatible with improvements in hepatic and renal blood flow.

Preliminary data from the PROFILE survival study, examining the ef-

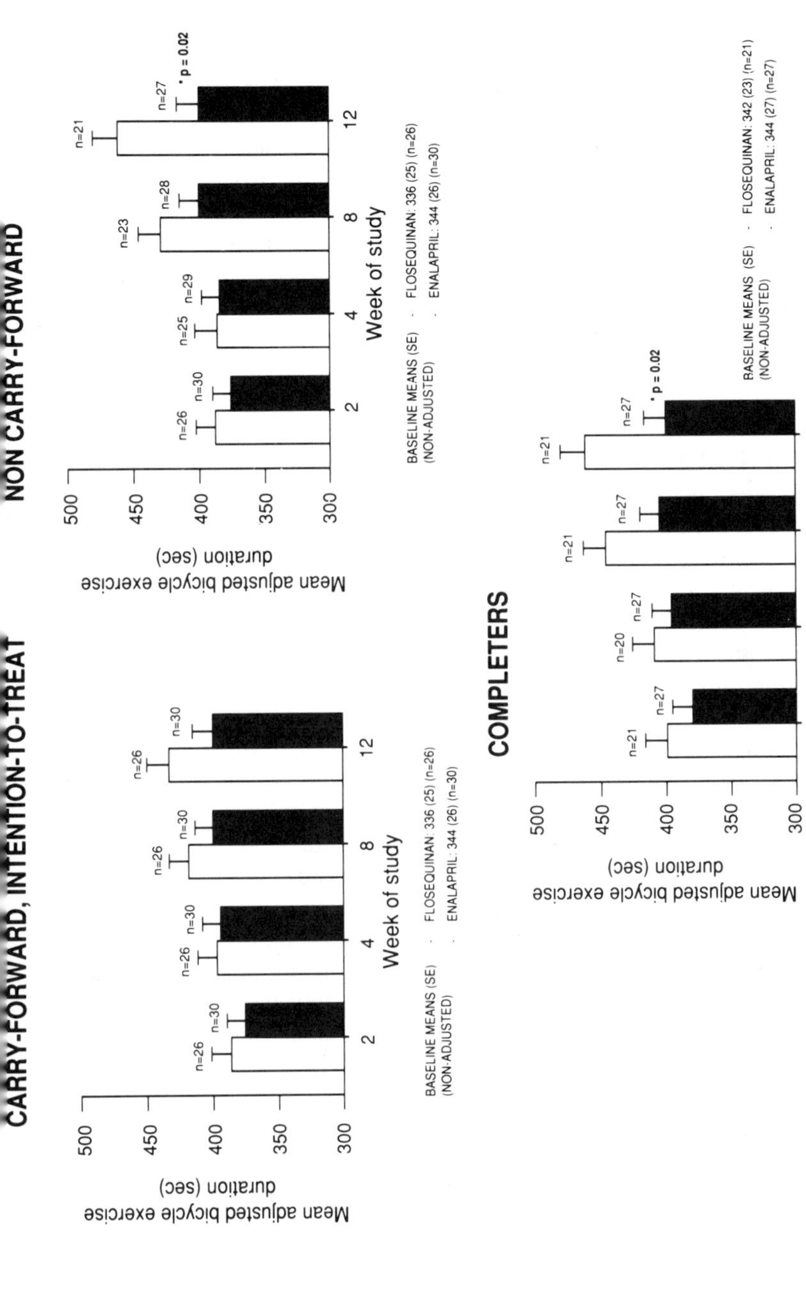

Figure 10 Comparison of the actions of flosequinan (open bars) and enalapril (solid bars) on exercise capacity in 61 patients with New York Heart Association Class III heart failure during repeated bicycle exercise evaluation. Data presented on intention-to-treat and for those completing the study. (From Ref. 75.)

fects of flosequinan compared to placebo in addition to conventional therapy (including ACE inhibition), has indicated an adverse effect on survival in patients treated with flosequinan 100 mg once daily (1-year survival: placebo—80.6%; flosequinan—73.0%). Excess mortality has not been seen in patients receiving flosequinan at 75 mg once daily (1-year survival: placebo—80.9%; flosequinan 80.3%), although at the time of the preliminary analysis the patient numbers in this latter group were not large enough to draw definite conclusions. Therefore, flosequinan 100 mg can no longer be recommended therapeutically and the safety/efficacy of lower doses (50 and 75 mg) is the subject of ongoing investigation.

POTASSIUM CHANNEL OPENERS

Cromakalim (BRL34915) is a benzopyran derivative consisting of a 50/50 racemic mixture, whose biological activity is primarily present in the negative isomer. Vascular smooth muscle relaxation is caused by opening of potassium channels, resulting in hyperpolarization of the resting membrane potential (79). Compounds with potassium channel–opening activity have been demonstrated to possess coronary vasodilator and systemic vasodilator effects but have relatively little action on veins. The combination of such systemic and coronary vasodilator activity would be expected to be beneficial in the treatment of ischemic heart disease and in heart failure.

The hemodynamic effects of cromakalim in a placebo-controlled study of 17 patients with ischemic disease were a 30% increase in cardiac output and a fall in vascular resistance and systemic arterial blood pressure (80). Left ventricular contractility (dp/dt) and stroke volume were unaltered. A small increase in the resting heart rate was observed.

Unlike nicorandil, cromakalim does not appear to increase intracellular cyclic GMP or to act via intracellular calcium modulation (81,82). Cromakalim also appears to have renal and peripheral (humoral) vasodilator actions. Therefore, agents of this class may be potentially of value in patients with heart failure. Further evaluation of their role in heart failure appears warranted.

CONCLUSION

Vasodilators are symptomatically effective in chronic heart failure; compared with diuretic therapy, they improve exercise capacity and hemodynamics and improve survival. Agents with balanced actions on the circulation appear preferable to drugs acting on the capacitance or resistance vessels alone, and compared with the ACE inhibitors, balanced vasodilation appears to result in better hemodynamic and exercise capacity but may not have as beneficial an impact on survival.

The role of such therapy therefore would appear to be as second-line treatment to ACE inhibitors or as an alternative when the latter are poorly tolerated. The possible benefit from the addition of balanced vasodilators to ACE inhibitors has yet to be defined.

REFERENCES

1. Braunwald E, et al. Am J Cardiol 1983; 51:603–605.
2. Smith WM. Am J Cardiol 1985; 55:3A–8A.
3. Likoff MJ, et al. Am J Cardiol 1987; 59:684–688.
4. The CONSENSUS Trial Study Group. N Engl J Med 1987; 316: 1429–1435.
5. Silke B. Cardiovasc Drugs Ther. In press.
6. Cohn JN. N Engl J Med 1977; 297:27–31.
7. Taylor SH, et al. Eur Heart J 1982; 3(suppl D):19–43.
8. Colucci WS. Ann Intern Med 1982; 97:67–77.
9. Taylor SH. In: Bussmann WD, Just H, eds. Vasoaktive Substanzen bei Herzinsuffizienz. Berlin/Heidelberg: Springer-Verlag, 1986:128–142.
10. Majid PA, et al. Lancet 1971; ii:719–724.
11. Nelson GIC, et al. J Cardiovasc Pharmacol 1984; 6:331–338.
12. Schwartz KM, et al. Clin Res 1980; 28:880A.
13. Franciosa JA. Prog Cardiovasc Dis 1981; 24: 319–330.
14. Silke B, et al. J Cardiovasc Pharmacol 1981; 3:329–355.
15. Silke B, et al. Br Heart J 1981; 46:663–670.
16. Elkayam UE, et al. Am J Cardiol 1979; 44:540–545.
17. Packer M, et al. Circulation 1979; 59:531–539.
18. Cohn JN, et al. N Engl J Med 1986; 314:1547–1552.
19. Magorien RD, et al. Am J Cardiol 1990; 65:638–643.
20. Packer M, et al. Am J Cardiol 1980; 45:655–660.
21. Verma SP, et al. J Cardiovasc Pharmacol. 1992; 20:274–281.
22. Massie B, et al. Circulation 1981; 63:269–278.
23. Packer M, et al. N Engl J Med 1980; 303:250–255.
24. Franciosa JA, et al. Am Heart J 1982; 104:587–594.
25. Packer M, et al. N Engl J Med 1982; 306:57–62.
26. Cohn JN, et al. N Engl J Med 1991; 325:303–310.
27. Abrams J. Am Heart J 1985; 110:216–224.
28. Rosen R, et al. Arch Int Pharmacodyn Ther 1987; 285: 226–237.
29. Williams DO, et al. Circulation 1975; 51:421–427.
30. Parker JO. Eur J Clin Pharmacol 1990; 38(suppl 1):S21–S25.
31. Packer M, et al. N Engl J Med 1987; 317:799–804.

32. Cowan JC, et al. Am J Cardiol 1987; 60:271–275.
33. Makhoul N, et al. Am J Cardiol 1990; 65:28J–31J.
34. DeMots H, et al. J Am Coll Cardiol 1989; 13:786–793.
35. Jonsson UE. Eur J Clin Pharmacol 1990; 38(suppl 1):S15–S19.
36. Levy WS, et al. Circulation 1989; 80(suppl II):II-214.
37. Sussex BA, et al. Circulation 1989; 80(suppl II):II-200.
38. Yusuf S, et al. Lancet 1988; i:1088–1092.
39. Franciosa JA, et al. Am J Cardiol 1980; 45:648–654.
40. Leier CV, et al. Circulation 1983; 67:817–822.
41. Kinoshita M, et al. Cardiovasc Drugs Ther 1990; 4:1078–1088.
42. Taira N, et al. Clin Exp Pharmacol Physiol 1979; 6:301–316.
43. Silke B, et al. Am J Cardiol 1989; 63:49J–55J.
44. Yokota M, et al. J Cardiovasc Pharmacol 1987; 10(suppl 8):S116–S122.
45. Kambara H, et al. J Cardiovasc Pharmacol 1987; 10(suppl 8):S104–S108.
46. Kambara H, et al. Am J Cardiol 1989; 21:56J–60J.
47. Kobayashi K, et al. J Cardiovasc Pharmacol 1987; 10(suppl 8):S109–S115.
48. Suryapranata K, et al. Am J Cardiol 1988; 61:292–297.
49. Yates DB. Am Heart J 1991; 121:974–983.
50. Lang D, et al. Eur J Pharmacol 1992; 226:259,264.
51. Richards NT, et al. Br J Pharmacol 1989; 98:734P.
52. Perreault CL, et al. Br J Pharmacol 1992; 106:511.
53. Resnick MS, et al. Br J Pharmacol 1991; 102:974–978.
54. Falotico R, et al. J Cardiovasc Pharmacol 1989; 14:412,418.
55. Greenberg S, et al. J Cardiovasc Pharmacol 1990; 15:900,910.
56. Corin WJ, et al. Am Heart J 1991; 121(2):537,540.
57. Riegger GAJ, et al. Cardiovasc Drugs Ther 1990; 4:1395–1402.
58. Frodsham G, et al. Eur J Pharmacol 1992; 211: 383,391.
59. Cowley AJ, et al. J Hypertens 1984; 2 (Suppl 2):547,549.
60. Scott RA, et al. Br J Clin Pharmacol 1991; 31:41–46.
61. Cowley AJ, et al. Br Med J 1988; 297:169–173.
62. Kessler PD, et al. Am Heart J 1987; 113:137–143.
63. Haas GJ, et al. Clin Cardiol 1990; 13:414–420.
64. Silke B, et al. Br J Clin Pharmacol 1987; 24:250P.
65. Elborn JS, et al. Br Heart J 1989; 61(4):331,335.
66. Elborn JS, et al. Br J Clin Pharmacol 1990; 29:519–524.
67. Schneeweiss A, et al. Cardiology 1989; 76(3):201,205.
68. Schneeweiss A, et al. Int J Cardiol 1989; 24(1):73,76.
69. Schneeweiss A, et al. Crit Care Med 1989; 17(9):879,881.
70. Hori M, et al. Hearts Vessels 1992; 7(3):133,140.
71. Packer M, et al. J Am Coll Cardiol 1993; (in press).
72. Pitt B. Circulation 1991; 84:4 (Suppl 2):1238A.
73. Cowley AJ, et al. Int J Cardiol 1993; 38:167,175.
74. Cowley AJ, et al. Circulation 1991; 84:4 (Suppl 2):1238A.
75. Silke B, et al. Eur Heart J 1992; 13:1092–1100.

76. Massie BM, et al. Circulation 1992; 86:4 (Suppl 1):2566A.
77. Tanaka T, et al. Jap J Nucl Med 1991; 28:241,246.
78. Elborn JS, et al. Chest 1992; 102:1155,1160.
79. Hamilton TC, et al. Br J Pharmacol 1986; 88:103–111.
80. Thomas P, et al. Br J Clin Pharmacol 1990; 19:325–331.
81. Cook NS, et al. J Cardiovasc Pharmacol 1988; 11:90–99.
82. Weir SW, et al. Br J Pharmacol 1986; 88:121–128.

10

ACE Inhibitors in the Treatment of Heart Failure

Peter Held and Karl Swedberg
Östra Hospital, University of Göteborg, Göteborg, Sweden

Heart failure is a complex clinical syndrome characterized by symptoms of dyspnea, fatigue, and peripheral edema. The high annual mortality associated with this syndrome has only recently been fully appreciated. The most important goal in the treatment of heart failure has traditionally been relief of symptoms, which has been accomplished by the use of diuretics and digitalis. Over the last two decades our knowledge of the underlying pathophysiology of heart failure has increased rapidly. A rather simple mechanistic view, concentrating on hemodynamic measurements, has been replaced by a more refined knowledge emphasizing the close interplay between hemodynamic changes and different compensatory mechanisms. The renin-angiotensin system plays a key role in the heart failure syndrome, and the development of the angiotensin converting enzyme (ACE) inhibitors made it possible to interact directly with this system. This has resulted in new approaches to treatment, and for the first time there are known data to support that medical treatment can improve prognosis. This chapter will focus on the clinical effects of the ACE inhibitors as reflected in the results of clinical trials. Properly conducted randomized and controlled trials are necessary to estimate the net effect of the balance between positive and negative effects. Recently, the results of several such large trials have become available, and the ACE inhibitors are now the best-documented class of drugs in the treatment of heart failure.

THE RENIN-ANGIOTENSIN SYSTEM IN HEART FAILURE

In the presence of left ventricular dysfunction, a number of important neurohormonal compensatory mechanisms are activated. The sympathetic nervous system is activated early and causes tachycardia, increased myocardial contractility, and peripheral vasoconstriction. Recent data indicate that activation of the sympathetic nervous system may occur even before the development of clinical heart failure and before activation of the renin-angiotensin system takes place (1).

The renin-angiotensin system is activated to varying degrees in mild to moderate and in severe heart failure. The degree of activation is proportional to the severity of disease (1,2). Renin release is stimulated by a reduction in serum sodium, decreased renal blood flow, and sympathetic stimulation, and probably by the use of diuretic drugs. Its most important effects are angiotensin II–mediated vasoconstriction and stimulation of aldosterone secretion. All the hormonal compensatory mechanisms aim to preserve vital organ perfusion but are, if long-standing, probably deleterious. The resulting increase in afterload and contractility may cause further depression of cardiac function and may perhaps precipitate myocardial ischemia in patients with coronary artery disease. Direct toxic effects on myocardial tissue from angiotensin II are also probable (3). Of particular interest is that survival is inversely related to the degree of activation of both the sympathetic nervous system and the renin-angiotensin system (2,4). The ACE inhibitors effectively reduce the conversion of angiotensin I to the vasoconstrictive angiotensin II, indirectly causing vasodilatation and decreased aldosterone secretion.

ACE INHIBITORS IN HEART FAILURE

Hemodynamic Effects

Treatment with vasodilators, including the ACE inhibitors, generally induces similar short-term changes in the patient with heart failure. Typically, there is an immediate decrease in arterial pressure and left ventricular filling pressure, while cardiac output increases to a varying degree. Heart rate often decreases slightly with ACE inhibitor treatment. These acute hemodynamic changes may be of importance in the immediate treatment of severe heart failure but cannot predict the long-term hemodynamic response (5). With ACE inhibitor treatment many patients do have sustained hemodynamic improvement, while a few will be found to have lost the early effects if repeated measurements are done after some months (6). Others who do not obtain immediate benefit will show beneficial changes during long-term treatment. The literature on the hemodynamic effects of ACE inhibitors contains, however, few randomized, controlled studies, and it is furthermore uncertain to which degree clinical improvement and effect on mortality are linked to these effects.

The regional distribution of blood flow is altered in heart failure, and this may be more important for symptoms than changes in central hemodynamics. In addition to the reduced renal blood flow, perfusion of the skin, working skeletal muscles, and the intestine is selectively reduced, while blood flow to the brain is preserved. It is reasonable to assume that a reduction in muscle blood flow is an important factor associated with the reduced exercise capability seen in heart failure (7). Conversely, an increase in working muscle blood flow is probably necessary to improve exercise capacity (8), although intrinsic changes in muscle function may also be of importance (9–11).

Several investigators have studied the effect of ACE inhibitors on limb blood flow at rest and during exercise. Short-term therapy has not been associated with any change in muscle blood flow, despite an increase in cardiac output (7,12,13). After continuous treatment for a couple of months, however, increase in maximal blood flow has been reported to occur (13). This discrepancy between early and late effects, in spite of immediate changes in cardiac output, may have several explanations. Vascular wall or tissue edema may take time to be corrected and might impair the ability of the peripheral arterial vessels to dilate. Similar findings have been reported in patients after heart transplantation, indicating that this may not be connected with the effects of the ACE inhibitors per se.

Cerebral blood perfusion is autoregulated within physiologic pressure limits. There are indications that ACE inhibitor treatment may shift the pressure-flow relation leftwards, i.e., that the minimal pressure for maintained perfusion is reduced (14). This may explain the surprisingly good tolerance to low systemic blood pressure that is often noticed among patients treated with ACE inhibitors.

Symptomatic Effects

Congestive heart failure is a clinical syndrome characterized by symptoms of dyspnea and fatigue at rest and during daily activities. One of the most important goals of therapy is to relieve the symptoms. There are different ways of measuring symptoms, but defining the most appropriate and clinically relevant measure is always problematic. It is clear that many patients improve symptomatically also when treated with placebo, indicating the absolute need for controlled trials. Measures of symptoms used in the ACE inhibitor trials vary from detailed quality of life questionnaires to simpler estimates of well-being and doctors' assessment of functional class according to the New York Heart Association (NYHA) classification.

There is overall good evidence of symptomatic relief from treatment with ACE inhibitors in heart failure of different severity. Several trials of captopril (15–17), enalapril (2,18–21), and lisinopril (22) have shown that NYHA class improves over time in comparison with placebo treatment. The improvement has often not been immediate and may take several weeks and sometimes months to become apparent (16,17). This is similar to the delayed improvement in exercise capacity reported in several trials (17,23). In spite of its theoretical appeal, the measurement of "quality of life" by different methods has not been universally successful. One of the earlier trials (18) reported clear improvement with captopril treatment, but others could not confirm this result. A subgroup within the CONSENSUS trial was evaluated by means of an extensive questionnaire. There were strong trends toward improvements in quality of life but no statistically significant findings (24). Quality of life evaluations in a mortality trial such as CONSENSUS face a particular problem, as many patients are lost from follow-up because of death. Preliminary data from the very carefully executed quality of life trial within the recent SOLVD trial (1) supports the view that it is difficult to demonstrate benefit. This should, however, not be taken as evidence of lack of effect of the treatment. It is possible that the methods used are not relevant or sensitive enough to measure important changes for the heart failure patient. A clear benefit of treatment in terms of a lesser need for hospitalizations (15,25) strongly indicates favorable and important symptomatic effect. Hospitalizations are frequent among patients with heart failure, and, in addition to the decrease in suffering, a reduction also has obvious implications for the cost of treatment.

Exercise Capacity

Exercise capacity in heart failure is reduced to a varying degree depending on the severity of disease. Although the clinical and practical relevance of measuring exercise capacity in sick patients can perhaps be questioned, exercise testing remains an important procedure in evaluating drugs for heart failure. The effect of ACE inhibitors in this respect has been studied in numerous trials, and overall, the available evidence supports the view that maximal exercise capacity does indeed improve with treatment. When studying the available results it is, however, evident that the generally held impression of a strong effect is perhaps not true. There are in fact only three or four trials (15,18,19), out of at least ten or 15 (15,17–23,26–31), that have reported a significant improvement to the active-treatment group compared with placebo treatment. Even those results are somewhat difficult to interpret, because, for example, of incomplete reporting of all randomized patients (17,32), and because of the use of different methods to analyze the results. Another problem inherent in long-term exercise trials is the possible imbalance caused by the mortality-reducing effect of the ACE inhibitor. This makes comparisons at the end of a trial difficult to interpret, since the groups may no longer be comparable. The trials that demonstrated an improvement are supported by a trend toward better exercise capacity in almost every reported study. Many of these trials reported "statistically significant" improvement but achieved this not by a comparison with the control group but by within-group comparison. This obviously misses the point of having a parallel placebo group. Many trials were small, however, and the lack of statistically significant differences may have been caused by low statistical power to detect a difference. Table 1 lists the available trials and their main results.

Neurohormonal Effects

As neuroendocrine activation is associated with worsening of heart failure and inversely related to prognosis, suppression of this activation may be of importance (33–35). In severe heart failure, ACE inhibitor therapy will reduce plasma levels of noradrenaline, angiotensin II, aldosterone, and atrial natriuretic peptide. It is likely, but has not been clearly demonstrated, that improvement in symptoms and in survival is related to this reduction in plasma hormone levels.

Effects on Survival

Symptomatic relief is an important and until recently the only achievable goal of heart failure treatment. Equally important is to find treatment that is able to reduce the extremely high long-term mortality. The ACE inhibitors are the only agents that have convincingly been shown to improve prognosis among these patients.

Since ACE inhibitors improve hemodynamics and factors associated with mortality such as ejection fraction (17), the hope was early raised that treatment would improve prognosis. An overview in 1987 of the mortality results available from the small trials supported this hope (36). The overview of about 1100 patients in 10 trials indicated a clear reduction in mortality. Data from mortality trials have, however, not become available until quite recently.

Three large trials testing the ACE inhibitor enalapril and with the primary objective of studying mortality have been conducted (25,37–38). Two of these compared enalapril with placebo treatment, while the third used the combination of hydralazine and isosorbide dinitrate in the control group.

Table 1 Exercise Capacity in Randomized, Controlled Trials[a]

Study (Ref.)	No. of patients	NYHA class	Daily dose	Bicycle (B) or treadmill (T)	Active treatment better (+) or worse (−) than placebo	Active treatment vs. placebo (*p*)
Enalapril						
Sharpe, 1984 (18)	36	II–III	10 mg	T	+	< 0.005
Jennings, 1984 (26)	12	III–IV	10–20 mg	B	+	NS
Creager, 1985 (23)	23	II–III	5–10 mg	B	+	< 0.05[b]
Franciosa, 1985 (27)	17	III–IV	5–20 mg	T	+	NS[b]
McGrath, 1985 (20)	25	II–III	10–20 mg	T	(+)	NS
Remes, 1986 (21)	24	II–IV	10–20 mg	B	+	NS
Cleland, 1985 (19)	20	II–IV	10–40 mg	T	+	$p < 0.01$
Rucinska, 1987 (30)	129	II–IV	5–20 mg	T	+	NS
	102	II–IV	5–20 mg	B	+	NS
Captopril						
Multicenter, 1983 (15)	92	II–III	75–300 mg	T	+	$p < 0.008$
Kramer, 1983 (28)	16	II–IV	150–300 mg	T	+	NS
Boccanelli, 1986 (29)	15	II–III	25–100 mg	T	−	NS
Captopril—Digoxin, 1988 (17)	204	I–III	75–150 mg	T	+	NS
Lisinopril						
Chalmers, 1987 (22)	72	II–IV	5–20 mg	T	+	$p < 0.01$
	42	II–IV	5–20 mg	B	+	NS
Ramipril						
Swedberg, 1991 (31)	223	II–III	1.25–10 mg	B	+	NS

[a]The interpretation of the results is complicated because the trials have not been analyzed in a similar way. In some trials, where an imbalance in exercise capacity was observed at baseline (e.g., 18) the absolute change from baseline in the treatment group was compared with the corresponding change in the placebo group. In other trials a pure between-group comparison at follow up was used irrespective of baseline differences (e.g., 15). The method used is probably the one that gives the most favorable result. The number of studies with statistically significant changes would probably be lower if the same method of analysis had been used in all trials.

[b]Part of the Rucinska (30) trial.

NYHA = New York Heart Association; NS = not significant.

The first to be reported was the multicenter Scandinavian CONSENSUS trial (36), planned to include 400 patients in NYHA functional class IV. The study was stopped early by the safety committee, when 253 patients had been randomized. At this time there was clear evidence of benefit from enalapril treatment (Table 2). After 6 months of treatment (primary end point), 44% of the patients in the placebo group compared with 26% in the enalapril group had died (40% reduction, $p < 0.002$). An important additional observation, subsequently confirmed in the recent Studies of Left Ventricular Dysfunction (SOLVD) trial (25), was that enalapril seemed to reduce deaths due to progressive heart failure but not sudden (presumed arrhythmic) deaths.

Only the most severely ill patients were included in CONSENSUS, while SOLVD (25) and V-HeFT II (38) studied mainly patients with milder disease. These trials also provided the first long-term results. SOLVD is the largest trial in heart failure conducted so far. The two arms of the trial divided the patients into two groups depending on whether they had symptomatic or asymptomatic left ventricular dysfunction (defined as ejection fraction below 35%). About 2500 symptomatic patients were randomized to enalapril or placebo and were treated for about 3½ years on average. Both men and women were included; 11% were in NYHA class I, 57% in class II, and 30% in class III. At the end of the treatment period, 39.7% of the patients in the placebo group compared with 35.2% in the enalapril group had died (16% reduction, one-sided $p < 0.0036$). The prevention arm of the trial randomized about 4200 patients with an ejection fraction < 35% to enalapril or placebo treatment. Preliminary results indicate that although there was a favorable trend in the enalapril group, with 8% lower mortality, this did not reach statistical significance. The combined data from both arms show a reduction in total mortality.

The V-HeFT II trial (38) randomized about 800 patients to enalapril or to treatment with a combination of hydralazine and isosorbide dinitrate. All patients were men, and the large majority were in NYHA class II and III. The statistical power of this trial was much lower than that of SOLVD, but the mortality results support the findings of the latter trial. After an average of 2.5 years of treatment, 32.8% of the enalapril-treated patients compared with 38.2% of the controls had died, a difference that did not quite achieve statistical significance ($p < 0.08$). The difference in mortality was, however, larger earlier in the trial than later, and after 2 years of treatment (primary objective) the difference of 28% was statistically significant. It is interesting to note that this figure is close to the 23% reduction found after 2 years in SOLVD.

One point of interest is that the patients treated with the combination of hydralazine and isosorbide dinitrate had a slightly better maximal ex-

Table 2 Mortality in Trials of ACE Inhibitors in Heart Failure

Trial (Ref.)	Mean treatment duration	NYHA class	No. deaths/no. randomized		
			Active treatment	Control	p
Overview 10 trials (34)	varying	varying	40/582 (6.9%)	58/542 (10.7%)	—[a]
CONSENSUS (35)	6 mon	IV	50/127 (39%)	68/126 (54%)	= 0.003
SOLVD (25)	3.5 yr	mainly I–III	452/1285 (35.2%)	510/1284 (39.7%)	= 0.0036[b]
V-HeFT (36)	2.5 yr	mainly II–III	132/403 (32.7%)	153/401 (38.2%)	= 0.08[c]

[a]No formal pooling of data performed.
[b]One-sided statistical test.
[c]$p = 0.016$ at 2 yr.
NYHA = New York Heart Association.

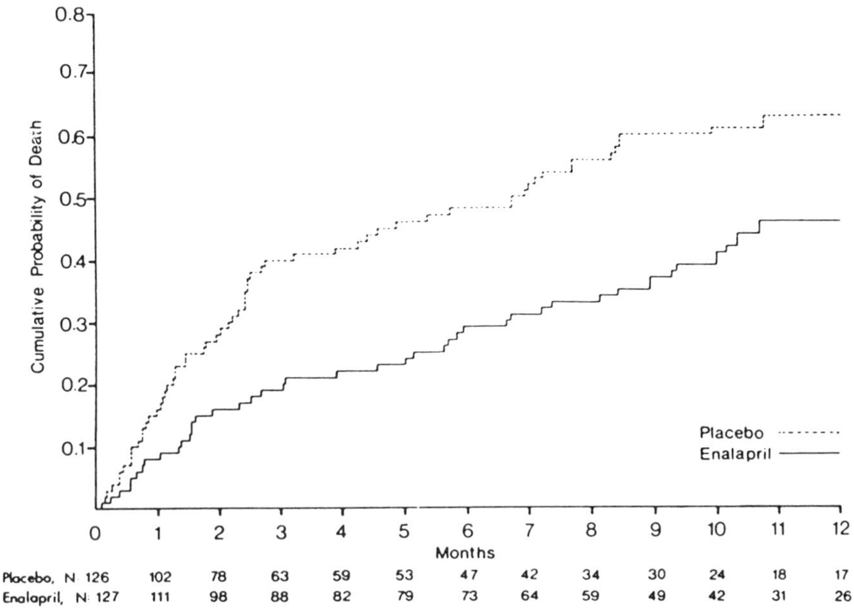

Figure 1 Cumulative mortality rate for up to 12 months in the CONSENSUS trial (35) including only patients in New York Heart Association class IV. At 6 months (primary end point) the mortality was 44% in the placebo group compared to 26% in the enalapril group ($p = 0.002$). Reproduced with permission.

ercise capacity and higher left ventricular ejection fraction than the enalapril-treated patients. This highlights the problems in relying only on intermediate or symptomatic end points when evaluating treatment efficacy.

Finally, it is noteworthy that in the recent large controlled clinical trial SAVE, treatment with captopril (50 mg t.i.d.), instituted between 3 and 16 days after an acute myocardial infarction, significantly improved survival and reduced the incidence of overt congestive heart failure in patients with a low ($< 40\%$) ejection fraction.

Important Side Effects

When it is carefully used, the clinically important side effects caused by ACE inhibition are few. Patients with heart failure have various clinical symptoms also without treatment, and a comparison with placebo treatment is necessary to get reliable data. Table 3 contains the most commonly reported side effects in the two largest placebo-controlled enalapril trials.

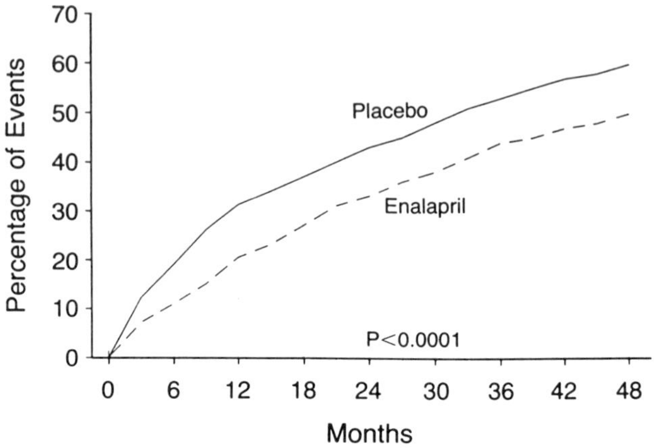

Figure 2 Percentage of events, defined as death or hospitalizations for congestive heart failure, occurring in the placebo and enalapril group in the SOLVD trial (25). The majority of the patients included were in New York Heart Association class II and III. Reproduced with permission.

The most commonly occurring problem is hypotension. In most patients the decrease in blood pressure is slight and clinically unimportant. One reason for this is probably that ACE inhibitors cause a change in the cerebral autoregulation, keeping cerebral blood flow unchanged and thus not causing symptoms (14). In some patients, and particularly among the more severely ill, hypotension may be more problematic. Most susceptible are patients in whom the renin-angiotensin system is highly activated, as reflected, for example, in low serum sodium levels. To avoid problems with hypotension, treatment in all patients should start at a low dose that is later titrated upward. In most cases, patients prone to develop hypotension will be identified after the first dose. Hospitalization to initiate treatment is needed only for patients with very low blood pressure or low serum sodium.

Renal dysfunction and hyperkalemia are the clinically most important side effects in addition to hypotension. Patients in whom the renin-angiotensin system is highly activated may develop a rapid increase in serum creatinine because of a drop in glomerular filtration pressure (GFP). As systemic blood pressure is important for GFP, patients with low systemic blood pressure treated with high doses of diuretics (activated renin-angiotensin system) are most susceptible and need careful monitoring. Great care should be taken when starting treatment in patients with seriously impaired renal function, and treatment should probably be avoided

Table 3 Most Commonly Reported Side Effects (%) in CONSENSUS (35) and in SOLVD (25)

	CONSENSUS		SOLVD	
	Placebo $N = 126$	Enalapril $N = 127$	Placebo $N = 1284$	Enalapril $N = 1285$
Hypotension	0	17[a]	NA	NA
Dizziness	4	13[b]	50	57
Acute myocardial infarction	4	4	4.1	3.1
Cough	0.8	3.1	31	37
Angioedema	0	0	4.1	3.8
Increased serum creatinine[c]	17	40[a]	7.7	10.7[a]
			(>177 μmol/L)	
Hyperkalemia[d]	6.3	19[a]	2.5	6.4[a]
	(any reported)		(≥5.5 mmol/L)	

[a] $p < 0.01$.
[b] $p < 0.05$.
[c] For CONSENSUS, any reported increase; for SOLVD, creatinine > 177 μmol/L.
[d] For CONSENSUS, any reported hyperkalemia; for SOLVD, potassium ≥ 5.5 mmol/L.
NA = not available.

if the serum creatinine level is above 250–300 μg/L. All patients should have serum creatinine and potassium checked within about a week of initiation of therapy and after changes of dose. Serum potassium may increase as a result of the reduction in aldosterone levels caused by treatment. For this reason, potassium supplementation and potassium-sparing diuretics should be used with great caution and are most often not needed.

Cough has been reported more often among patients treated with ACE inhibitors, but the incidence varies and should be related to that of the placebo groups. A dry, irritating cough is probably experienced by 10% to 15% of patients. In some, dose reduction may reduce the cough, but for most of these patients the ACE inhibitor has to be withdrawn. The reason for the cough is unclear, but effects on bradykinin degradation have been suggested.

Patient Selection and Implications

Treatment with ACE inhibitors has until recently been confined to the most severely affected patients in NYHA class IV and perhaps class III. Patients in class I and II have most often not been treated, although they constitute the large majority of those with heart failure. With the results of the recently published SOLVD (25) and V-HeFT II (38) trials added to the previous CONSENSUS (37) experience, enalapril has definitely been proven to reduce mortality among all classes of heart failure patients. Benefit with regard to symptoms has also been well documented. The conclusion that emerges from these studies is therefore that a large majority of heart failure patients with systolic dysfunction will benefit and should be treated.

ACE inhibitors are relatively expensive, and a decision to extend treatment to milder cases will inevitably have cost implications. The data from SOLVD demonstrating a lesser need for hospitalizations do, however, indicate that there is also a cost-reducing effect. The net cost will probably compare favorably with that of many other generally accepted medical interventions, such as treatment for moderate hypertension. It therefore seems reasonable to recommend the combination of an ACE inhibitor and a diuretic agent as standard treatment for heart failure with systolic dysfunction.

REFERENCES

1. Francis GS, Benedict C, Johnstone DE, et al. Comparison of neuroendocrine activation in patients with left ventricular dysfunction with and without congestive heart failure. A substudy of the studies of left ventricular dysfunction (SOVLD). Circulation 1990; 82:1724–1729.
2. Swedberg K, Eneroth P, Kjekshus J, Wilhelmsen L, for the CONSENSUS Study Group. Hormones regulating cardiovascular function in patients with severe congestive heart failure and their relation to mortality. Circulation 1990; 82:1730–1736.
3. Weber KT, Janicki JS. Angiotensin and the remodelling of the myocardium. Br J Clin Pharmacol 1989; 28:141S–150S.
4. Nicklas JM, Benedict C, Johnstone DE, et al. Relationship between neurohumoral profile and one year mortality in patients with CHF and/or LV dysfunction (abstr). Circulation 1991; 84:II-468.
5. Franciosa JA. Effectiveness of long-term vasodilator administration in the treatment of chronic left ventricular failure. Prog Cardiovasc Dis 1982; 24: 319–330.
6. Packer M, Medina N, Yusak M, Meller J. Hemodynamic patterns of response during long-term captopril therapy for severe chronic heart failure. Circulation 1983; 68:803–812.
7. Wilson JR, Martin JL, Schwartz D, Ferraro N. Exercise intolerance in patients with chronic heart failure: role of impaired nutritive flow to skeletal muscle. Circulation 1984; 69:1079–1087.
8. Mancini DM, Davis L, Wexler JP, Chadwick B, LeJemtel TH. Dependence of enhanced maximal exercise performance on increased peak skeletal muscle

perfusion during long-term captopril therapy in heart failure. J Am Coll Cardiol 1987; 10:845–850.
9. Massie B, Conway M, Yonge R, et al. Skeletal muscle metabolism in patients with congestive heart failure: relation to clinical severity and blood flow. Circulation 1987; 76:1009–1019.
10. Mancini DM, Ferraro N, Tuchler M, Chance B, Wilson JR. Detection of abnormal calf muscle metabolism in patients with heart failure using phosphorus-31 nuclear magnetic resonance. Am J Cardiol 1988; 62:1234–1240.
11. Buller P, Jones D, Poole-Wilson PA. Direct measurement of skeletal muscle fatigue in patients with chronic heart failure. Br Heart J 1991; 6520–6524.
12. Kugler J, Maskin C, Frishman H, Sonnenblick EH, LeJemtel TH. Regional and systemic metabolic effects of angiotensin-converting enzyme inhibition during exercise in patients with severe heart failure. Circulation 1982; 66: 1256–1261.
13. Drexler H, Banhardt U, Meinertz T, Wollschläger H, Lehman M, Just H. Contrasting peripheral short-term and long-term effects of converting enzyme inhibition in patients with congestive heart failure. Circulation 1989; 79: 491–502.
14. Paulson OB, Jarden JO, Godtfredsen J, Vorstrup S. Cerebral blood flow in patients with congestive heart failure treated with captopril. Am J Med 1984; 76(5B):91–95.
15. Captopril Multicenter Research Group. A placebo-controlled trial of captopril in refractory chronic congestive heart failure. J Am Coll Cardiol 1983; 2: 755–763.
16. Bussman W-D, Störger H, Hadler N, et al. Long-term treatment of severe chronic heart failure with captopril: a double-blind, randomized, placebo-controlled, long-term study. J Cardiovasc Pharm 1987; 9(suppl 2):S50–S60.
17. The Captopril-Digoxin Multicenter Research Group. Comparative effects of therapy with captopril and digoxin in patients with mild to moderate heart failure. *JAMA* 1988; 259:539–544.
18. Sharpe DN, Murphy J, Coxon R, Hannan SF. Enalapril in patients with chronic heart failure: a placebo-controlled, randomized, double-blind study. Circulation 1984; 70:271–278.
19. Cleland JGF, Dargie HJ, Ball SG, et al. Effects of enalapril in heart failure: a double-blind study of effects in exercise performance, renal function, hormones, and metabolic state. Br Heart J 1985; 54:305–312.
20. McGrath BP, Arnolda L, Matthews PG, et al. Controlled trial of enalapril in congestive heart failure. Br Heart J 1985; 54:405–414.
21. Remes J, Nikander P, Rehnberg S, et al. Enalapril in chronic heart failure, a double blind placebo-controlled study. Ann Clin Res 1986; 18:124–128.
22. Chalmers JP, West MJ, Cyran J, et al. Placebo-controlled study of lisinopril in congestive heart failure: a multicenter study. J Cardiovasc Pharmacol 1987; 9(suppl 3):S89–S97.

23. Creager MA, Massie BM, Faxon DP, et al. Acute and long-term effects of enalapril on the cardiovascular response to exercise and exercise tolerance in patients with congestive heart failure. J Am Coll Cardiol 1985; 6:163–170.
24. Wiklund I, Swedberg K. Methodological problems in analyzing quality of life data in severe congestive heart failure. J Clin Res Pharmacoepidemiol 1991; 5:265–273.
25. The SOLVD Investigators. Effect of enalapril on survival in patients with reduced left ventricular ejection fractions and congestive heart failure. N Engl J Med 1991; 325:293–302.
26. Jennings G, Kiat H, Nelson L, et al. Enalapril for severe heart failure. A double blind study. Med J Aust 1984; 141:723–726.
27. Franciosa JA, Wilen MM, Jordan RA. Effects of enalapril, a new angiotensin-converting enzyme inhibitor, in a controlled trial in heart failure. J Am Coll Cardiol 1985; 5:101–107.
28. Kramer BL, Massie BM, Topic N. Controlled trial of captopril in chronic heart failure: a rest and exercise hemodynamic study. Circulation 1983; 67: 807–816.
29. Boccanelli A, Zachara E, Liberatore SM, Carboni GP, Prati PL. Addition of captopril versus increasing diuretics in moderate but deteriorating heart failure: a double blind comparative trial. Postgrad Med J 1986; 62(suppl 1):184–187.
30. Enalapril Congestive Heart Failure Investigators. Long-term effects of enalapril in patients with congestive heart failure: a multicenter, placebo-controlled trial. Heart Failure 1987; 3:102–107.
31. Swedberg K, Amtorp O, Gundersen T, Remes J, Nilsson B. Is maximal exercise testing a useful method to evaluate treatment of moderate heart failure (abst). Circulation 1991; 84:II-57.
32. Newman TJ, Maskin CS, Dennick LG, et al. Effects of captopril on survival in patients with heart failure. Am J Med 1988; 84(suppl 3A):140–144.
33. Cohn JN, Levine TB, Olivari MT, et al. Plasma norepinephrine as a guide to prognosis in patients with chronic congestive heart failure. N Engl J Med 1984; 311:819–823.
34. Swedberg K, Eneroth P, Kjekshus J, Snapinn S, for the CONSENSUS Trial Study Group. Effects of enalapril and neuroendocrine activation on prognosis in severe congestive heart failure (follow-up of the CONSENSUS trial). Am J Cardiol 1990; 66:40D–45D.
35. Dzau VJ, Colucci WS, Hollenberg NK, Williams GH. Relation of the renin-angiotensin-aldosterone system to clinical state in congestive heart failure. Circulation 1981; 63:645–651.
36. Furberg CD, Yusuf S. Effect of drug therapy on survival in chronic congestive heart failure. Am J Cardiol 1988; 62:41A–45A.
37. The Cooperative North Scandinavian Enalapril Survival Study Group. Effects of enalapril on mortality in severe congestive heart failure. Results of the

Cooperative North Scandinavian enalapril survival study (CONSENSUS). N Engl J Med 1987; 316:1429–1435.
38. Cohn JN, Johnson G, Ziesche S, et al. A comparison of enalapril with hydralazine–isosorbide dinitrate in the treatment of chronic congestive heart failure. N Engl J Med 1991; 325:303–310.

11

β-Adrenoceptor Agonists and Partial Agonists for Heart Failure

Derek G. Waller
Southampton General Hospital, Southampton, United Kingdom

Michael K. Davies
Queen Elizabeth Hospital and University of Birmingham, Birmingham, United Kingdom

INTRODUCTION

Activation of the sympathetic nervous system occurs early in the course of heart failure (see Chap. 3). The failing heart derives benefit from an increase in heart rate and contractility that attempts to maintain cardiac output. These cardiac effects are mediated predominantly by β-adrenoceptors, but sympathetic activation also has potentially detrimental actions on the peripheral circulation through stimulation of α-adrenoceptors.

β-ADRENOCEPTOR STIMULATION IN HEART FAILURE

Selective β-adrenoceptor stimulation appears to offer a means of capitalizing on the advantages of sympathetic stimulation, while avoiding some of the less desirable peripheral vascular effects. If successful, the improvement in cardiac performance should suppress endogenous catecholamine drive and reduce the detrimental vasoconstrictor effects. However, excessive cardiac stimulation by catecholamines may provoke myocardial necrosis (1,2) or potentially serious arrhythmias (3,4).

The primary abnormality in heart failure is a loss of functioning myocardium leading to a fall in cardiac output. Superficially, inotropic therapy—enhancing the contractile performance of the remaining myocardium—might appear as an attractive therapeutic concept. However, the use of inotropes in chronic heart failure has been disappointing, and salutary lessons continue to be learned (see Chaps. 15). An important consideration for the use of β-adrenoceptor agonists is the reduced β-adrenoceptor density in patients with heart failure, which impairs the heart's ability to respond adequately not only to endogenous catecholamines but also to exogenously administered β-adrenoceptor agonists. This has been confirmed both in vitro and in vivo, with patients who had significant β-adrenoceptor down-regulation showing grossly impaired contractile responses to exogenous dobutamine (5–8). The degree of this impairment correlates with the degree of β-adrenoceptor down-regulation (7). Any treatment regimen that enhances β-adrenoceptor stimulation (either via direct β-adrenoceptor agonism or indirectly via increasing compensatory sympathetic tone) is likely to accelerate down-regulation of β-adrenoceptors and deterioration in myocardial function. Studies have confirmed rapid β-adrenoceptor down-regulation following exposure to agonists in vitro and in vivo in humans and in animals (9–12).

This loss of β-adrenoceptor function accounts for tachyphylaxis leading to rapid tolerance (over 24–72 h), which has been observed with virtually all β-adrenoceptor agonists in heart failure. The majority of β-adrenoceptor agonists are available only for intravenous use, and despite intensive research corresponding oral forms are still lacking. This further restricts their application to acute heart failure or as intermittent therapy in chronic heart failure.

The Pharmacological Basis of β-Adrenoceptor Partial Agonist Activity

The structure of the β-adrenoceptor has been described in detail in Chapter 3. The extent of the response of the β-adrenoceptor to an agonist is determined first by the affinity of the molecule for the receptor and additionally by its ability to "recruit" transducer G_s proteins and therefore to amplify the response within a single receptor complex. A molecule that initiates coupling with a high efficiency will demonstrate potent agonist activity. Antagonist molecules bind to the receptor but do not initiate coupling with the G protein. The interaction of agonists and antagonists with the receptor is reversible and competitive; the success of an antagonist in maintaining receptor blockade will depend on its affinity for the receptor; compounds with low affinity will be readily displaced when the concentration of a competing high-affinity agonist increases.

Partial agonists usually demonstrate high affinity for a receptor and therefore have the potential to deny access to the natural agonists adrenaline and noradrenaline. However, they initiate receptor coupling with low efficiency and produce a submaximal tissue response. Different partial agonist molecules show varying degrees of efficiency of receptor coupling and consequently different amounts of agonist activity. The degree of partial agonist activity (PAA) is expressed as a percentage of the maximal response produced by a full agonist. For the β-adrenoceptor, comparisons are usually made with isoprenaline. Quantifying the degree of PAA is complex, since the methodology applied to humans produces data that are difficult to interpret. Studies using animal tissues show considerable interspecies variation, and their relevance to human responses is often unclear (13).

Clinical Significance of Partial Agonist Activity: Potency and Selectivity

A molecule with β-adrenoceptor PAA will submaximally stimulate the receptors that it occupies, while making them unavailable for endogenous catecholamine stimulation. Consequently, when there is low sympathetic nervous tone, such a molecule acts as a weak agonist and mimics a higher level of sympathetic stimulation. As endogenous sympathetic activity increases, agonist molecules will exceed the concentration required to achieve the level of stimulation produced by the partial agonist molecule. The drug then begins to behave as a receptor blocker. The point at which effective blockade ensues is determined by the degree of PAA; a compound with a high degree of PAA may produce stimulation close to that achieved by maximum sympathetic stimulation. Such a molecule will behave as an agonist in most clinical situations. Conversely, a weak partial agonist more closely resembles a β-adrenoceptor blocker in its clinical effects. Thus, the degree of PAA has a profound influence on the hemodynamic profile of a drug and on its use in patients with impaired myocardial contractility (14).

The importance of receptor selectivity of β-adrenoceptor antagonists in determining the unwanted effects of this class of drugs is widely appreciated. Equally important to the clinical use of partial agonists in heart failure is the relative selectivity of the agonist activity. Most experience in heart failure involves compounds with β_1-selective agonist and antagonist properties. There are theoretically both advantages and disadvantages in using molecules with β_2-selective or nonselective partial agonist activity, but few data have been published on the use of such compounds in patients with impaired left ventricular function. This may be due in part to concern that excessive β_2-adrenoceptor stimulation can produce serious arrhythmias (15) while contributing less inotropic support for the heart than β_1-adrenoceptor stimulation.

β_1-Adrenoceptor Partial Agonists in Heart Failure

Although the number of β_1-adrenoceptors is reduced in heart failure, they still mediate the majority of the cardiac stimulation produced by catecholamines. Stimulation of β_2- and α-adrenoceptors also increases myocardial contractility, but the receptors have low affinity for agonist binding, and uncoupling of β_2-adrenoceptors in the failing heart reduces their ability to generate intracellular cyclic AMP by some 30% (16).

β_1-adrenoceptor stimulation by partial agonist drugs has two potentially beneficial actions. First, it provides submaximal stimulation of receptors, which produces a positive inotropic response when endogenous sympathetic activity is low. Second, the antagonist activity will prevent excessive cardiac stimulation when sympathetic tone is high. As discussed above, the point at which the drug begins to behave as an antagonist will be determined by its degree of PAA.

Prenalterol was one of the first β-adrenoceptor partial agonists to be used in heart failure. However, its agonist activity is not β_1-selective, and it has a high level of PAA at β-adrenoceptors (approximately 65%) (17). It therefore acts as a full agonist at most physiological levels of sympathetic tone. Of the β_1-selective partial agonists, the PAA of xamoterol is about 43% (18), which approximates to the level of sympathetic activity that accompanies moderate levels of exercise in healthy volunteers. Epanolol demonstrates about 20% PAA (19) and acts as an effective β-adrenoceptor antagonist even during mild exercise. It has not been studied in the failing heart. Cicloprolol has an intermediate degree of PAA at about 30% (17). Most data for this group of drugs in patients with impaired ventricular function have been obtained using xamoterol.

β-Adrenoceptor Partial Agonists and Adrenoceptor Regulation

Since β-adrenoceptor partial agonists act as antagonists when endogenous catecholamine levels are high, they have the potential to limit receptor down-regulation in heart failure. When Kowalski et al. (20) subcutaneously infused isoprenaline into rats, they demonstrated that after 6 days the cardiac ventricular β_1-adrenoceptor density was reduced by an average of 43%. Those receptors still available at the cell surface also showed uncoupling from adenylate cyclase. In another group of rats xamoterol was infused at twice the concentration of isoprenaline, yet had no effect on receptor density or sensitivity. In vitro studies by Limas and Limas (21) demonstrated that internalization of cell membrane β-adrenoceptors from rat cardiac myocytes occurred to a similar degree after both isoprenaline and xamoterol. However, xamoterol inhibited down-regulation of β-adrenoceptors when given with isoprenaline. Thus in heart failure, which predisposes to receptor down-regulation, xamoterol may reduce the detrimental effects of endogenous catecholamines on receptor numbers and sensitivity. However, coadministration of xamoterol and isoprenaline in the same model did not abolish receptor down-regulation (22).

There are few data on adrenoceptor regulation by partial agonists in humans. Watanabe et al. (23) found that xamoterol up-regulated β_2-adrenoceptor numbers on peripheral blood lymphocytes in both healthy volunteers and patients with heart failure. The significance of such changes for cardiac β-adrenoceptors is unknown. However, these findings were not confirmed in a preliminary report of the effect of xamoterol for 2 weeks in healthy volunteers, in whom numbers of lymphocyte β_2-adrenoceptors and their responsiveness to isoprenaline were unaffected by treatment. Infusion of the nonselective β-adrenoceptor agonist isoprenaline produced a similar fall in diastolic blood pressure (mainly a β_2-adrenoceptor effect) before and after xamoterol, but the systolic blood pressure increase and tachycardia were attenuated after xamoterol, indicating effective β_1-adrenoceptor blockade (24).

NONSELECTIVE β-ADRENOCEPTOR FULL AGONISTS

Noradrenaline and Adrenaline

These are potent naturally occurring catecholamines with powerful, nonselective effects at α- and β-adrenoceptors. They may be useful in certain acute situations such as following surgery and in many forms of shock (including that produced by toxins or anaphylaxis). However, their clinical applications are severely restricted by marked positive chronotropic effects, a propensity to precipitate ventricular arrhythmias, and effects on peripheral vascular tone. In heart failure their use has been largely superseded by the development of inotropes with much lesser chronotropic and vascular effects.

Isoprenaline

Isoprenaline has potent β_1- and β_2-adrenoceptor agonist effects. Despite powerful inotropic properties it has no place in the management of patients with heart failure because of its marked peripheral vasodilatory, chronotropic, and arrhythmogenic effects.

Dobutamine

Dobutamine is a synthetic sympathomimetic amine providing a combination of α-, β_1-, and β_2-agonist effects. It is a racemic mixture whose α_1-agonist effects reside primarily with the *l* isomer and its potent β_1- and β_2-agonist effects with the *d* isomer. It produces a hemodynamic profile of marked inotropism with mild peripheral vasodilatation (because of a balance of α and β_2 effects) and little chronotropic effect. It is markedly less arrhythmogenic than dopamine and noradrenaline. In the absence of any dopaminergic receptor activity it does not selectively increase renal blood flow. These properties make it the "gold standard" agonist against which other compounds with potential inotropic properties are evaluated. It is effective in acute heart failure and frequently used in combination with dopamine (Chap. 13) to obtain a concomitant improvement in renal blood flow.

In common with other β_1-adrenoceptor full agonists, no oral form of the drug exists, and this limits its potential in chronic heart failure therapy. However, both intermittent and continuous dobutamine infusions during the course of chronic heart failure have been evaluated (25,26). Initially encouraging results indicated that hemodynamic improvement was maintained for a number of weeks following a short (72-h) course of intravenous dobutamine (27). However, this enthusiasm for intermittent infusions has been tempered by reports that such therapy is associated with an unacceptably high mortality (28,29). Dobutamine has been shown to induce β-adrenoceptor down-regulation and rapid tolerance (12,30). Interestingly, it has been suggested that the effects on β-adrenoceptor function can be mitigated by the use of higher doses over longer periods of time (12). The degree of receptor loss is smaller than with lower doses, and it has been postulated that exogenous dobutamine in this situation is sufficient to turn off endogenous sympathetic drive, with a net beneficial effect on the level of β-adrenoceptor stimulation. However, the longer-term effects of high-dose, prolonged dobutamine infusion in the management of heart failure await clarification.

Dobutamine has also been used in the investigation of β-adrenoceptor function in heart failure, both in vitro and in vivo. The impaired myocardial contractile response to dobutamine parallels the level of β-adrenoceptor down-regulation (5–8). Dobutamine infusions have also been used as a prognostic indicator to determine cardiac reserve in patients with severe heart failure. An inadequate response (in terms of increases in cardiac output above basal levels of 1 W) delineates patients with a high mortality (31,32). It is likely that the response in this situation reflects the level of residual β-adrenoceptor function. Dobutamine increases myocardial oxygen demands and enhances regional perfusion abnormalities in ischemic heart disease (33–35). This suggests a further reason for caution when considering inotropic support in patients with heart failure, since in most cases (75%) the underlying etiology is ischemic heart disease.

β_2-ADRENOCEPTOR FULL AGONISTS

Pirbuterol

Pirbuterol is a β_2-adrenoceptor agonist with both vasodilatory and positive inotropic properties. Acute therapy results in significant improvements in cardiac index, stroke volume index, and radionuclide ejection fraction, associated with a significant fall in left ventricular filling pressure and systemic vascular resistance (11,36). Although long-term symptomatic improvement and improved exercise performance have been reported with chronic oral therapy, other studies have shown that rapid hemodynamic tolerance occurs. In addition, enhanced β-adrenoceptor down-regulation has been documented with the use of pirbuterol, with restoration to pretreatment levels on withdrawal of the drug (11). Furthermore, the use of chronic pirbuterol therapy may be associated with an adverse effect on mortality. In a study of 63 patients with moderate to severe heart failure, Dawson et al. (37) reported that the 3-month mortality was 32%. Of the 20 patients who died, 16 were receiving pirbuterol at the time of death. The risk of increased mortality and the development of tolerance have prevented this drug from being adopted for the treatment of patients with heart failure.

Salbutamol and Terbutaline

Salbutamol and terbutaline are two other predominantly β_2-adrenoceptor agonist drugs that have been investigated for the treatment of patients with heart failure. Both agents produce acute hemodynamic improvements primarily through vasodilatation. Intravenous and oral salbutamol have been used in the acute treatment of patients with severe heart failure (38–40) and have produced improvements in both systolic and diastolic function (40). Although beneficial long-term hemodynamic effects have also been reported following chronic oral therapy, this has been associated with a propensity to serious arrhythmias (41). Inhaled and intravenous terbutaline have been shown to have beneficial effects in small groups of patients (42,43). However, the drugs have adverse effects on potassium kinetics, with the potential to induce hypokalemia. Neither drug has gained a recognized place in routine therapy, and there is a paucity of long-term studies in significantly large groups of patients. The hemodynamic profile of either drug offers little advantage over conventional inotropes with or without combined vasodilator therapy.

Dopexamine

This is a dopamine analogue with dopaminergic and β_2-adrenoceptor agonist activity but without α- or β_1-agonist effects (44). It should, therefore, provide many of the useful hemodynamic effects of dopamine—i.e., increases in contractility and renal blood flow—but even at higher doses produce vasodilatation rather than vasoconstriction. Improvements in contractility may be largely reflex as a result of vasodilatation, although direct β_2-agonist effects at the myocardial level could also contribute. Theoretically, a β_2-adrenoceptor agonist may be particularly efficacious in heart failure, as β_2-adrenoceptors are thought to be down-regulated to a lesser extent than β_1-adrenoceptors (see Chap. 3). This selective sparing may make β_2-adrenoceptor stimulation particularly important for inotropic responsiveness in heart failure. However, selective receptor preservation may be specific to certain etiologies and observed only in heart failure that is secondary to congestive cardiomyopathic disease, not in ischemic heart failure (45). If β_2-adrenoceptors are not subject to down-regulation, tachyphylaxis to chronic dopexamine therapy should not occur. However, conflicting reports leave this issue unresolved. Both rapid tachyphylaxis (45–48) and lack of tolerance (49) have been reported. One problem with the interpretation of these data is that dopexamine enhances sympathetic tone and may produce tolerance via further β_1-adrenoceptor down-regulation (50,51).

The lack of any oral preparation of dopexamine, the modest improvements in inotropic state and diuretic effect, and the common problem of tachycardia and ventricular arrhythmias with larger doses significantly limit its applications in the management of heart failure. Profound vasodilatation may also produce significant adverse effects in some patients by excessive lowering of ventricular filling pressure.

β_1-ADRENOCEPTOR PARTIAL AGONISTS

Prenalterol

Although prenalterol is a selective β_1-adrenoceptor partial agonist, it has 65% to 80% of the maximum agonist activity of isoprenaline and behaves as a full agonist in almost all clinical situations. In its oral form it has been shown to have inotropic and reflex vasodilatory effects when acutely administered to patients with moderate and severe heart failure (52,53). Improvements in cardiac index and stroke volume index are associated with a fall in systemic vascular resistance in a dose-dependent manner (52). Improvements in exercise tolerance during chronic therapy have been reported and have been attributed to the beta-blocking capacity of this drug when sympathetic tone is high, attenuating exercise-induced increases in heart rate and reducing exercise double product (54). This may be of particular importance in maintaining left ventricular function during exercise in the setting of heart failure due to ischemic heart disease. However, tolerance to the hemodynamic effects occurs during long-term use of prenalterol. In a study of 16 patients with severe heart failure, the initial beneficial inotropic and vasodilatory effects were significantly attenuated after 3 months of oral therapy (55). Further receptor down-regulation and reduced efficacy during chronic therapy, as a result of the predominant β-adrenoceptor agonism of the drug, would be consistent with these observations. Prenalterol has been withdrawn because of side effects in animals.

Xamoterol

Adrenoceptor Selectivity and Agonist Activity

Early studies in dogs suggested that xamoterol was highly selective for β_1-adrenoceptors (49). Receptor-binding studies have confirmed a weak affinity for β_2-adrenoceptors. Cook et al. (56) demonstrated by differential radioligand displacement in isolated animal tissues that the selectivity of xamoterol for β_1-adrenoceptors was about 40 times greater than for β_2-adrenoceptors. In other studies its affinity for β_2-adrenoceptors was 100 times lower than for β_1-adrenoceptors (57,58).

The selectivity of xamoterol was supported by studies in healthy humans by Jennings et al. (59). After autonomic blockade with prazosin, atropine, and clonidine, xamoterol produced a rise in heart rate and mean arterial blood pressure, with a 24% increase in cardiac output. By contrast, isoprenaline increased heart rate but decreased mean arterial pressure (the latter a consequence of β_2-adrenoceptor–mediated vasodilatation). The degree of partial agonist activity shown by xamoterol could not be precisely determined in this study, since the increase in heart rate produced by isoprenaline was not maximal. However, the authors suggested an estimate of between 30% and 60%. It has also been shown that the increase in sleeping heart rate produced by xamoterol is unaffected by specific β_2-adrenoceptor inhibition (60) and that xamoterol does not reduce the bronchodilatation, skeletal muscle tremor, or fall in blood pressure in response to the β_2-selective agonist terbutaline (61). However, it did increase airways resistance in two of the asthmatic subjects studied, indicating some measure of β_2-adrenoceptor blockade.

The degree of PAA of xamoterol has been assessed from the chronotropic effect of the drug in atrial tissue from a variety of species. From these results the agonist activity has been estimated to be equal to or less than 55% of that produced by isoprenaline (57,62,63). In anesthetized dogs, the PAA was found to be 43% (49) and 50% (48). The applicability of such observations to humans is uncertain, since relative agonist and antagonist potency and selectivity vary among species and tissues (64).

Lemoine et al. (65) reported that while xamoterol had an 18 times greater affinity for β_1-adrenoceptors in the feline heart, in human ventricular membrane β_1-selectivity was 30 times greater. Of interest in these studies was the finding that the activation of receptor-bound adenylate cyclase by xamoterol was blocked by the β_1-adrenoceptors selective antagonist CGP 20,712A, but was unaffected by the β_2-selective antagonist ICI 118,551. It is therefore apparent that xamoterol acts principally as a β_1-adrenoceptor partial agonist and exhibits only weak antagonist properties at β_2-adrenoceptors.

Dose-Response Relationships

Xamoterol is a hydrophilic molecule that is poorly absorbed from the gut, leading to an average systemic bioavailability of about 5% (66). About 9% of the drug is absorbed after oral dosing, but almost half is inactivated by first-pass metabolism in the gut wall to the sulfate conjugate. Despite this low bioavailability, intersubject variability is relatively small, resulting in predictable blood concentrations after oral dosing. Elimination of xamoterol is largely by the kidney, which accounts for about three-quarters of total body clearance (67); since renal clearance is higher than glomerular filtration rate, tubular secretion probably contributes to elimination (68). The elimination half-life of the drug is therefore dependent on the level of renal function. In healthy young volunteers, this is about 16 h (59), increasing to 27 h in elderly subjects as a consequence of mild renal impairment (69). Patients with heart failure and normal renal function eliminate xamoterol at the same rate as young volunteers (67).

The relationship between the plasma xamoterol concentration and contractile performance of the left ventricle has been examined in patients with ischemic heart failure (70). Cumulative doses of xamoterol were given to 24 patients, and a dose-related increase in the rate of pressure change in the left ventricle at a developed pressure of 40 mm Hg ($(dP/dt)/DP_{40}$) was demonstrated. It was calculated from these data that the mean plasma xamoterol concentration found 12 h after a dosing schedule of 200 mg twice daily (71) would produce 75% of the maximum observed response, while the peak concentration 1 h post-dose equated to 90% of the maximum. Measurement of systolic time intervals in healthy volunteers indicated that a maximum positive inotropic response was achieved after a 100-mg oral dose, but that higher doses produced a more sustained improvement. In patients with heart failure, there was a sustained decrease in total electromechanical systole (an index of inotropic effect) throughout the 12-h dose interval with doses of 100, 200, and 300 mg twice daily (71). Such observations provide a rational basis for the most widely used dosage regimen of 200 mg twice daily, but assume that the magnitude of improvement in systolic contractility directly correlates with clinical benefit. Such an assumption has not been validated with other therapies in heart failure: hemodynamic improvement and clinical response are not always associated (72).

Hemodynamic Effects of Xamoterol

The partial agonist properties of xamoterol confer on it a hemodynamic profile that clearly differentiates the drug from pure β-adrenoceptor antagonists. These are most clearly seen at rest, however, whereas in the presence of high levels of sympathetic tone (such as are found during exercise), the antagonist properties of the drug determine the cardiac responses.

Resting Hemodynamics Systolic contractility is improved by xamoterol in patients with left ventricular impairment. Both oral and intravenous xamoterol produce increases in cardiac index of 15% to 30% (73–77). This results from increased stroke volume with a small (10%) rise in heart rate. The increase in cardiac output appears to be greater in those patients with the lowest initial ejection fractions (76). Peripheral vascular resistance is reduced, consistent with a reflex response to the increase in cardiac output and blood pressure rather than a direct vasodilator action of xamoterol. Various investigators have examined the mechanism of improvement in cardiac function in greater detail. Xamoterol produces a significant increase in global resting systolic contractility (+LV dP/dt_{max}) of 20% to 35% (76,78) with an associated increase in ejection fraction (73,76). When it was given to patients with ischemic heart disease and regional ventricular dysfunction, contraction of abnormal segments improved (76). Although improvement in contractility undoubtedly contributes to the beneficial effects of xamoterol, considerable attention has been given to its influence on diastolic function. Many patients with heart failure have a normal ejection fraction and well-preserved systolic contractility. A poor correlation between abnormal systolic function and exercise capacity has been emphasized in several studies (79). The closer correlation between elevated left ventricular filling pressure and a reduced ability to exercise suggests that the diastolic performance of the heart may be the most important determinant of clinical status. Xamoterol lowers left ventricular end-diastolic pressure in a dose-dependent manner after acute administration (80), which could be a consequence of either enhanced systolic function or improved diastolic relaxation. However, an independent effect on diastolic function is shown by the ability of xamoterol to shorten the peak rate of decrease of pressure ($-$LV dP/dt$_{max}$) and to shorten the time constant of the isovolumic pressure decrease during the first 40 ms after $-$LV dP/dt$_{max}$ (78).

Both the systolic and the diastolic effects of xamoterol at rest are consistent with its β_1-adrenoceptor agonist properties. Patients with heart failure have reduced ventricular distensibility, in part because of impaired diastolic relaxation (79). This results in an upward shift of the left ventricular diastolic pressure-volume relationship and a rise in filling pressure. The reduced rate of pressure decay in diastole reflects impaired calcium reuptake by the sarcoplasmic reticulum. This is a process that requires more energy than myocardial contraction and, like the contractile process, is enhanced by intracellular cyclic AMP. β-Adrenoceptor stimulation, unlike therapy with glycosides, improves both contractile function and diastolic relaxation by increasing cyclic AMP generation (81).

Exercise Hemodynamics During exercise, β-adrenoceptor blocking properties of xamoterol become apparent, with a 10% to 15% reduction in the rate of rise in heart rate (75,82,83). The acute effects of xamoterol on myocardial function during graded exercise have been studied in patients with mild to moderate left ventricular dysfunction after myocardial infarction. Systolic contractility (+LV dP/dt$_{max}$) was significantly increased to 25% and 50% of maximum exercise capacity but not significantly different from placebo at 75% and maximum exercise (78). Left ventricular relaxation was also improved; the peak $-$LV dP/dt was reduced at 25% of maximum exercise (although no different from placebo at higher exercise levels), while the time constant of relaxation (T_1) was shorter at 50% of maximal exercise (with a favorable trend at 25%). Global ejection fraction increases during exercise after xamoterol compared with placebo, with a restoration of response even when absent prior to treatment (83,84). The changes in contractility and diastolic relaxation increase stroke volume during exercise, maintaining cardiac output at maximum exercise despite a reduced heart rate (77).

These changes in cardiac function can produce a reduction in left ventricular filling pressure during exercise (85), although this has not always been demonstrated (77).

The improvements in cardiac function produced by xamoterol have been reported in patients with impaired left ventricular function due to a variety of etiologies, including ischemic and dilated cardiomyopathy.

Recent studies have also suggested that similar benefits in right ventricular function can be produced in congestive heart failure (86) and in pulmonary heart disease (87). This action of xamoterol may be important in the improvement of exercise tolerance, which may partly depend on right ventricular performance.

Hemodynamics in Severe Heart Failure An early report of the acute effects of xamoterol in patients with congestive heart failure suggested that the β-adrenoceptor blocking action of xamoterol might produce adverse effects in patients with severe heart failure. Detry et al. (85) found that although resting cardiac function was improved, cardiac output was decreased during exercise. Such an effect is more consistent with blockade than with stimulation of β-adrenoceptors. They suggested that xamoterol could be detrimental in patients who rely on a high degree of sympathetic tone to maintain cardiac output, i.e., those with severe heart failure. Such a possibility was supported by observations in individual patients of hemodynamic deterioration after intravenous xamoterol (73,88,89).

Later data suggested that in certain situations xamoterol improves hemodynamic function, even in patients with severely impaired left ventricular contractility. These studies have involved patients who were hemodynamically stable in New York Heart Association (NYHA) class II–III heart failure during treatment with ACE inhibitors. Systolic blood pressure was increased after the addition of xamoterol to captopril (90), while in a further study additional improvements in cardiac function were demonstrated (91). The latter investigation showed an increase in systolic and diastolic function similar to those reported in milder degrees of heart failure. End-systolic volume index was reduced, consistent with the rise in ejection fraction. Left ventricular end-diastolic pressure at rest was reduced by 54%. The results contrast with the clinical effects of xamoterol in patients with severe heart failure, which are discussed later.

Effects on Myocardial Metabolism A major concern when using drugs with positive inotropic effects is the risk of increasing metabolic demand and exhausting energy stores. In a group of patients with ischemic heart disease, xamoterol had no effect on coronary blood flow, arterial lactate concentration, or myocardial lactate consumption. During a cold pressor test, there was a trend to a decrease in myocardial lactate extraction, but this did not reach statistical significance (76). In a subsequent study of 36 patients with left ventricular dysfunction, lactate extraction was improved at rest after xamoterol (92), suggesting a favorable effect on aerobic metabolism.

By contrast, in a more recent study of patients with idiopathic dilated cardiomyopathy, intravenous xamoterol produced an increase in both myocardial blood flow and oxygen consumption without a change in stroke volume or cardiac output (93). These observations suggest a reduction in myocardial efficiency after xamoterol in this group of patients, although the data were markedly influenced by unfavorable effects in two or three individuals. However, other studies have not found any increase in myocardial oxygen consumption despite improved myocardial performance in angina (94), ischemic left ventricular dysfunction (76,94), or dilated cardiomyopathy (73). The balance of evidence suggests that there is no detrimental effect of xamoterol on myocardial metabolism in most situations and that the efficiency of aerobic metabolism is often enhanced both at rest and during exercise.

It is possible that any increased oxygen demand produced by β_1-adrenoceptor stimulation at rest or during mild exercise is offset by other effects of xamoterol. In particular, reduced end-diastolic wall stress will augment effective myocardial perfusion, and reduced systolic wall stress will lower oxygen demand (76).

Effects on Arrhythmias A second important consideration of inotropic therapy in heart failure is the potential for enhancing or generating arrhythmias (96). Sudden death is common in heart failure, and lethal rhythm disturbances are believed to be responsible for many of these events. Stimulation of cardiac β-adrenoceptors is arrhythmogenic, while β-adrenoceptor antagonists inhibit rhythm disturbances provoked by endogenous catecholamines (4). In 13 patients with NYHA class II–III heart failure, 24-h Holter monitoring did not show any significant arrhythmogenic effect with xamoterol. However, the numbers of ventricular premature beats were extremely variable in this study, and no episodes of ventricular tachycardia occurred during treatment with placebo or xamoterol (82). A similar study in 26 patients also indicated a lack of effect on arrhythmias (97). In this study, small numbers of multiform ventricular ectopics, couplets, and runs of ventricular tachycardia were found with equal frequency during treatment with xamoterol or placebo. In severe heart failure (NYHA class III or IV despite treatment with an ACE inhibitor), the incidence of ventricular premature beats, couplets, and nonsustained ventricular tachycardia was similar in 76 patients treated with xamoterol and 30 patients who received placebo (98).

In other situations, xamoterol has been shown to have an antiarrhythmic action. In patients with poor left ventricular function and recurrent sustained ventricular tachycardia, xamoterol used as an adjuvant therapy to amiodarone reduced spontaneous ventricular tachycardia on exercise and suppressed ventricular tachycardia during programmed stimulation (99). Xamoterol may also be useful in atrial fibrillation as sole therapy (100) or in combination with digoxin (101,102) by reducing both tachycardia on exercise and resting bradycardias. Atrial fibrillation is frequently associated with heart failure (103), and this action of xamoterol may be beneficial. However, exercise tolerance in patients with atrial fibrillation is not always improved by xamoterol, despite its beneficial effects on ventricular rate (102).

Effects on Myocardial Ischemia A high proportion of patients with heart failure have impaired ventricular function as a consequence of ischemic heart disease. Exercise performance may be reduced by ischemia leading to failure of diastolic relaxation and increasing left ventricular end-diastolic pressure. Antianginal actions of xamoterol have been shown in two small studies, presumably reflecting the β-adrenoceptor antagonist effect of the drug during exercise. In the first study, intravenous xamoterol reduced ST-segment depression and improved exercise performance by 26% (94). In the other there was a significant decrease in ST-segment depression at peak exercise after single oral doses of xamoterol (104). Coronary blood flow and myocardial oxygen consumption during atrial pacing are increased in parallel by xamoterol in patients with coronary artery disease (105). The antianginal effects of xamoterol may contribute to its efficacy in ischemic heart failure; large-scale studies have confirmed a reduction in chest pain during everyday activities, and chest pain was also less likely to limit exercise (106).

Clinical Efficacy Xamoterol has been studied in several large trials in patients with all grades of severity of heart failure. Analyses have been published of individual studies and also of data pooled from several studies using similar protocols. Subgroup analyses have been retrospectively performed on pooled patient groups, despite a lack of randomization for these characteristics.

Mild-to-Moderate Heart Failure. Four large studies, three multicenter and one single-center, have explored the efficacy of xamoterol in patients with NYHA class II and III heart failure. The protocols differed only in the formal exercise test employed: two used graded treadmill exercise, the others a bicycle ergometer. Xamoterol was given at a dosage of 200 mg twice daily for 3 months; in all studies twice as many patients were randomized to xamoterol as to placebo. Two studies also randomized patients to receive digoxin as a comparator.

Patients could receive a maximum diuretic dose of 80 mg furosemide (or equivalent), but the only permitted vasodilator therapy was long-acting nitrates. Several end points were used, and these are discussed below.

A total of 617 patients received xamoterol and 300 placebo in the four trials. Retrospective subset analyses included patients with cardiomegaly on chest x-ray (cardiothoracic ratio > 0.52, xamoterol n = 184, placebo n = 85) (107), xamoterol monotherapy (xamoterol n = 290, placebo n = 135) (108), and patients aged over 65 years (xamoterol n = 200, placebo n = 116) (109,110).

Clinical signs and symptoms: The pooled data from the four studies revealed significant reductions in the signs of heart failure; these included edema, lung crepitations, added heart sounds, raised jugular venous pressure, and hepatomegaly (109). Clinical signs showed improvement similar to that found with digoxin (111). Symptoms of breathlessness and fatigue were improved by xamoterol, and during formal exercise testing patients were less likely to stop because of breathlessness. The antianginal and antiarrhythmic effects of xamoterol were supported by a reduced incidence of chest pain or rhythm disturbances as reasons for terminating exercise.

In the patients treated with xamoterol monotherapy, pulmonary crepitations and hepatomegaly were significantly reduced, as were breathlessness and tiredness (108). In the subgroup with cardiomegaly, breathlessness was significantly improved, and a trend towards decreased tiredness was also found (107). Results from the subset of patients over 65 years old were also similar to those in the pooled data analysis (110).

Exercise tolerance: In the combined patient group, there was a 37% increase in exercise capacity, compared with 18% seen with placebo (109). In the published comparison with digoxin, the improvement after xamoterol was 33%, compared with 5% on placebo. The improvement after digoxin was 17%, not significantly greater than with placebo and significantly less than with xamoterol (111). Subset analyses showed that patients with cardiomegaly, those using xamoterol monotherapy, and the older patients had benefit similar to that seen in the pooled patient group (107,108,110).

Quality of life: There is considerable interest in the measurement of quality of life in heart failure as an index of global improvement in well-being. In the studies with xamoterol, attempts were made to quantify improvements in quality of life using 11 Likert questions. These focused on aspects of life that were valued by the patients, concentrating on quantifying symptoms, the ability to perform daily activities, and mood. An aggregate score of "life values" was generated from the Likert questions; these showed significant improvement after xamoterol compared with placebo (106). The validity of these measures as an index of improvement in heart failure is not yet well established (112), but the data suggest that xamoterol may have a useful impact on global well-being as well as improving exercise tolerance in a formal graded exercise test.

Long-term response to xamoterol: Most of the efficacy data for xamoterol were derived from studies of 3 months' duration or less. The importance of confirming sustained benefit with xamoterol is underlined by the potential for tolerance with full β-adrenoceptor agonists.

Pouleur et al. (113) performed a study with a similar design in 14 patients with ischemic left ventricular function treated with xamoterol for a mean of 51 months. Similar dose-dependent decreases of left ventricular end-diastolic pressure, peak +LV dP/dt, and +[LV dP/dt]/DP_{40} were found after intravenous xamoterol both before and after long-term treatment. Diastolic function also showed benefit with enhancement of rate of decrease in isovolumic pressure, indicating that improved relaxation was also maintained. The same investigators have also reported that, compared with placebo, peak ventricular filling rate was increased and mean diastolic filling pressure was reduced after 3 months of treatment with xamoterol (114).

Kayanakis et al. (115) examined cardiac performance in an open study involving 18 patients treated for 1 year. Resting cardiac index was improved by 13% at 3 months and maintained at 12% above baseline after 12 months. Pulmonary wedge pressure showed a sustained reduction of 20%. In association with this there was a 27% increase in exercise duration at 3 months that was maintained at 12 months.

A further study has assessed exercise tolerance after 18 months of treatment with xamoterol. Twenty-one patients (one NYHA class III, the others class II) with ischemic heart failure were treated with xamoterol or placebo for 4 weeks each in a double-blind, cross-over study. Eighteen "responders" continued treatment for 18 months, after which they received xamoterol or placebo again for 4 weeks each in a randomized, cross-over study. The 14 patients who completed the study showed a reduced exercise tolerance on placebo at the end of the study compared with entry. After xamoterol, the increase in exercise tolerance was similar at both time points (116).

It can be concluded from these studies that the benefits of xamoterol in NYHA class II–III heart failure are not only demonstrable after 3 months' treatment but persist during long-term therapy. This supports independent observations that β-adrenoceptor down-regulation is not likely to impair the response to treatment.

Severe Heart Failure. Xamoterol acts as a β-adrenoceptor antagonist at the high levels of sympathetic tone that are found in patients with the most severe degrees of heart failure. Introduction of a full β-adrenoceptor antagonist at high doses in this situation removes the sympathetic drive to the failing myocardium and can lead to profound clinical deterioration. It has, however, been shown that if these drugs are introduced at very low doses, they can be well tolerated. In such patients, careful dose titration often produces improvement in functional status, which is presumed to reflect adrenoceptor up-regulation (117). Using full doses of a β-adrenoceptor partial agonist in patients with severe heart failure therefore carries the risk of producing adverse hemodynamic effects.

Early experience with intravenous xamoterol suggested that this might indeed be the case. Reports of hemodynamic deterioration in individual subjects suggested that a low ejection fraction or high circulating noradrenaline concentrations predisposed to this effect (118,119). However, more encouraging evidence of improvements in cardiac function was provided by a study carried out in patients with NYHA class II–III heart failure, despite treatment with diuretics and ACE inhibitors (91). The longer-term benefits of xamoterol in such patients were investigated in a recent multicenter study (98). At enrollment, patients were in NYHA class III or IV heart failure despite treatment with diuretics and ACE inhibitors. Xamoterol 200 mg twice daily was given to 352 patients and placebo to 164 patients, and follow-up continued for 13 weeks. Xamoterol did not improve physical signs of heart failure or exercise duration. Symptomatic improvement in breathlessness was found, however, in comparison with placebo. This study was not designed to examine mortality, but more deaths occurred among those patients randomized to receive xamoterol than among those treated with placebo. However, several of these occurred some time after xamoterol had been withdrawn. In severe heart failure, xamoterol acted predominantly as an antagonist during the daytime (reducing daytime heart rate) and as an agonist at night. Premature death could reflect either of these actions. Early deterioration after introduction of xamoterol could be due to pump failure produced by beta-blockade. Alternatively, the agonist activity of the drug might provoke lethal arrhythmias. However, a subgroup of patients were examined by 48-h Holter monitoring, and no increase in arrhythmias was found during treatment with xamoterol. The mode of death and the temporal relationship to introduction of the drug were not fully reported, so that the cause of death remains speculative. Measurements of plasma catecholamines in a subgroup of patients in this study showed mean noradrenaline levels of 650–750 pg/ml. It has previously been shown that xamoterol begins to act as an antagonist at endogenous noradrenaline levels of 450–500 pg/ml (120). It seems most likely, therefore, that giving xamoterol in this situation was equivalent to introducing a large dose of a β-adrenoceptor antagonist, with consequent deleterious effects. It is perhaps worth contrasting these data with evidence from the study in milder heart failure, in which no trend to premature death was found at either 1- or 4-year follow-up (121,122).

The results from treatment of severe heart failure raise important questions about the use of xamoterol. The principal concern is the ability of physicians to identify accurately patients with milder disease who may benefit from the drug.

Cicloprolol

The literature about the use of cicloprolol in heart failure is small compared with that concerning xamoterol. Intravenous cicloprolol was compared with atenolol in a dose-response study involving patients with ischemic heart disease and reduced cardiac reserve. Cicloprolol increased resting left ventricular ejection fraction and reduced end-diastolic volume. Although there was a trend to a lower filling pressure, this was not significant (123). During supine bicycle exercise there was an attenuation of exercise tachycardia and of the increase in cardiac index. Cardiac performance was enhanced at rest and less depressed on exercise in comparison with atenolol, but these effects were less marked than those produced by xamoterol. A second single-dose intravenous study with cicloprolol in patients with impaired cardiac function produced essentially similar results (124).

It is not known how these effects will translate into clinical response in patients with heart failure. However, since the greater partial agonist activity of xamoterol produces only a modest increase in myocardial contractility, the prospects for cicloprolol do not appear promising.

CONCLUSIONS

The prolonged use of full β-adrenoceptor agonists in chronic heart failure will probably be limited by receptor down-regulation and loss of responsiveness. A useful short-term inotropic effect can be obtained with dobutamine in acute heart failure and in combination with dopamine to dilate renal arterioles. Dobutamine is widely used to provide temporary myocardial support. In severe chronic heart failure, infusions of dobutamine for up to 72 h may produce prolonged benefit. However, the risks of metabolic exhaustion of the myocardium and the potential for producing serious arrhythmias can limit the usefulness of this approach.

The concept of using a β-adrenoceptor partial agonist in chronic heart failure is more attractive. β_1-Adrenoceptor–selective compounds hold the greatest promise, and on theoretical grounds the modest (43%) partial agonist activity of xamoterol provides a near-optimal balance between agonist and antagonist activity. The drug appears to prevent the down-regulation of β-adrenoceptors that reduces the effectiveness of pure agonists during long-term treatment.

Administration of xamoterol produces modest improvements in both systolic and diastolic function in the failing heart that are maintained during long-term use. In patients with less severe forms of myocardial dysfunction, these improvements are accompanied by the ability to exercise more and a subjective reduction in breathlessness and, to a lesser extent, fatigue. In this group of patients, assessments of the effect of treatment on well-being suggest that xamoterol improves the ability to undertake tasks that they value.

In more severe heart failure the results are less encouraging. Despite evidence of potentially useful hemodynamic responses, exercise tolerance is unchanged by xamoterol when it is added to therapy with diuretics and ACE inhibitors. A small excess of deaths in the group of patients treated with xamoterol, compared with those given placebo, raises the question of safety in severe heart failure.

Current data suggest that xamoterol has a role in the treatment of patients with less severe forms of heart failure. It improves exercise performance when added to diuretics and may also be useful as sole therapy in some patients. Benefits may be greatest in those with ischemic etiology, in whom diastolic dysfunction can be prominent and impaired coronary flow contributes to limitation of exercise capacity. In these patients the β-adrenoceptor antagonist properties of xamoterol could prove particularly useful.

REFERENCES

1. Rona G, Chappel CI, Balazs T, Gantry R. An infarct-like myocardial lesion and other toxic manifestations produced by isoproterenol in the rat. Arch Pathol 1959; 67:443–455.
2. Cruickshank JM, Degante JP, Kuurne T, Vincent JL, Dwyer GN, Haynes Y, Kytha J, Carruthers ME, Patel S. Reduction of stress-catecholamine-induced cardiac necrosis by β_1-selective blockade. Lancet 1977; 2:585–589.
3. Bigger JT. Why patients with congestive heart failure die: arrhythmias and sudden death. Circulation 1987; 75(suppl IV):16–23.
4. Upward JW, Waller DG, George CF. Class II antiarrhythmic agents. Pharmacol Ther 1988; 37:81–109.
5. Fowler MB, Laser JA, Hopkins GL, Minobe W, Bristow MR. Assessment of the β-adrenergic receptor pathway in the intact failing human heart: progressive β-receptor down regulation and specific pharmacologic subsensitivity to agonist response. Circulation 1986; 74:1290–1302.
6. Bristow MR, Ginsburg R, Fowler M et al. β_1 and β_1 adrenergic receptor subpopulations in normal and failing human ventricular myocardium: coupling of both receptor subtypes to muscle contraction and selective β_1 receptor down regulation in heart failure. Circ Res 1986; 59:297–309.
7. Hohm M, Beuckelmann D, Brown L et al. Reduction of beta adrenoceptor density and evaluation of positive inotropic responses in isolated diseased human myocardium. Eur Heart J 1988; 9:844–852.
8. Ginsburg R, Bristow M, Billingham ME et al. Study of the normal and failing isolated human heart: decreased response of failing heart to isoproterenol. Am Heart J 1983; 106:535–540.

9. Galant SP, Duriseti L, Underwood S, Insel PA. Decreased beta adrenergic therapy. N Engl J Med 1978; 299:315–322.
10. Bristow MR, Sandoval AB, Gilbert EM, Deisher T, Minobe W, Rasmussen R. Myocardial alpha and beta adrenergic receptors in heart failure: is cardiac derived norepinephrine the regulatory signal? Eur Heart J 1988; 9(suppl H):35–40.
11. Colucci WS, Alexander RW, Williams GH et al. Decreased lymphocyte beta adrenergic receptor density in patients with heart failure and tolerance to the beta adrenergic agonist pirbuterol. N Engl J Med 1981; 305:185–190.
12. Bristow MR, Port JD, Hershberger RE, Gilbert EM, Fieldman AM. The β-adrenoceptor receptor-adenylate cyclase complex as a target for therapeutic intervention in heart failure. Eur Heart J 1989; 10(suppl B):45–54.
13. Cruickshank JM. Measurement and cardiovascular relevance of partial agonist activity (PAA) involving β_1- and β_2-adrenoceptors. Pharmacol Ther 1990; 46:199–242.
14. Waller DG. β-adrenoceptor partial agonists: a renaissance in cardiovascular therapy? Br J Clin Pharmacol 1990; 30:157–171.
15. Mettauer B, Rouleau J-C, Burgess JH. Detrimental arrhythmogenic and sustained beneficial hemodynamic effects of oral salbutamol in patients with chronic congestive heart failure. Am Heart J 1985; 109:840–847.
16. Bristow MR, Ginsburg R, Umans V, Fowler M, Minobe W, Rasmussen R, Zera P, Menlover R, Shah P, Jamieson S, Stinson EB. β_1- and β_2-adrenoceptor receptor subpopulations in non failing and failing human ventricular myocardium: coupling of both receptor subtypes to muscle contraction and selective β_1-receptor down-regular in heart failure. Circ Res 1987; 59:297–309.
17. Hadfield SE, Slee S-J, Snow HM. The cardiovascular pharmacology of xamoterol, cicloprolol, prenalterol and pindolol in the anaesthetised dog. Br J Clin Pharmcol 1989; 28:78s–81s.
18. Nuttall A, Snow HM. The cardiovascular effects of ICI 118,587: a β_1-adrenoceptor partial agonist. Br J Pharmacol 1982; 77:381–388.
19. Smith H, Halliday SE, Earl DCN, Stribling D. Effects of selective (beta$_1$ and beta$_2$) and non-selective beta-adrenoceptor antagonists on the cardiovascular and metabolic responses to isoproterenol: comparison with ICI 141,292. J Pharmacol Exp Ther 1983; 226: 211–216.
20. Kowalski MT, Haworth D, Lü X, Thomson DS, Barnett DB. Comparison of the effects of xamoterol and isoprenaline on rat cardiac beta-adrenoceptors: studies of function and regulation. Br J Pharmacol 1990; 99:27–30.
21. Limas CJ, Limas C. Effect of xamoterol on the reversible cycling of cardiac β-adrenoceptors. Circulation 1989; 80(suppl 11):11–18.
22. Barnett D, Lü X. Effects of co-administration of xamoterol and isoprenaline on rat ventricular beta-adrenoceptor down regulation. Br J Pharmacol 1989; 98:732P.
23. Watanabe K, Hirokawa Y, Suzuki K, Shibata A, Tsuchinashi H, Nagatomo T. The increase in β-adrenergic receptors in lymphocytes following treatment with xamoterol. Jpn J Clin Pharmacol Ther 1988; 19:555–561.

24. Schlieper P, Khamssi M. The effects of epanolol and xamoterol on human β_1- and β_2-adrenoceptors. In vitro and in vivo studies. Arch Pharmacol 1989; 339(suppl.):R94.
25. Leier CV, Webel J, Bush CA. The cardiovascular effects of the continuous infusion of dobutamine in patients with severe heart failure. Circulation 1977; 56:468–472.
26. Unverferth DV, Magorien RD, Lewis RP, Leier CV. Long term benefits of dobutamine in patients with congestive cardiomyopathy. Am Heart J 1980; 100:622–630.
27. Liang CS, Sherman LG, Doherty JU, Wellington K, Lee VW, Hood WB. Sustained improvement of cardiac function in patients with congestive heart failure after short term infusion of dobutamine. Circulation 1984; 69: 113–119.
28. Dies F, Krell MJ, Whitlow P et al. Intermittent dobutamine in ambulatory outpatients with chronic cardiac failure. Circulation 1986; 74(suppl II); 11–38.
29. Krell MJ, Kline EM, Bates ER et al. Intermittent ambulatory dobutamine infusions in patients with severe congestive heart failure. Am Heart J 1986; 112:787–791.
30. Unverferth DV, Blandford M, Kates RE, Leier CV. Tolerance to dobutamine after a 72 hour continuous infusion. Am J Med 1980; 69:262–266.
31. Tan LB. Cardiac pumping capability and prognosis in heart failure. Lancet 1986; ii:1360–1363.
32. Tan LP, Littler WA. Measurement of cardiac reserve in cardiogenic shock: implications for prognosis and management. Br Heart J 1990; 64:121–128.
33. Berthe C, Pierard LA, Hiernaux M et al. Predicting the extent and location of coronary artery disease in acute myocardial infarction by echocardiography during dobutamine infusion. Am J Cardiol 1986; 58:1167–1172.
34. Mannering D, Cripps T, Leech G, Mehta N, Valentine H, Gilmour S, Bennett ED. The dobutamine stress test as an alternative to exercise testing after acute myocardial infarction. Br Heart J 1988; 59:521–526.
35. Pierard LA, Berthe C, Albert A, Carlier J, Kulbertus HE. Haemodynamic alterations during ischaemia induced by dobutamine stress testing. Eur Heart J 1989; 10:783–790.
36. Awan NA, Evenson MK, Needham KE, Evans TO, Hermanovich J, Taylor CR, Amsterdam E, Mason DT. Hemodynamic effects of oral pirbuterol in chronic severe heart failure. Circulation 1981; 63:96–101.
37. Dawson JR, Canepa-Anson R, Kuan P, Reuben SR, Poole-Wilson PA, Sutton GC. Symptoms, haemodynamics and exercise capacity during long-term treatment of chronic heart failure. Br Heart J 1983; 50:282–289.
38. Fowler MB, Timmis AD, Chamberlain DA. Synergistic effects of a combined salbutamol-nitroprusside regimen in acute myocardial infarction and severe left ventricular failure. Br Med J 1980; 280:435–437.
39. Fowler MB, Timmis AD, Crick JP, Vincent R, Chamberlain DA. Comparisons of haemodynamic responses to dobutamine and salbutamol in cardiogenic shock after acute myocardial infarction. Br Med J 1982; 284:73–76.

40. Sharma B, Goodwin JF. Beneficial effects of salbutamol on cardiac function in severe congestive cardiomyopathy. Circulation 1978; 58:449–460.
41. Mettauer B, Rouleau JL, Burgess JH. Detrimental arrhythogenic and sustained beneficial hemodynamic effects of oral salbutamol in patients with chronic heart failure. Am Heart J 1985; 109:840–847.
42. Slutsky R. Hemodynamic effects of inhaled terbutamine in congestive heart failure patients without lung disease. Beneficial cardiotonic and vasodilator beta-agonist properties evaluated by catheterisation and radionuclide angiography. Am Heart J 1981; 101:556–560.
43. Wang RYC, Tse TF, Yu DYC, Lee PK, Chow MSS. Beneficial hemodynamic effects of intravenous terbutamine in patients with severe heart failure. Am Heart J 1982; 104:1016–1021.
44. Brown RA, Dixon J, Farmer JB et al. Dopexamine: a novel agonist at peripheral dopamine receptors and β_2 adrenoceptors. Br J Pharmacol 1985; 85:599–608.
45. Brodde OE, Zerkowski HR, Borst HG, Maier W, Michel MC. Drug- and disease-induced changes of human cardiac β_1 and β_2 adrenoceptors. Eur Heart J 1989; 10(suppl B):38–44.
46. Murphy JJ, Hampton JR. Failure of dopexamine to maintain haemodynamic improvement in patients with chronic heart failure. Br Heart J 1988; 60: 45–49.
47. Colardyn FA, Vandenbogaerde JF. Use of dopexamine hydrochloride in intensive care patients with low output left ventricular heart failure. Am J Cardiol 1988; 62:68c–72c.
48. Bohm M, Reuschel-Janetschek E, Erdmann E. Lack of sustained hemodynamic effects of the β_2 adrenoceptor agonist dopexamine in end-stage congestive heart failure. Am J Cardiol 1990; 65:395–396.
49. Svenson G, Strandberg LE, Lindvall B, Erhardt L. Haemodynamic response to dopexamine hydrochloride in post-infarction heart failure: lack of tolerance after continuous infusion. Br Heart J 1988; 60:489–496.
50. Smith GW, O'Connor SE. An introduction to the pharmacologic properties of Dopacard (dopexamine hydrochloride). Am J Cardiol 1988; 62:9c–17c.
51. Goldberg LI, Bass AS. Relative significance of dopamine receptors, beta adrenoceptors and norepinephrine uptake inhibition in the cardiovascular actions of dopexamine hydrochloride. Am J Cardiol 1988; 62:37c–40c.
52. Petch MC, Wisbey C, Ormerod O, Scot C, Goodfellow RM. The acute haemodynamic effects of oral prenalterol in severe heart failure. Br Heart J 1984; 52:49–52.
53. Hendry NG, Comerford MB, Besterman EMM. A dose response study with oral prenalterol in patients with chronic congestive cardiac failure. Clin Cardiol 1984; 7:23–28.
54. Glover DR, Wathen CG, Murray RG, Petch MC, Muir AL, Littler WA. Are the clinical benefits of oral prenalterol in ischaemic heart failure due to beta blockade? Br Heart J 1985; 53:208–215.

55. Lambertz H, Meyer J, Erbel R. Long-term hemodynamic effects of prenalterol in patients with severe congestive heart failure. Circulation 1984; 69:298–305.
56. Cook N, Richardson GH, Barnett DB. Comparison of the β_1 selective affinity of heart prenalterol and Corwin demonstrated by radioligand binding. Eur J Pharmacol 1984; 98:407–412.
57. Malta E, Mian MA, Raper C. The in vitro pharmacology of xamoterol (ICI 118,587). Br J Pharmacol 1985; 85:179–187.
58. Gurden JM, Apperley GH, Drew GM. A comparison of the properties of prenalterol and Corwin at β_1- and β_2-adrenoceptors in vitro. J Auton Pharmacol 1989; 9:79–91.
59. Jennings G, Bobik A, Oddie C, Restall R. Cardioselectivity, kinetics, hemodynamics and metabolic effects of xamoterol. Clin Pharmacol Ther 1984; 35:594–603.
60. McCaffrey PM, Riddell JG, Shanks RG. The selectivity of xamoterol, prenalterol and salbutamol as assessed by their effects in the presence and absence of ICI 118,551. J Cardiovasc Pharmacol 1988; 11:543–551.
61. Löfdahl C-G, Svedmyr N. Effects of xamoterol (ICI 118,587) in asthmatic patients. Br J Clin Pharmacol 1984; 18: 597–601.
62. Hattori Y, Sakuma I, Nakao Y, Kanno M. Pharmacological analysis of the cardiac actions of xamoterol, a β-adrenoceptor antagonist with partial agonistic activity, in guinea-pig heart: evidence for involvement of adenylate cyclase system in its cardiac stimulant actions. J Pharmacol Exp Ther 1987; 242:1077–1085.
63. Vigholt-Sorensen E, Nielsen-Kudsk F. Size and combined myocardial pharmacodynamics of xamoterol, isoprenaline and g-strophantin in the isolated rabbit heart. Eur J Pharmacol 1986; 125:363–371.
64. Kenakin TP, Beck D. In vitro studies on the cardiac activity of prenalterol with reference to use in congestive cardiac failure. J Pharmacol Exp Ther 1982; 220:77–85.
65. Lemoine H, Bilski A, Kaumann AJ. Xamoterol activates β_1-adrenoceptors in mammalian myocardium: comparison of its affinity for β_1- and β_2-adrenoceptors coupled to the adenylate cyclase in feline and human ventricle with positive inotropic effects. J Cardiovasc Pharmacol 1989; 13:105–117.
66. Marten TR, Bourne GR, Miles GS, Shuker B, Rankine HD, Dutka VN. The metabolism of ICI 118,587, a partial agonist of β_1-adrenoceptors, in mice, rats, rabbits, dogs and humans. Drug Metab Dispos 1984; 12: 652–660.
67. Vigholt-Sorensen E, Faergeman O, Day M, Bastain W. Pharmacokinetics of xamoterol after intravenous and oral administration to patients with chronic heart failure. Eur J Clin Pharmacol 1988; 35:183–185.
68. Bastain W, Boyce MJ, Stafford LE, Morton PB, Clarke DA, Marlow HF. Pharmacokinetics of xamoterol after intravenous and oral administration to volunteers. Eur J Clin Pharmacol 1988; 34:469–473.

69. Scott AK, Webster J, Petrie JC, Bastain W. The effect of age and cardiac failure on xamoterol pharmacokinetics. Br J Clin Pharmacol 1988; 25: 163–168.
70. Marlow HF, Hine FL, Snow HM, Pouleur H, Rousseau MF. Relationship between positive inotropic responses and plasma concentrations of xamoterol in middle-aged and elderly populations. Br J Clin Pharmacol 1990; 29: 511–518.
71. James MA, Papouchado M, Channer KS, Jones JV, Marlow HF, Bastain W, Barker NP, Harry JD, Wardleworth AG. The effect of oral dosing of xamoterol on systolic time intervals in man and xamoterol plasma concentrations in heart failure patients. Br J Clin Pharmacol 1990; 29:447–453.
72. Franciosa JA, Dunkman WB, Leddy CL. Hemodynamic effects of vasodilators and long-term response in heart failure. J Am Coll Cardiol 1984; 3:1521–1530.
73. Amende I, Simon R, Hood WP, Lichtlen PR. Die akute wirkung des kardioselektiven beta-1-partiellen agonisten, corwin, auf die ventrikelfunktion und den myokardialen sauerstoffverbrauch bei patienten mit dilativer kardiomyopathie. Z Kardiol 1986; 75:291–295.
74. Kayanakis J-G, Snow M. One year of Corwin therapy in cardiac failure. Cardiovasc Drugs Ther 1987; 1:256.
75. Molajo AO, Bennett DH. Effect of xamoterol (ICI 118,587), a new β_1-adrenoceptor partial agonist, on resting haemodynamic variables and exercise tolerance in patients with left ventricular dysfunction. Br Heart J 1985; 54:17–21.
76. Rousseau MF, Pouleur H, Vincent MF. Effects of a cardioselective $beta_1$ partial agonist (Corwin) on left ventricular dysfunction and myocardial metabolism in patients with previous myocardial dysfunction. Am J Cardiol 1983; 51:1267–1274.
77. Virk SJS, Davies MK. Effects of xamoterol on resting and exercise haemodynamics in patients with chronic heart failure. Br J Clin Pharmacol 1989; 28:15s–22s.
78. de Feyter PJ, Serruys PW, Suryapranata H. Improvement of left ventricular contractility and relaxation with the β_1-adrenergic receptor partial agonist xamoterol at rest and during exercise in patients with post infarction left ventricular dysfunction. Circulation 1990; 81(suppl 111):99–106.
79. Packer M. Abnormalities of diastolic function as a potential cause of exercise intolerance in chronic heart failure. Circulation 1990; 81(suppl 111):78–86.
80. Pouleur H, Hanet C, Rousseau MF. Clinical experience with xamoterol in patients with severe systolic and diastolic dysfunction. Eur Heart J 1990; 11(suppl. A):33–38.
81. Little WC, Rassi A, Freeman GL. Comparison of effects of dobutamine and ouabain on left ventricular contraction and relaxation in closed-chest dogs. J Clin Invest 1987; 80:613–620.
82. Erlemeier H-H, Kupper W, Bleifeld W. Exercise capacity, arrhythmias, humoral and chemical parameters during long-term therapy with xamoterol. Int J Cardiol 1990; 28:197–208.

83. Vigholt-Sorensen E, Faergeman O, Snow M. Effects of xamoterol, a β_1-adrenoceptor partial agonist, in patients with ischaemic dysfunction of the left ventricle. Br Heart J 1989; 62:335–341.
84. Bostrom P-A, Johansson BW, Lecerof H, Lilja B, Torp A. Effect of xamoterol on exercise capacity and left ventricular function in angina pectoris and in dilated cardiomyopathy. J Intern Med 1989; 226:331–335.
85. Detry J-MR, Decoster PM, Brassieur LA. Haemodynamic effects of 'Corwin' (ICI 118,587), a new cardioselective β-adrenoceptor partial agonist. Eur Heart J 1983; 4:584–591.
86. Raigoso J, Rousseau MF, Van Mechelen H, Van Eyll C, Pouleur H. Changes in left ventricular function during inotropic stimulation: Importance of the right ventricular response. Eur Heart J 1990; 11(suppl):53.
87. Oliver RM, Fleming JS, Waller DG. The effect of xamoterol on right ventricular function in pulmonary heart disease. Eur J Cardiol 1991; In Press.
88. Bhatia SJS, Swedberg K, Chatterjee K. Acute hemodynamic and metabolic effects of ICI 118,587 (Corwin), a selective beta_1 agonist, in patients with dilated cardiomyopathy. Am Heart J 1986; 111:692–696.
89. Simonsen S. Haemodynamic effects of ICI 118,587 in cardiomyopathy. Br Heart J 1983; 51:654–657.
90. McAlpine HM, Henderson F, Dargie H. Addition of xamoterol to captopril in severe chronic heart failure. Eur J Clin Pharmacol 1989; 36:A71.
91. Pouleur H, Hanet C, Rousseau MF. The efficacy and safety of chronic oral administration of xamoterol to patients with severe heart failure treated with ACE inhibitors. Br J Clin Pharmacol 1989; 28:82s–83s.
92. Rousseau MF, Pouleur H, Hanet C, Cheron P, Marlow HF. Effects of xamoterol on exercise tolerance and left ventricular function in ischaemic heart disease (abstr). 10th World Congress of Cardiol 1986;
93. Thierfelder L, Holubarsch C, Hasenfuss G, Weiss HW, Just H. Influence of xamoterol on hemodynamics and myocardial energetics in patients with idiopathic dilated cardiomyopathy. Circulation 1989; 80(suppl II):177.
94. Detry J-MR, Decoster PM, Buy J-J, Rousseau MF, Brassieur LA. Antianginal effects of Corwin, a new beta-adrenoceptor partial agonist. Am J Cardiol 1984; 53:439–443.
95. Sakai O, Fujita M, Sasayama S, Asanoi H, Nakajima H, Yokawa S. Effect of xamoterol on myocardial energetics in man. Jpn Circ J 1988; 52:149–154.
96. Katz AM. Potential deleterious effects of inotropic agents in the therapy of chronic heart failure. Circulation 1986;73(suppl III):III-184–III-190.
97. Virk S, Qiang F, Murray G, Littler WA, Davies MK. The effect of xamoterol on arrhythmias in patients with mild to moderate heart failure. Cardiovasc Drugs Ther 1989; 3(suppl 2):639.
98. The Xamoterol in Severe Heart Failure Study Group. Xamoterol in severe heart failure. Lancet 1990; 336:1–6.
99. Paul V, Griffith M, Ward DE, Camm AJ. Adjuvant xamoterol or metoprolol in patients with malignant ventricular arrhythmia resistant to amiodarone. Lancet 1989; ii:302–305.

100. Ang EL, Chan WL, Cleland JGF, Moore D, Krikler SJ, Alexander NDE, Oakley CM. Placebo controlled trial of xamoterol versus digoxin in chronic arterial fibrillation. Br Heart J 1990; 64:256–260.
101. Molajo AO, Coupe MO, Bennett DH. Effect of Corwin (ICI 118,587) on resting and exercise heart rate and exercise tolerance in digitalised patients with chronic atrial fibrillation. Br Heart J 1984; 52:392–395.
102. Lewis RV, McMurray J, McDevitt DG. Effects of atenolol, verapamil and xamoterol on heart rate and exercise tolerance in digitalized patients with chronic atrial fibrillation. J Cardiovasc Pharmacol 1989; 13:1–6.
103. Kannel WB, Abbott RD, Savage DD, McNamara PM. Epidemiologic features of chronic atrial fibrillation: the Framingham study. N Engl J Med 1982; 306:1018–1022.
104. Barrios L, Geboers J, Piessens JH, de Geest H. Effects of xamoterol, a new beta-adrenoceptor partial agonist in patients with angina pectoris. Eur J Clin Pharmacol 1986; 29:667–691.
105. Simonsen S. The effects of xamoterol and pacing on myocardial blood flow and metabolism in patients with coronary artery disease. Eur Heart J 1990; 11(suppl A):61.
106. Blackwood R, Marlow HF. Xamoterol in the management of patients with exertional breathlessness and fatigue due to cardiac disease. J Am Coll Cardiol 1988; 11:143A.
107. The European "Corwin" Study Group. Xamoterol in mild to moderate heart failure: a subgroup analysis of patients with cardiomegaly but no concomitant angina pectoris. Br J Clin Pharmacol 1989; 28:67s–96s.
108. Timewell RM, Stark RD, Marlow HF and The European "Corwin" Study Group. Xamoterol monotherapy in heart failure. Eur Heart J 1990; 11(suppl A):62–64.
109. Marlow HF. Review of clinical experience with xamoterol. Effects on exercise capacity and symptoms in heart failure. Circulation 1990; 81(suppl III):93–99.
110. Wray R and The European Corwin Study Group. The efficacy of xamoterol (Corwin) in elderly patients with heart failure. Eur Heart J 1988; 9(suppl 1):171.
111. The German and Austrian Xamoterol Study Group. Double blind placebo-controlled comparison of digoxin and xamoterol in chronic heart failure. Lancet 1988; 1:489–493.
112. Waller DG. The effect of drug treatment on quality of life in mild to moderate heart failure. Drug Safety 1991; 6:241–246.
113. Pouleur H, Etienne J, Van Mechelen H, Gurne O, Rousseau MF. Effects of the β_1-adrenergic receptor partial agonist xamoterol in left ventricular diastolic dysfunction—an evaluation after 1–6 years of oral therapy. Circulation 1990; 81(suppl III):87–92.
114. Pouleur H, van Eyle C, Cheron P, Hanet C, Charlier AA, Rousseau MF. Changes in left ventricular filling dynamics after long-term xamoterol therapy in ischemic left ventricular dysfunction. Heart Failure 1986; 2:176–184.

115. Kayanakis J-G, Courtault L, Fauvel JM, Bourahowe JP, Snow HM. Changes in exercise tolerance and resting haemodynamics during long-term treatment of heart failure with xamoterol. Eur Heart J 1990; 11(suppl A):52–53.
116. Vigholt-Sorensen E, Faergeman O. Ischaemic left ventricular failure: evidence of sustained benefit after 18 months treatment with xamoterol. Br Heart J 1990; 64:186–189.
117. Heilbrunn SM, Shah P, Bristow MR, Valantine HA, Ginsburg R, Fowler MB. Increased β-receptor density and improved hemodynamic response to catecholamine stimulation during long-term metoprolol therapy in heart failure from dilated cardiomyopathy. Circulation 1989; 79:483–490.
118. Ikaheimo MJ, Takkunes JT. The effects of $beta_1$-adrenoceptor partial agonist ICI 118,587 on left ventricular function in patients with coronary heart disease. Int J Cardiol 1984; 5:339–349.
119. Kawamoto H, Murakami R, Ohta T, Shimada R, Morioka S, Moriyami K. Acute and chronic effects of ICI 118,587 ("Corwin") in patients with chronic heart failure. Jpn Circ J 1987; 51:918.
120. Sato H, Inoue M, Matsuyama T, Ozaki H, Shimazu T, Takeda H, Ishida Y, Kamada T. Hemodynamic effects of the β_1-adrenoceptor partial agonist xamoterol in relation to plasma levels during exercise in patients with left ventricular dysfunction. Circulation 1987; 75:213–220.
121. Waller DG. Long-term studies of xamoterol in heart failure. Br J Clin Pharmacol 1989; 28(suppl 1):53–58S.
122. Marlow HF, Lewis JA. Effects of xamoterol on mortality in mild to moderate heart failure. Eur Heart J 1990; 11(abstr. suppl):132.
123. Silke B, Verma SP, Sharma SK, Frais MA, Reynolds G, Taylor SH. Comparative effects of atenolol and cicloprolol on cardiac performance in coronary heart disease. J Cardiovasc Pharmacol 1989; 13:155–161.
124. Rigaud M, Hamoir V, Chabanier A, Neveux E, Cazor JL, Bardet J, Bourdarias JP. Effects hémodynamiques en repos at à l'effort d'un nouvel agent bêta-agoniste partiel (cicloprolol) dans l'insuffisance cardiaque modérée. Arch Mal Coeur 1988; 81:1251–1258.

12

The Paradox of β-Adrenergic Blockers for the Management of Congestive Heart Failure

Eric J. Eichhorn
University of Texas Southwestern and
Dallas Veterans Administration Medical Centers,
Dallas, Texas

Man is an embodied paradox, a bundle of contradictions.—Charles Caleb Colton

INTRODUCTION

Congestive heart failure is a progressive disorder of systolic and/or diastolic ventricular dysfunction that results in reduced forward flow and/or elevated filling pressures. In dilated cardiomyopathy due to ischemic or nonischemic etiologies, the resultant systolic and diastolic dysfunction result in pulmonary and systemic congestion and activation of compensatory mechanisms to help maintain blood pressure and oxygenation (1–3). These compensatory mechanisms are mediated through the cardiac and aortic baroreceptors and sympathetic nervous system (1,2,4,5). The result of constant adrenergic stimulation is a state of vasoconstriction and high adrenergic tone (1–4). Although such stimulation provides the heart and circulation with short-term benefits, and despite the activation of some peripheral counterregulatory (vasodilator) mechanisms, such as atrial naturetic factor (6) and prostaglandin E_2 (7), that help to offset long-term vasoconstriction (1), the long-term consequences are those of progressive ventricular dysfunction and further stimulation of adrenergic drive (Fig. 1).

Two pieces of information suggest that neurohormonal activation plays a major role in determining the survival of patients with congestive heart

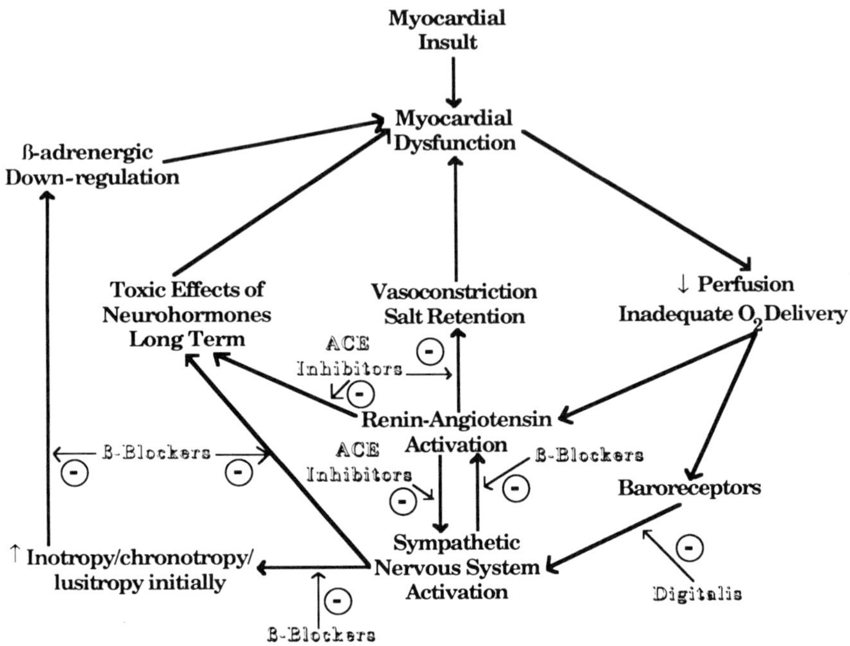

Figure 1 After a myocardial insult, ventricular dysfunction results in activation of the neurohormonal pathways, the renin-angiotensin system, and the sympathetic nervous system. These pathways are antagonized by angiotensin converting enzyme inhibitors, β-adrenergic blockers, and digitalis preparations. These neurohormonal antagonists break the cycle and retard further myocardial dysfunction with additional concomitant neurohormonal activation.

failure (1). First, both plasma catecholamines (8–10) and plasma renin activity (11) are activated in proportion to the severity of ventricular dysfunction and functional impairment present in patients with heart failure. Left ventricular dysfunction itself has been shown to be prognostically important in congestive heart failure (12–14). Thus, by transitive inference, as left ventricular dysfunction worsens and as norepinephrine increases, the more prognostically unfavorable the outcome. This has indeed been shown to be the case (15–17). Plasma norepinephrine has been shown to be an important prognostic marker for determining survival among these patients (Fig. 2) (15). In patients with severe ventricular dysfunction, plasma norepinephrine provides prognostic information independent of hemodynamic and ejection fraction indexes (1,15). This latter piece of data suggests that norepinephrine may play a more active adverse role in determining

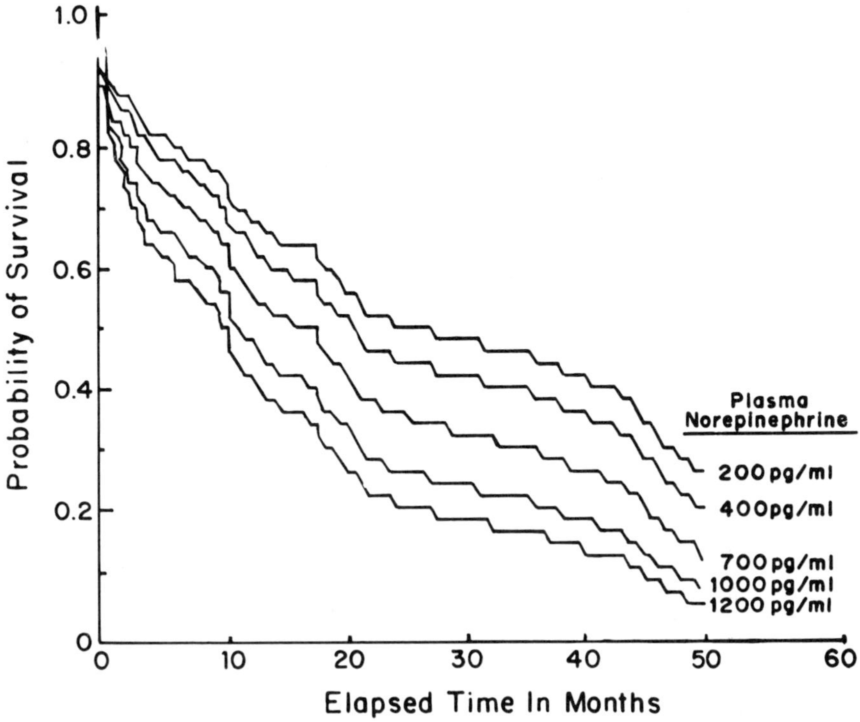

Figure 2 Predicted survival curves based on initial measurement of plasma norepinephrine. (From Ref 15.)

survival rather than just being a marker of left ventricular dysfunction. Likewise, hyponatremia, which reflects the activation of the renin-angiotensin system (11,18–20), is a prognostic marker for survival in patients with severe heart failure (1,21).

The second piece of evidence that neurohormonal activation is prognostically important comes from the beneficial effect on survival seen when neurohormonal antagonists are administered (22–25). With the advent of angiotensin converting enzyme (ACE) inhibitors, we finally had an intervention that drastically reduced neurohormonal activation and its long-term consequences. Use of such an agent has been shown to improve survival (25) as well as result in long-term improvements in ventricular performance (17,26–34). Use of direct vasodilators (such as prazosin, minoxidil, and hydralazine) that do not reduce but often amplify neurohormonal activation results in no long-term hemodynamic benefit when these agents are used alone (35–44). Although reduction of afterload acutely permits improved systolic performance, these older vasodilators such as hydralazine, minoxidil, nitroprusside, and prazosin are subject to long-term development of tolerance, which stimulates opposing forces such as reflex vasoconstriction, increases circulating catecholamines, and activates the renin-angiotensin-aldosterone axis, resulting in fluid retention and a return to baseline loading conditions (36,44). Additionally, the Veterans Administration cooperative study showed no survival benefits from the direct vasodilator prazosin, but some survival benefit from hydralazine given with isosorbide dinitrate (45). The preliminary results from the second Veterans Administration cooperative study suggest that such a survival benefit is less than that of ACE inhibitors (183). In addition, it is not clear if the survival benefit to this treatment was due to hydralazine or isosorbide dinitrate. Thus, long-term hemodynamic and survival benefit appears to occur predominantly with agents that antagonize neurohormonal activation, and β-adrenergic blockade may be another means by which to block the long-term consequences of neurohormonal activation on the heart.

The use of agents such as ACE inhibitors and β-adrenergic blockers, which have been classically used to lower blood pressure and reduce inotropy and chronotropy, respectively (46–52), seems paradoxical when they are proposed for use in patients who are hypotensive and have low cardiac output at baseline. Therefore, these agents have required years to gain acceptance. However, it must be remembered that the sympathetic nervous system and renin-angiotensin system evolved in man over thousands of years to protect him acutely from volume loss (1,3). As a long-term solution to congestive heart failure, activation of these systems results chronically in adverse consequences of which progressive myocardial damage may be the result. Worsening left ventricular dysfunction in turn increases the activation of these neurohormonal systems, and a vicious cycle is established (Fig. 1). The use of beta-blockers, ACE inhibitors, and digitalis preparations (which have recently been shown to alter baroreceptor sensitivity and reduce sympathetic discharge) (53) breaks the cycle. However, ACE inhibitors and beta-blockers must be instituted carefully, so as not to quickly withdraw neurohormonal support, which could result in systemic and pulmonary congestion and/or cardiovascular collapse. This is the paradox of these agents. In order to derive long-term benefit, one must withdraw short-term support (adrenergic drive).

HISTORICAL PERSPECTIVE: THE EARLY BETA-BLOCKER TRIALS

In 1975, in a small pilot study, Waagstein and associates (22) reported that β-adrenergic blockade given to seven patients with congestive cardiomyopathy resulted in clinical improvement in their condition and improved echocardiographic indexes of ventricular function. A subsequent study by this same group of 28 patients placed on open-label beta-blockade suggested that ejection fraction and clinical improvement resulted from β-adrenergic blockade (54). They also reported that in 15 patients who were taken off beta-blockers, clinical deterioration resulted (55). These studies were the first to suggest that beta-blockade could be beneficial for heart failure. However, these studies were initially met with substantial skepticism. Subsequently, in two case reports of patients with heart failure and sinus tachycardia, low-dose beta-blockade resulted in an improvement in symptoms and exercise tolerance (56).

In 1985, Engelmeier and associates (57) randomized 25 patients to metoprolol (n = 9) or placebo (n = 16) in a double-blind, randomized trial. Twelve of the patients assigned to placebo were crossed over to metoprolol in an open-label design after 1 year. These crossover patients were compared to 16 similar subjects treated with standard therapy. Metoprolol-treated patients had improvement in mean exercise capacity by an average of 3 mets and in functional classification. The patients without beta-blocker therapy did not improve. Additionally, improvement in radionuclide ejection fraction from 0.13 ± 0.06 to 0.21 ± 0.10 was seen in the metoprolol group at 1 year ($p < 0.02$) but was not seen in the placebo group. Thus, data were mounting that beta-blockade resulted in hemodynamic and functional improvement.

In addition to improving hemodynamic status, two small trials of beta-blockade (23,24) have suggested that such agents may reduce mortality in congestive heart failure, although the size of both these trials precludes conclusive evidence of a beneficial effect on survival. In the first trial (23), 24 patients with congestive cardiomyopathy were given either alprenolol, metoprolol, or practolol, and survival was compared with that in a comparable group who were selected retrospectively. A significant survival benefit was seen at 1, 2, and 3 years in the group receiving beta-blockers (Fig. 3). In the trial by Anderson and colleagues (24), 50 patients were randomized prospectively to metoprolol or standard therapy. By intention to treat, there were no differences in survival. However, as several of the deaths were of patients who were treated initially with beta-blockers but did not tolerate the treatment (and dropped out), there was a trend (p = 0.12) favoring beta-blocker treatment (Fig. 3).

In addition to these small survival studies, a subgroup analysis of the effect of propranolol after acute myocardial infarction in patients with and without heart failure participating in the Beta Blocker Heart Attack Trial (BHAT) (58) documented a similar reduction in overall mortality in patients with and without heart failure when compared with a placebo population. However, there was a striking 47% reduction in sudden death

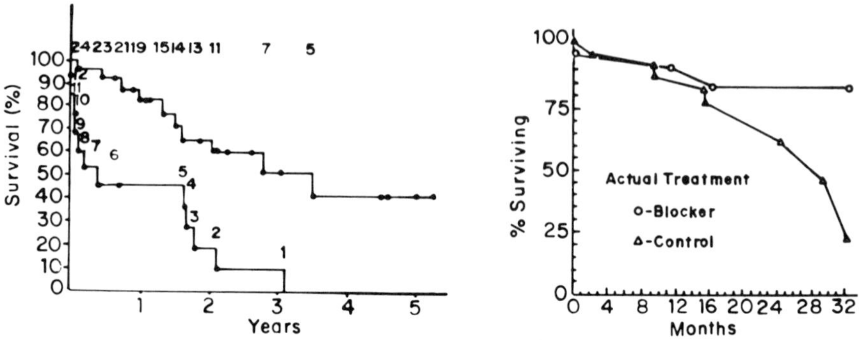

Figure 3 Survival curves from two small trials of β-adrenergic blockers. The top graph depicts the survival for a group of patients selected retrospectively who were treated with digitalis and diuretics (lower curve) versus patients treated with digitalis, diuretics, and β-adrenergic blockers (upper curve). The difference between the curves is significant ($p < 0.01$). (From Ref. 23.) The graph on the right shows survival curves by actual treatment method for control and beta-blockade groups. The difference in curves trended toward but did not reach significance. (From Ref. 24.)

among the heart failure patients as compared with 13% among the patients without heart failure. These data suggested a beneficial effect of beta-blockade on mortality, and perhaps on lethal arrhythmias.

In contrast to a beneficial long-term effect on ventricular function and possibly survival with beta-blockers, β-adrenergic agonists have shown no benefit, and have even produced worsening of myocardial ischemia and ventricular arrhythmias in patients with congestive heart failure (59–65). This is exemplified by the results of a recent trial using the partial β-agonist xamoterol (66). In this trial, by intention-to-treat analysis, 9.1% of the xamoterol-treated patients and 3.7% of the placebo-treated patients died within 100 days of randomization. Use of β-adrenergic blocking agents with intrinsic sympathomimetic activity may account for the lack of beneficial effect seen in another early beta-blocker trial (67).

Two beta-blocker trials (67,68) have shown no significant benefit from these agents. However, these trials assessed patients after only 1 month of therapy and may not have allowed enough time to achieve clinical improvement.

NEUROEFFECTOR PATHWAYS IN CARDIAC MUSCLE

In order to understand several of the proposed benefits of beta-blockers, one must first understand the derangements that occur in the β-adrenergic neuroeffector pathway. The heart receives sympathetic innervation from postganglionic nerve endings (69,70) that primarily release the neurotransmitter norepinephrine. Approximately 70% to 80% of synaptic cleft norepinephrine is reaccumulated in the nerve terminal, while the remainder is enzymatically metabolized either within the neural junction or in the circulation (69). Previous investigators have found a good correlation between sympathetic nerve traffic and plasma norepinephrine in congestive heart failure (2), which may be due to both endogenous norepinephrine release and sympathetically mediated adrenal medulla release into the circulation.

Human ventricular myocardium is primarily a β-adrenergic organ, in contrast to other species such as the rat, which has a mixture of β- and α_1-adrenergic receptors (69,71–73). Human myocardium contains proportionally many fewer α_1 than β receptors (69,71). In addition, human myocardium contains proportionally more β_2-receptors than that of many other species (71,74,75). The β_1- and β_2-receptor nucleotide sequences do not cross-hybridize with one another (76). Thus, β_1- and β_2 receptors are produced from separate genes, and their properties are not due to post-transcriptional modification of a single gene product. In normal healthy myocardium, the β_1 population comprises 77% of all β-receptors, while the β_2 population comprises 23% (74).

Norepinephrine has a higher affinity for cardiac β_1-adrenoceptors than either β_2- or α_1-receptors (77,78). Thus, high sympathetic activity will promote primarily β_1-stimulatory effects on the heart while promoting α_1 vasoconstrictive effects on the peripheral circulation (79). Hormonal release of norepinephrine and epinephrine by the adrenal medulla results in both β_1 and β_2 stimulation of the myocardium as well as α_1-mediated peripheral vasoconstriction.

In addition, β_1-adrenergic stimulation activates the renin-angiotensin system through renin release from the juxtoglomerular apparatus (80). Activation of this pathway acts in five ways (81–83): (1) direct vasoconstriction is mediated primarily through angiotensin II; (2) sodium retention is mediated via aldosterone and distal tubule reabsorption and reduced glomerular filtration; (3) angiotensin II may play a role in the development of myocardial hypertrophy in congestive heart failure, as angiotensin II receptors are present in the heart (84,85) and receptor stimulation induces protein synthesis in vitro (86); (4) angiotensin I (87) and II (84) may be weak inotropes in congestive heart failure; and (5) angiotensin II is known to act at the presynaptic terminal (88,89) to block neuronal reuptake of norepinephrine (89) and enhance norepinephrine biosynthesis (90). Thus, both the sympathetic nervous system and the renin-angiotensin system act in concert to amplify their release, and so there is crossover neurohormonal activation. Additionally, recent evidence has suggested that angiotensin II itself may have some cardiotoxic properties (91). Therefore, its prolonged activation in congestive heart failure may result in adverse consequences.

The myocyte cell surface contains many membrane bound receptors, including β_1, β_2, α_1, vasoactive intestinal peptide (VIP), histamine, somatostatin, muscarinic (M_2), and adenosine receptors (92). These receptors act through two elucidated pathways to transduce the neuroeffector stimulation of the receptor into a biological signal (69,92): (a) the receptor–G protein–adenylate cyclase complex (RCG) and (b) the phosphoinositide transmembrane signaling system.

The α_1 and muscarinic agonists mediate their signal through their receptors coupled to a yet-unidentified G protein and phospholipase C (69,92). This enzyme cleaves phosphatidyl inositol 4,5-biphosphate to produce two intracellular messengers: inositol 1,4,5-triphosphate (IP_3) and 1,2-diacylglycerol (DAG) (93–100). The former effects Ca^{2+} mobilization from sarcoplasmic reticulum to produce transient inotropic effects, while the latter activates protein kinase C, which effects slow channel Ca^{2+} flux, and a more sustained inotropic effect (93–100). Protein kinase C may also act as feedback inhibition of α_1 and perhaps β effects within the cell (94,101). As α_1-receptor density is low in human myocardium (69,78,102) and as α_1-agonists are weak inotropes (69,78,102), this pathway is relatively unimportant in human myocardium as compared with the β-adrenergic system. Although α_1-agonists may play a role in peripheral vasoconstriction in congestive heart failure, lack of long-term efficacy for reducing systemic vascular resistance and afterload when prazosin (an α_1-antagonist) is given to heart failure patients (103,104) suggests the role of α_1-agonists is minor. In addition, norepinephrine inhibition in patients with severe heart failure results in little or no change in hemodynamics (including heart rate, pulmonary wedge pressure, stroke volume, and systemic vascular resistance) during a 48-h infusion of metyrosine (α-methyl-*p*-tyrosine) (105). As norepinephrine's affinity for the α_1-receptor in human myocardium is weak as compared with the β_1-receptor (69), there appears to be little alteration in the α_1 cell surface receptor density in congestive heart failure despite high levels of endogenous norepinephrine (69,78,106). However, as α_1 stimulation (107,108), as well as angiotensin II (86), may be important for the development of myocyte hypertrophy, this pathway may play a role in congestive heart failure.

As β-agonist stimulation is a potent inotropic and chronotropic stimulus to the heart, this pathway is very influential in the failing heart (69,92,109). The β_1- and β_2-receptors act independently through a membrane-bound receptor–G_s (stimulatory guanine nucleotide binding protein)–adenylate cyclase complex (RCG) to transduce the signal from the neurohormone to a biological effect (69,92,110–112). The G proteins serve to amplify the β-agonist signal 100-fold. In addition, the RCG complex performs two tasks. It activates adenylate cyclase, which converts ATP to cyclic AMP, and it directly activates cardiac calcium channels independently of cyclic AMP (69,92,113). Cyclic AMP increases the activity of protein kinases that phosphorylate several intracellular proteins (69,92,114–117). Sarcolemmal protein phosphorylation results in slow channel Ca^{2+} influx (118). Phospholamban, a protein located within the sarcoplasmic reticulum, is likewise phosphorylated, resulting in increased cytosolic Ca^{2+} flux through activation of Ca^{2+}-ATPase (114,119,120). In addition, the inhibitory subunit of troponin is phosphorylated (121,122). Phosphorylation of these intracellular proteins results in positive chronotropic, inotropic, and lusitropic effects (69,92).

ABNORMALITIES OF NEUROEFFECTOR PATHWAYS IN CONGESTIVE HEART FAILURE

In the failing human heart, myocardial (tissue) norepinephrine is depleted (123), while coronary sinus norepinephrine exceeds arterial levels (124,125), suggesting net norepinephrine release by the heart. The primary defect in norepinephrine equilibrium appears to be decreased cardiac neuronal uptake per unit of interstitial space (69,126). Although norepinephrine release is mildly decreased, it is not decreased as much as uptake. Because norepinephrine uptake is decreased, norepinephrine spillover increases and augments sympathetic drive, despite the fact that myocardial tissue levels are decreased. However, despite the increase in local and systemic norepinephrine concentrations, norepinephrine does not appear to be important for maintaining resting cardiac function in heart failure. Cardiac performance does not appear to be affected by reserpine (127) pretreatment in normal hearts or metyrosine (α-methyl-*p*-tyrosine) (105) pretreatment in hearts that are failing. That norepinephrine is acutely effective for maintaining pressure homeostasis in the presence of hypovolemia (i.e., is an effective inotrope and pressor) yet chronically plays little role in maintaining cardiac function seems paradoxical. The explanation for this phenomenon may be found in the postsynaptic β-receptor regulation. Acute changes in presynaptic norepinephrine are met with transient responses. In contrast, chronic elevations in presynaptic norepinephrine, due to decreased uptake, may result in postsynaptic β-receptor alterations (down-regulation) that decrease the sensitivity to this neurotransmitter and lessen its impact on normal function. However, because of the increased long-term presence of presynaptic norepinephrine in congestive heart failure, adverse phenomena may occur.

As mentioned, norepinephrine acts in the heart primarily as a β_1-agonist, and to a lesser degree as a weak β_2- and α_1-agonist. Thus, in the presence of high adrenergic tone due to congestive heart failure, the β_1 pathway is most affected (Fig. 4). The concentration of β_1-receptors in failing human myocardium is reduced (down-regulated) by approximately 50% to 60% without a change in receptor affinity (72,74,128,129). As the human heart contains few or no "spare β-receptors" (128), down-regulation of β-receptors results in a reduction in maximal isoproterenol-mediated adenylate cyclase stimulation (Fig. 5) (74,92). This also results in subsensitivity to β_1-agonist stimulation with an agent such as denopamine (a selective β_1-agonist) (74,92). Although the concentration of β_2-receptors is not reduced in the failing heart, there is subsensitivity to selective β_2-agonists such as zinterol (i.e., zinterol produces a submaximal muscle tension response in vitro) (74,92). These data suggest the β_2-receptor is mildly uncoupled to the effector system. However, as can be seen in Figure 4, in congestive heart failure the β_2-receptor subpopulation assumes a more prominent role in eliciting agonist support. Thus, in congestive heart failure, the β-receptors are decreased (β_1) and uncoupled (β_2) from the effector system. The fact that cardiac venous norepinephrine levels and coronary sinus norepinephrine levels correlate inversely and significantly ($r = 0.73$ for central venous, 0.66 for coronary sinus, both $p < 0.05$) with β-adrenergic receptor

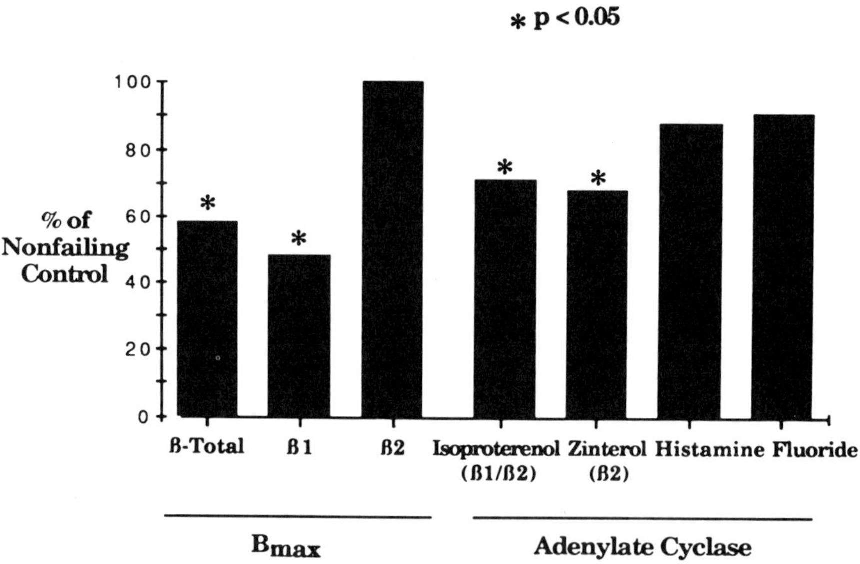

Figure 4 Effect of heart failure on β-receptor density and adenylate cyclase responses in nonfailing and failing human left ventricles, with data expressed as percentage of values in nonfailing hearts. (From Ref. 92.)

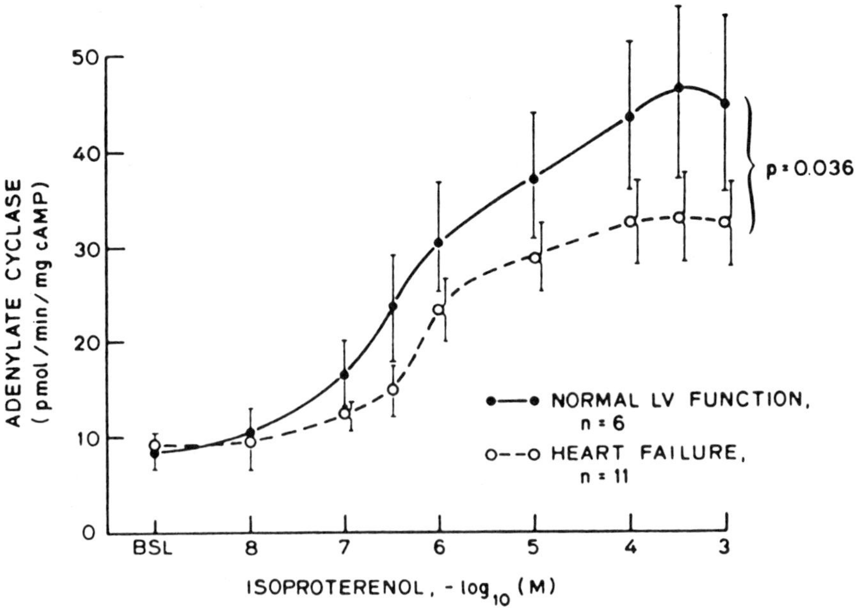

Figure 5 *L*-isoproterenol-stimulated adenylate cyclase activity (mean ± SEM) in left ventricles from normally functioning hearts (n = 6) (solid circles) and failing hearts (n = 11) (open circles). (From Ref. 128.)

density in right ventricular biopsy specimens suggests that norepinephrine is the mediator of the down-regulation of β-receptors (73,92).

Recent data have suggested a postreceptor defect(s) in the G protein system in the setting of congestive heart failure. An increase in the amount of G_i detected by ADP ribosylation catalyzed by the toxin from Bordetella pertussis has been detected in human hearts (130–132) in patients with congestive heart failure. Subsequent studies with cDNA probes have suggested an increase in the encoding of α_{i3} by mRNA in failing compared with nonfailing hearts (133). While studies of animal myocardium (134–136) and human lymphocytes (137) have suggested a decrease in guanine nucleotide regulatory protein (G_s) in heart failure, a small decrease (138) or none (130,131,135) in G_s has been found in human myocardium. These data suggest a decrease in the G_s/G_i activity ratio, and suggest a defect not only in β-adrenergic receptor density in congestive heart failure, but also in the G regulatory proteins that couple the neurohormonal signal to the effector system.

The effector system downstream appears to be intact in congestive heart failure. Forskolin (139), which directly increases adenylate cyclase activity, produces a similar contractile response in vitro for tissues isolated from failing and nonfailing hearts, suggesting a functional enzyme in congestive heart failure. Additionally, calcium infusion evokes a maximal inotropic response in patients with idiopathic dilated cardiomyopathy, whereas these patients have a submaximal response to the β-agonist dobutamine (Fig. 6) (129,140). An inverse relation exists between resting plasma norepinephrine and the contractile response to dobutamine infusion, suggesting progressive subsensitivity to β-agonist stimulation in congestive heart failure (140). These data suggest that the effector system is intact in congestive heart failure, while there are alterations in the β-receptors and perhaps the G_s regulatory protein complexes.

EFFECT OF β-ADRENERGIC BLOCKADE ON HEMODYNAMICS, EXERCISE CAPACITY, AND β-RECEPTOR DENSITY

Recent studies of β-adrenergic blockade have both better elucidated its salutary effect and provided some clues to how, mechanistically, it may provide benefit. Heilbrunn and associates (141) examined 14 patients with dilated cardiomyopathy who were treated with open-label metoprolol for

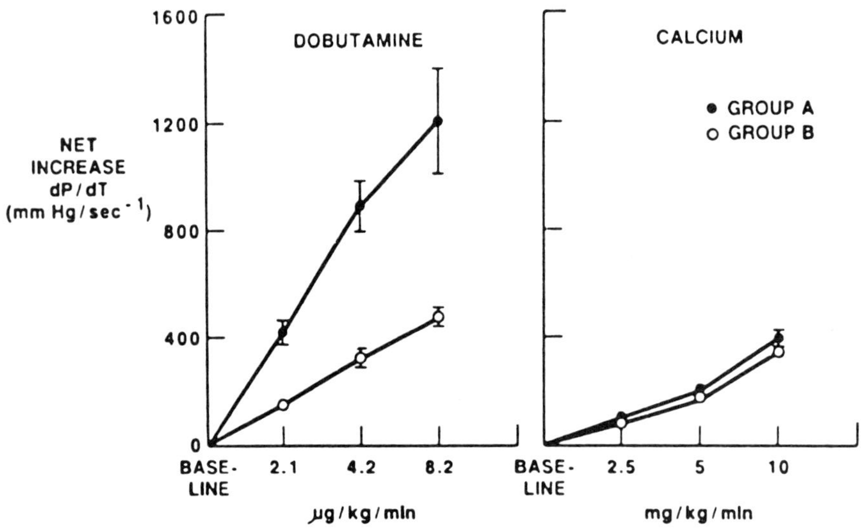

Figure 6 Peak dP/dt responses to dobutamine and calcium gluconate in patients with ejection fractions > 40% (group A) and patients with idiopathic dilated cardiomyopathy and ejection fractions <20% and a 50% reduction in β-receptor density (group B). (From Ref. 129.)

6 months. Treatment resulted in an increase in left ventricular ejection fraction from 0.26 ± 0.03 to 0.39 ± 0.03 (p = 0.005), a reduction in heart rate from 94 ± 5 to 69 ± 4 min^{-1} (p = 0.001), and an increase in stroke work from 27 ± 4 to 43 ± 3 g-m/m^2 (p = 0.002). In addition, response to graded doses of the β-agonist dobutamine was examined. As can be seen in Figure 7, inotropic and chronotropic responsiveness to dobutamine was increased after metoprolol therapy. To explain this finding of increased sensitivity to a β-agonist, the β-adrenergic receptor density and K_d was examined from right ventricular biopsies obtained before and after therapy in nine of the patients. The receptor density increased from 39 ± 7 to 80 ± 12 fmol/mg protein (p = 0.005) (Fig. 8), while there was no significant change in K_d (from 27.7 ± 3.5 to 21.8 ± 4.8, p = NS). These data suggest "up-regulation" of the β-receptors, especially the β_1-receptors, which are down-regulated by neurohormonal stimulation, although β_1-receptors were not specifically measured in this study.

A recent study from Waagstein and associates (142) examined the effect of open-labeled metoprolol on 33 patients with dilated cardiomyopathy. Seven of 33 patients (21%) were intolerant of therapy. Of the 26 patients who survived more than 6 months on therapy, 24 improved their functional

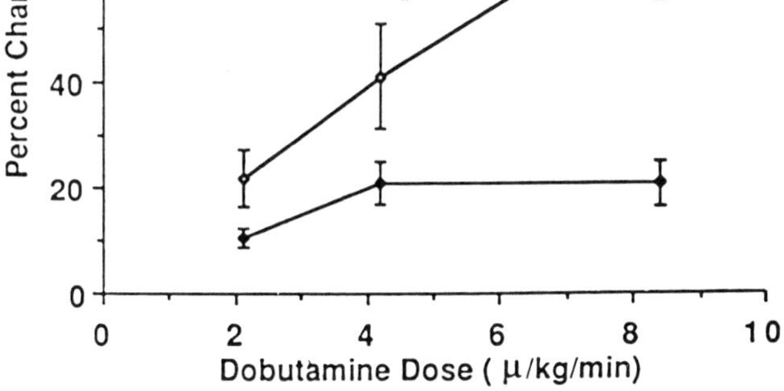

Figure 7 Plot of percent increment in peak left ventricular dP/dt compared with baseline at entry and baseline at 6 months of metoprolol therapy during dobutamine infusion. Values were obtained during atrial pacing at 110 beats/min and represent mean ± SEM; n = 8 patients. (From Ref. 141.)

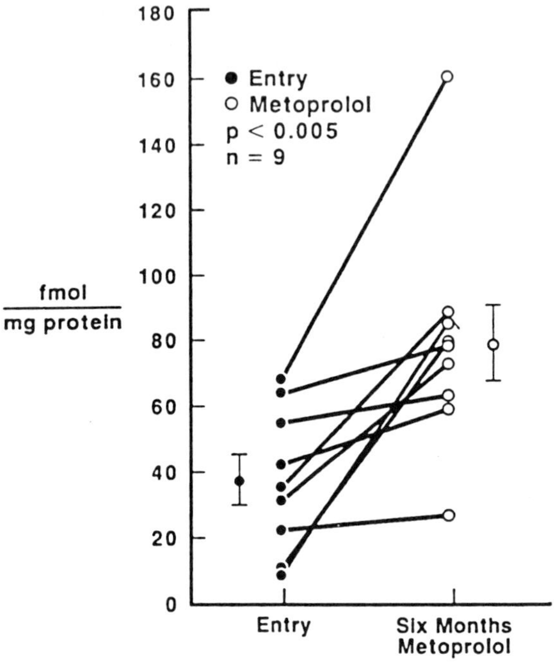

Figure 8 Plot of myocardial β-adrenergic receptor density (fmol/mg protein) measured at entry and after 6 months of metoprolol therapy. Data represent mean ± SEM; n = 9 patients. (From Ref. 141.)

class. Metoprolol was withdrawn from 24 patients, with clinical deterioration in 16 (67%). Hemodynamic evaluation of 22 patients on long-term metoprolol therapy revealed a decrease in heart rate, systemic and pulmonary vascular resistance, mean pulmonary capillary wedge pressure, left ventricular end-diastolic pressure, and pulmonary artery mean pressure, and an increase in systolic blood pressure, cardiac index, and left ventricular stroke work. In addition, echocardiographic indexes of left ventricular end-diastolic dimension decreased, as did the grade of mitral regurgitation. Ejection fraction decreased in the patients who underwent metoprolol withdrawal. In nine patients, β-adrenergic receptor density was determined from analysis of right ventricular biopsies. Before therapy, there was a decreased number of receptors in comparison with normal controls. However, long-term therapy up-regulated the receptors from 30.3 ± 2.9 to 49.0 ± 7.1 fmol/mg protein ($p < 0.05$). These data supported the findings of Heilbrunn (141) and suggested (1) that β-blockade improves hemodynamics after treatment and withdrawal results in clinical deterioration and (2) that β-receptor density is increased after therapy.

A new β-adrenergic blocker, bucindolol, has recently been developed (143–148). This agent is a nonselective β-antagonist equipotent to propranolol, with mild vasodilatory action (143,144,146,147). Although a small amount of intrinsic sympathomimetic activity has been noted in some in situ model system studies, this drug appears to have no such intrinsic activity in humans (148). A double-blind comparison of bucindolol plus standard therapy (n = 13) versus placebo plus standard therapy (n = 9) in 24 patients was recently completed by Gilbert and associates (144). A test dose of bucindolol 12.5 mg was given acutely, and was tolerated in 23 of 24 patients (96%). The acute hemodynamic response to bucindolol in these 23 patients was evaluated before long-term blinded randomization. Heart rate, systemic vascular resistance, and mean arterial pressure fell with the test dose, but mean pulmonary capillary wedge pressure, cardiac index, and stroke work did not change. Long-term therapy resulted in improvements in left ventricular ejection fraction, cardiac index, and left ventricular stroke work, while mean pulmonary capillary wedge pressure and heart rate fell. Although New York Heart Association functional class fell in the bucindolol group, exercise time did not change in either the placebo or bucindolol group. In addition, maximum oxygen consumption fell from 20.1 ± 1.3 to 18.1 ± 1.2 ml O_2/kg/min (p = 0.051) in the bucindolol group. However, β-adrenergic blockers have long been known to blunt maximum oxygen consumption in normal subjects (149). In patients with heart failure, this effect may be augmented despite improvements in hemodynamics. In addition, beta-blockade inhibits glycogen breakdown and lipolysis in skeletal tissue (149,150). This effect may result in limited substrate availability and could adversely affect maximum oxygen consumption.

Our laboratory has recently completed an open-label trial of bucindolol in patients with congestive heart failure (143). Fifteen male patients, aged 32 to 62 years (50 ± 11 years, mean ± SD), in New York Heart Association functional class II–IV, entered the trial. Seven of the 15 patients who entered the trial were in functional class III or IV. All patients had a radionuclide ventriculographic left ventricular ejection fraction less than 0.45 at entry. Twelve of the patients had dilated nonischemic cardiomyopathy, while three had ischemic cardiomyopathy. Angiotensin converting enzyme inhibitors were allowed, but were not changed during the trial or during the 2 months before entry. Other medications, except for diuretics, were unchanged during the trial. Bucindolol was titrated over 4 to 5 weeks from 12.5 mg b.i.d. to 100 mg b.i.d. No patient, including those with a left ventricular ejection fraction less than 0.15, was forced to discontinue therapy because of side effects or worsening congestive failure. When this study (143) and the study by Gilbert and colleagues (144) are compared with the study by Waagstein and associates (142), the data suggest that bucindolol is acutely tolerated better than metoprolol in patients with compromised ventricles. However, a direct comparison has yet to be performed. Cardiac catheterization included assessment of end-systolic elastance (Ees); ejection fraction and volumes; peak +dP/dt; peak −dP/dt; T (tau), the time constant of exponential isovolumic pressure fall; and myocardial oxygen consumption and coronary flow. These measurements were made at baseline and after atrial pacing to match pre- and postdrug heart rates. Pressure-volume assessments and Ees were determined from analysis of simultaneously acquired digital ventriculograms interfaced with micromanometer pressure signals. These results can be found in Tables 1 and

Table 1 Hemodynamic Changes After 3 Months of Therapy with Oral Bucindolol (Mean + S.D.)

	Pre-treatment	Post-treatment	p value
Heart rate (min^{-1})	82 ± 20	73 ± 11	0.059
Cardiac output (l/min)	5.0 ± 1.5	5.8 ± 1.6	0.0043
Stroke volume (ml)	64 ± 25	82 ± 28	0.0009
Mean PA (mm Hg)	30 ± 12	21 ± 9	0.0029
LV peak systolic (mm Hg)	109 ± 17	120 ± 26	0.023
Ao end-systolic (mm Hg)	90 ± 12	98 ± 18	0.049
LVEDP (mm Hg)	19.0 ± 7.5	14.8 ± 4.8	0.021
PVR ($dyn/s/cm^{-5}$)	196 ± 176	131 ± 103	0.034
SVR ($dyn/s/cm^{-5}$)	1318 ± 406	1183 ± 290	0.17
CSF (ml/min)	109 ± 44	116 ± 53	0.53
Myocardial O_2 difference (vol %)	11.9 ± 1.2	11.6 ± 1.6	0.24
Myocardial O_2 consumption (ml/min)	11.6 ± 4.4	12.3 + 4.9	0.77
Myocardial O_2 extraction (%)	68 ± 6	65 ± 6	0.086
LV stroke work index ($g\text{-}m/m^2$)	34 ± 13	47 ± 19	0.0059
LV minute work (kg-m/min)	5.5 ± 2.2	7.0 ± 2.6	0.0096
Myocardial efficiency (%)	28 ± 18	30 ± 14	0.75

PA = pulmonary arterial; LV = left ventricular; Ao = aortic; EDP = end-diastolic pressure; PVR = pulmonary vascular resistance; SVR = systemic vascular resistance; CSF = coronary sinus blood flow. (Reprinted by permission of author and American Heart Association, Inc.; Circulation 1990; 82: 473–483.)

Table 2 Volumetric and Contractility Changes After 3 Months of Therapy with Oral Bucindolol at Matched Paced Heart Rates (Mean ± S.D.)

	Pre-treatment Pacing	Post-treatment Pacing	p value
Heart rate (min^{-1})	99 ± 16	98 ± 15	0.34
Ao end-systolic pressure (mm Hg)	91 ± 12	97 ± 19	0.107
Peak + dP/dt (mm Hg/s)	895 ± 172	1055 ± 265	0.014
LVEDV (ml)	257 ± 92	228 ± 98	0.041
LVESV (ml)	205 ± 95	170 ± 96	0.0047
LVEF	0.23 ± 0.12	0.29 ± 0.14	0.0071
Ees (mm Hg/ml)	0.60 ± 0.40	1.11 ± 0.45	0.0049

Ao = aortic; LV = left ventricular; EDV = end-diastolic volume; ESV = end-systolic volume; EF = ejection fraction; Ees = end-systolic elastance. (Reprinted by permission of author and American Heart Association, Inc.; Circulation 1990; 82: 473–483.)

2. After 3 months of bucindolol therapy, heart rate fell mildly, but the fall did not reach statistical significance. There was a significant increase in cardiac output, left ventricular stroke work, minute work, and stroke volume despite falls in left ventricular end-diastolic pressure and volume. As afterload, as reflected by aortic end-systolic pressure, increased, this increase in stroke volume and stroke work must be interpreted as a shift in the Frank-Starling relation due to increased contractility after therapy with bucindolol. This is further supported by an increase in Ees from 0.60 ± 0.40 mm Hg/ml to 1.11 ± 0.45 mm Hg/ml after therapy ($p < 0.005$) (Fig. 9). There was an upward shift in the $+dP/dt_{max}$–end-diastolic volume relation ($p = 0.0005$) (Fig. 10). In addition, left ventricular ejection fraction increased despite increased end-systolic pressures and lower end-diastolic volumes. This increase in ejection fraction was due primarily to a decrease in left ventricular end-systolic volume. In addition to improvements in contractility, myocardial relaxation was improved by chronic beta-blockade therapy. This was demonstrated by a reduction in tau from 92 ± 17 to 73 ± 11 ms ($p = 0.0013$) at matched heart rates. As can be seen in Figure 11, the relationship of tau to end-systolic pressure at matched paced heart rates demonstrates a downward shift of the relationship ($p = 0.014$). This suggests improved myocardial relaxation.

The myocardial chamber stiffness constant (slope of the relationship of the natural logarithm of left ventricular end-diastolic pressure versus left ventricular end-diastolic volume) decreased nonsignificantly from 0.020 ±

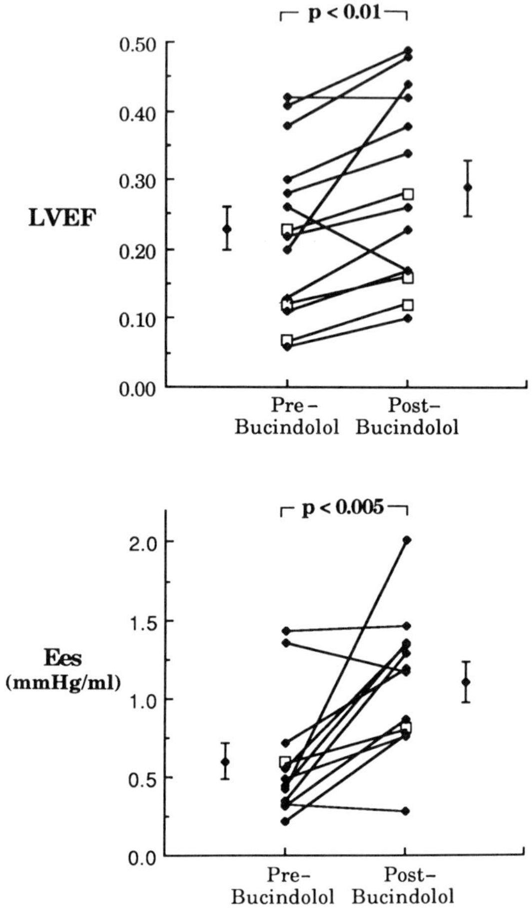

Figure 9 The changes in left ventricular ejection fraction (LVEF) and end-systolic elastance (Ees) are shown (mean ± SEM). Patients with an ischemic etiology for their left ventricular dysfunction are represented by open squares, while patients with nonischemic cardiomyopathies are represented by closed diamonds. There was an increase in left ventricular ejection fraction ($p < 0.01$) with beta-blocker therapy (top panel). In the group with no coronary artery disease, there was an increase in ejection fraction ($p < 0.025$). The end-systolic elastance derived from the end-systolic pressure-volume relationship is shown for each of the patients (bottom panel). There was a significant increase in end-systolic elastance ($p < 0.005$). This suggests myocardial contractility was improved with bucindolol therapy. (From Ref. 143.)

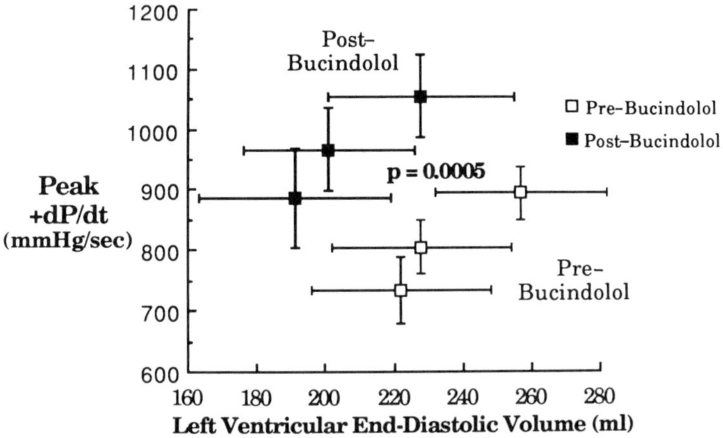

Figure 10 The peak $+dP/dt_{max}$–left ventricular end-diastolic volume relationship is shown for the pre- and post-bucindolol states (mean ± SEM). The three pre- and post-bucindolol points represent the mean group values at either pacing baseline, after a small dose of nitroprusside, or after a larger dose of nitroprusside. There was a significant upward and leftward shift in this relationship ($p < 0.01$) after therapy with bucindolol, demonstrating, in a relatively load-independent fashion, improved myocardial contractility. (From Ref. 143.)

0.026 to 0.013 ± 0.010 ($p = 0.51$), suggesting no change in overall left ventricular stiffness.

Pulmonary artery pressures and pulmonary resistance decreased from 196 ± 176 to 131 ± 103 dyn/s/cm^{-5} ($p = 0.034$). Systemic vascular resistance did not change (from 1318 ± 406 to 1183 ± 290 dyn/s/cm^{-5}; $p = 0.17$).

Coronary sinus blood flow, myocardial oxygen difference, and oxygen consumption did not change with beta-blocker therapy. Myocardial oxygen extraction trended down, while myocardial efficiency did not change (28% ± 18% pretreatment versus 30% ± 14% post-treatment; p = NS). As mechanical work increased without an increase in oxygen consumption, we hypothesize that one mechanism of improvement may have been a shift in substrate utilization from fatty acids to glucose. It has long been known that fatty acids and glucose provide the major substrates for myocardial energy metabolism and that excess utilization of free fatty acids by the heart increases myocardial oxygen consumption (151–153). Several experimental observations suggest that fatty acid substrate utilization by the heart is less efficient than that of glucose. In the oxygen-limited heart, high

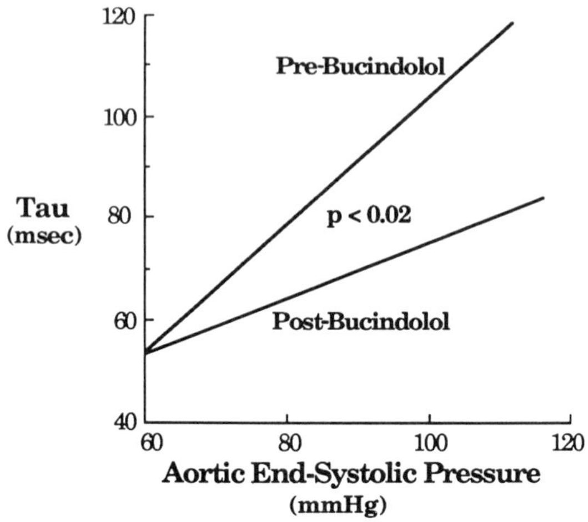

Figure 11 Improvements in isovolumic relaxation as manifest by a reduction in the tau–end-systolic pressure relation at matched heart rates (tau = the time constant of exponential isovolumic pressure fall). Each line represents the mean slope and intercept of this relationship before and after therapy with bucindolol. There was a downward shift in this relationship after therapy with a β-adrenergic blocker ($p < 0.02$), demonstrating improved myocardial relaxation. (From Ref. 143.)

concentrations of free fatty acids depress myocardial performance (151,154). This effect is presumably due to the increased need for oxygen in the presence of fatty acid metabolism. In addition, the increase in plasma fatty acids at rest has been shown to have no effect on myocardial oxygen consumption (155). However, when oxygen consumption is increased by atrial pacing or stress, myocardial oxygen consumption is increased disproportionately in the presence of infused lipids and heparin as compared to a control state (155). Catecholamines stimulate release and utilization of fatty acids (151,155) and inhibit insulin-induced glucose transport by skeletal muscle (156,157). Conversely, propranolol increases insulin sensitivity while increasing blood free fatty acids in diabetic rat skeletal muscle (156). This suggests β-adrenergic stimulation plays a role in substrate uptake and utilization in heart failure. As congestive heart failure is a state of increased adrenergic stimulation, with elevated sympathetic nerve traffic and increased plasma norepinephrine levels (1–4,15), lipolysis and glycogenolysis are both stimulated (158). In the dog, myocardial oxygen consumption, which is increased by β-agonist stimulation, is further increased by a β-stimulated increase in (i.e., a shift to) fatty acid utilization (152).

As myocardial work does not change or decreases when there is a shift from glucose to fatty acid utilization, this shift represents a reduction in myocardial efficiency (152). Support for this hypothesis comes from one of the early beta-blocker trials (159), in which lactate extraction increased with beta-blocker therapy. This suggests increased pyruvate utilization for oxidative phosphorylation.

EFFECT OF β-ADRENERGIC BLOCKADE ON NEUROHORMONAL ACTIVATION

Our laboratory recently examined the effect of chronic beta-blockade with bucindolol on plasma renin activity and norepinephrine levels in 15 patients with dilated cardiomyopathy (160). Supine plasma renin activity fell with bucindolol therapy from 11.6 ± 13.4 to 4.3 ± 4.1 ng/ml/h (p = 0.044), while plasma norepinephrine was unchanged, from 403 ± 231 to 408 ± 217 (p = 0.95), with beta-blockade with bucindolol. Seven of the patients underwent myocardial catecholamine assessment with MIBG (I-123 metaiodobenzylguanidine) scintigraphy (160,161). Regional MIBG uptake was unchanged (from 56.6 ± 21.7 to 54.7 ± 23.2 counts/voxel, p = NS) after bucindolol therapy, suggesting that the major defect in myocardial norepinephrine kinetics, adrenergic uptake, was unchanged with therapy (160). Although plasma norepinephrine did not change with therapy, heart rate tended to decrease, suggesting the presence of beta-adrenergic antagonism at the receptor level. Despite the fact that these patients were on ACE inhibitors, recent research has suggested alternative enzyme systems that might convert angiotensin I to angiotensin II (162). Thus, reduction of plasma renin, even in the presence of ACE inhibitors, may provide more complete deactivation of this pathway. Thus, neurohormonal activation was reduced with bucindolol. The reduction in plasma renin appears soon after beta-blocker administration, unless ventricular decompensation occurs (163). Despite reductions in plasma renin activity and the presence of β-adrenergic blockade, the response of renin or norepinephrine levels to chronic bucindolol therapy did not predict which patients had improved in hemodynamic status ($\chi^2 = 0.37$ for renin, $\chi^2 = 0.82$ for norepinephrine). As these variables did not correlate well with improvement, we infer that β-adrenergic antagonists may improve left ventricular function by mechanisms other than just attenuation or blockade of neurohormonal activation. However, reduction in neurohormonal activation may be beneficial in the long term. Reduction of β-adrenergic stimulation may be beneficial to the heart in a number of ways: (1) by inhibiting the direct toxic effects of catecholamines (164–166) and angiotensin II (91) on the myocardium; (2) by shifting substrate utilization from fatty acids to glucose (143), thus improving efficiency and energy utilization; (3) by reducing ventricular arrhythmias (1,58) (and the incidence of ventricular fibrillation), which may be provoked by sympathetic stimulation; and (4) by promoting up-regulation of beta$_1$-receptors and recoupling of beta$_2$-receptors, which may provide inotropic responsiveness to stress or exercise (69,72,92,128,129,141,142). In contrast to our study, other investigators (144) have documented a reduction in plasma norepinephrine levels after treatment with bucindolol. More extensive studies are needed to define the effect of beta-blockade on reflex sympathetic activity.

THEORIES AS TO WHY β-ADRENERGIC THERAPY IS BENEFICIAL

Several explanations have been set forth why beta blockade should theoretically work in congestive heart failure. The most likely explanations include the following.

1. Catecholamines have been shown to be deleterious to the heart in both animal models and in humans (164,166). The human heart "protects" itself from the effects of norepinephrine by down-regulating the receptors most affected, the β_1-receptors (69,74,92). Blockade of the effects of catecholamines at the receptor level with β-antagonists may provide more complete protection from the long-term effects of this neurohormone. Indeed, upregulation of β_1-receptors seen in several studies after administration of metoprolol (141,142) suggests decreased effective norepinephrine stimulation.

2. β_1-receptors are up-regulated after beta-blocker therapy (69,72,74,92,128,129,141,142). Although the importance of this finding is only now being elucidated, there is "resensitizing" of the β-receptors to β-agonists (as shown by Heilbrunn, Fig. 7). Despite improved sensitivity to β-agonists, up-regulation of β-receptors cannot explain the improvements seen at rest in the studies by Eichhorn and colleagues (143) and Waagstein and associates (142). In these studies, heart rate fell from predrug baseline, suggesting the presence of blocked (not stimulated) β-receptors, yet ventricular function improved. In addition, β-receptor up-regulation occurs within hours to days of beta-blocker administration, while clinical improvement may take several months to occur (167). Finally, no relation exists between changes in β-receptor density after administration of beta-blockers and the clinical response to treatment (141,167). Thus, other mechanisms may exist to explain ventricular improvement with long-term beta-blocker administration. However, despite this evidence against β-receptor up-regulation as a mechanism of ventricular improvement with beta-blockers, there may be improved response to stress and exercise with

β-receptor upregulation, as endogenous catecholamines may increase in these states (69,92).

3. As previously mentioned, catecholamines are known to shift substrate utilization from glucose to fatty acids, which may reduce the efficiency of the heart (143,151–158). β-Adrenergic blockade may shift substrate utilization back to glucose, thus increasing myocardial efficiency. This may also result in increased energy for synthetic and reparative processes and calcium mobilization (168,169). The latter may result in improved relaxation and contraction.

4. Beta-blockade may result in inhibition of sympathetically mediated vasoconstriction via prostaglandins and renin release (168). As mentioned, angiotensin II may have some direct cardiotoxic properties (91), which would be inhibited by beta-blockers. As angiotensin (86), and perhaps norepinephrine (107,108), may have some potential for inducing protein synthesis and myocardial hypertrophy, the long-term effect of beta-blockers on ventricular remodeling has yet to be elucidated.

5. In addition to improved hemodynamics due to the previously mentioned factors, a very important effect of beta-blockers is their ability to reduce sudden death, especially after a myocardial infarction (58,170–172). In pooled data from randomized trials encompassing 18,000 postinfarct patients, the average reduction in all-cause mortality as compared with placebo was about 20%, and the reductions in sudden death were about 30% (170). While the ability to reduce sudden death and ventricular fibrillation cannot be directly extrapolated to non-postinfarct patients, the data are very suggestive of a beneficial effect of beta-blockers. This may in part explain the beneficial survival trends seen in the early beta-blocker trials (23,24).

TITRATION OF BETA-BLOCKERS IN CONGESTIVE HEART FAILURE

As the failing heart depends on neurosympathetic stimulation to maintain cardiac output, acute withdrawal of this sympathetic tone by full-dose ACE inhibitor or beta-blocker therapy can result in decompensation or circulatory collapse. Neurosympathetic tone must be withdrawn slowly. Thus, small doses of beta-blockers should be instituted initially and titrated slowly. We suggest the following regimens for metoprolol and bucindolol titration in compensated congestive failure:

1. Metoprolol 6.25 mg orally twice daily for 1 week followed by a doubling of the dose every week (as tolerated) until 50 mg orally two or three times daily is reached, or until symptoms appear.

2. Bucindolol 12.5 mg orally twice daily for 1 week followed by a doubling of the dose every week (as tolerated) until 100 mg orally two times daily is reached, or until symptoms appear.

The patients who are most likely to deteriorate after initiating beta-blockade are those who are most dependent on adrenergic drive to maintain circulation (1,58). These patients tend to have the most marked cardiac dilatation, the highest heart rates, and highest plasma norepinephrine levels. In patients with these characteristics or with decompensated heart failure, smaller initial doses may be used by dilutional techniques with weekly titration, either as described above or at a slightly slower rate. It must be emphasized that despite very beneficial results thus far, this promising form of therapy may not be beneficial in all patients and is still somewhat untested on a widespread basis. Thus, the utmost care must be used when initiating therapy.

FUTURE DIRECTIONS

New beta-blockers have recently been introduced, including carvedilol (173,174), which is a nonselective beta-blocker (with predominant β_1-antagonism) and vasodilating activity like bucindolol. Another agent, xamoterol, has been touted as a beta-blocker with intrinsic sympathomimetic activity (i.e., a partial agonist) and has been used to treat congestive heart failure (66,175–178). As partial agonists act differently from most beta-blockers (indeed, some may act more as agonists than as antagonists), and since concerns about possible adverse effects of xamoterol on survival have recently been raised (66), this topic will not be covered in this chapter. In any case, the optimal agent for the treatment of congestive heart failure has not yet been determined. Recent in vitro data suggest a selective β_1-adrenergic blocker may enhance coupling of β_2-adrenoceptors to adenylate cyclase, perhaps because of changes at the level of Gs and/or Gi proteins (179). If this is also true in vivo, nonselective β-adrenergic blockers may not have advantages over selective beta-blockade. This has yet to be determined.

Recent evidence has suggested that β-adrenergic receptors are linked to sodium channels via a G_s protein (71,180). The implications of this pathway have yet to be elucidated.

The effect of beta-blockers on survival in congestive heart failure has yet to be conclusively determined, although earlier studies suggested a beneficial effect (23,24). The fact that beta-blockers reduce neurohormonal activation (160) (like ACE inhibitors) also suggests the possibility of a beneficial effect on survival (1,181). A prospective, double-blind, randomized trial has yet to answer this very important question, although a current trial, Metoprolol in Dilated Cardiomyopathy (MDC) (181), may provide some answers.

Recent evidence has emerged to suggest that the effect of beta-blockade on ischemic and on nonischemic dilated cardiomyopathy is different (182). This may be due to differences in skeletal support (i.e., fibrosis, scarring, remodeling) or differences in the response of the neuroeffector systems. In addition, it is unclear if beta-blockers are most beneficial if the patient is treated early or late in the course of heart failure. Future research may help to elucidate which patients to treat and when to intervene.

REFERENCES

1. Packer M, Lee WH, Kessler PD, Gottlieb SS, Bernstein JL, Kukin ML. Role of neurohormonal mechanisms in determining survival in patients with severe chronic heart failure. Circulation 1987; 75(suppl IV):IV-80–92.
2. Leimbach WN, Wallin BG, Victor RG, Aylward PE, Sundolf G, Mark AL. Direct evidence from intraneural recordings for increased central sympathetic outflow in patients with heart failure. Circulation 1986; 73:913–919.
3. Francis GS, Goldsmith SR, Olivari MT, Levine TB, Cohn JN. The neurohormonal axis in congestive heart failure. Ann Intern Med 1984; 101:370–377.
4. Packer M. Neurohormonal interactions and adaptations in congestive heart failure. Circulation 1988; 77:721–730.
5. Packer M, Lee WH, Medina N, Yushak M. Altered baroreflex response to the systemic vasoconstriction induced by oxygen inhalation in heart failure (abstr). Circulation 1987; 75(suppl IV):IV-357.
6. Laragh JH. Atrial natriuretic hormone, the renin-aldosterone axis, and blood pressure-electrolyte homeostasis. N Engl J Med 1985; 313:1330–1340.
7. Dzau VJ, Packer M, Lilly LS, Swartz SL, Hollenberg NK, Williams GH. Prostaglandins in severe heart failure: relation to activation of the renin-angiotensin system and hyponatremia. N Engl J Med 1984; 310:347–352.
8. Thomas JA, Marks BH. Plasma norepinephrine in congestive heart failure. Am J Cardiol 1978; 41:233–243.
9. Francis GS, Goldsmith SR, Cohn JN. Relationship of exercise capacity to resting left ventricular performance and basal plasma norepinephrine levels in patients with congestive heart failure. Am Heart J 1982; 104:725–731.
10. Levine TB, Francis GS, Goldsmith SR, Simon AB, Cohn JN. Activity of the sympathetic nervous system and renin-angiotensin system assessed by plasma hormone levels and their relation to hemodynamic abnormalities in congestive heart failure. Am J Cardiol 1982; 49:1659–1666.
11. Dzau VJ, Colucci WS, Hollenberg NK, Williams GH. Relation of the renin-angiotensin-aldosterone system to clinical state in congestive heart failure. Circulation 1981; 63:645–651.

12. Franciosa JA, Wilen M, Ziesche S, Cohn JN. Survival in men with severe chronic left ventricular failure due to either coronary heart disease or idiopathic dilated cardiomyopathy. Am J Cardiol 1983; 51:831–836.
13. Unverferth DV, Magorien RD, Moeschberger ML, Baker PB, Fetters JK, Leier CV. Factors influencing the one-year mortality of dilated cardiomyopathy. Am J Cardiol 1984; 54:147–152.
14. Schwarz F, Mall G, Zebe H, Schmitzer E, Manthey J, Scheurlen H, Kubler W. Determinants of survival in patients with congestive cardiomyopathy: quantitative morphologic findings and left ventricular hemodynamics. Circulation 1984; 70:923–928.
15. Cohn JN, Levine TB, Olivari MT, Garberg V, Lura, D, Francis GS, Simon AB, Rector T. Plasma norepinephrine as a guide to prognosis in patients with chronic congestive heart failure. N Engl J Med 1984; 311:819–823.
16. Cohn JN, Rector T, Olivari MT, Levine TB, Francis GS. Plasma norepinephrine, ejection fraction and maximal oxygen consumption as prognostic variables in congestive heart failure (abstr). Circulation 1985; 72(suppl III):III-285.
17. Creager MA, Faxon DP, Halperin JL, Melidossian CD, McCabe CH, Schich EC, Ryan TJ. Determinants of clinical response and survival in patients with congestive heart failure treated with captopril. Am Heart J 1982; 104:1147–1154.
18. Levine TB, Franciosa JA, Vrobel T, Cohn JN. Hyponatremia as a marker for high renin heart failure. Br Heart J 1982; 47:161–166.
19. Brown JJ, Davies DL, Johnson VW, Lever AF, Robertson JIS. Renin relationships in congestive cardiac failure, treated and untreated. Am Heart J 1970; 80:329–342.
20. Packer M, Medina N, Yushak M. Relation between serum sodium concentration and the hemodynamic and clinical responses to converting enzyme inhibition with captopril in severe heart failure. J Am Coll Cardiol 1984; 3:1035–1043.
21. Lee WH, Packer M. Prognostic importance of serum sodium concentration and its modification by converting-enzyme inhibition in patients with severe chronic heart failure. Circulation 1986; 73:257–267.
22. Waagstein F, Hjalmarson A, Varnauskas E, and Wallentin I: Effect of chronic beta-adrenergic receptor blockade in congestive cardiomyopathy. Br Heart J 1975; 37:1022–1036.
23. Swedberg K, Waagstein F, Hjalmarson A, Wallentin I: Prolongation of survival in congestive cardiomyopathy by beta receptor blockade. Lancet 1979; 1:1374–1376.
24. Anderson JL, Lutz JR, Gilbert EM, Sorenson SG, Yanowitz FG, Menlove RL, Bartholomew M: A randomized trial of low-dose beta-blockade therapy for idiopathic dilated cardiomyopathy. Am J Cardiol 1985; 55:471–475.
25. The CONSENSUS trial study group. Effects of enalapril on mortality in severe congestive heart failure: results of the Cooperative North Scandan-

avian Enalapril Survival Study (CONSENSUS). N Engl J Med 1987; 316:1429–1435.
26. Chatterjee, K, Rouleau, J, Parmley WW. Captopril in congestive heart failure: improved left ventricular function with decreased metabolic cost. Am Heart J 1982; 104:1137–1146.
27. The Captopril Multicenter Research Group. A cooperative multicenter study of captopril in congestive heart failure: hemodynamic effects and long-term response. Am Heart J 1985; 110:439–447.
28. Sharpe DN, Murphy J, Coxon R, Hannon SF. Enalapril in patients with chronic heart failure: a placebo-controlled, randomized, double-blind study. Circulation 1984; 70:271–278.
29. Cody FS, Couit AB, Schaer GL. Evaluation of a long-acting converting enzyme inhibitor (enalapril) for the treatment of congestive heart failure. J Am Coll Cardiol 1983; 1:1154–1159.
30. Fitzpatrick D, Nicholls MG, Inkram H, Espiner EA. Haemodynamic, hormonal, and electrolyte effects of enalapril in heart failure. Br Heart J 1983; 50:163–169.
31. DiCarlo L, Chatterjee K, Parmley WW, Swedberg K, Atherton B, Curran D, Cucci M. A new angiotensin converting enzyme inhibitor in chronic heart failure: acute and chronic hemodynamic evaluations. J Am Coll Cardiol 1983; 2:865–871.
32. Turini GA, Weber B, Brunner HR. The renin-angiotensin system in refractory heart failure: clinical hemodynamic and hormonal effects of captopril and enalapril. Eur Heart J 1983; 4:189–197.
33. Awan NA, Mason DT. Vasodilator therapy of severe congestive heart failure: the special importance of angiotensin-converting enzyme inhibition with captopril. Am Heart J 1982; 104:1127–1136.
34. Ader R, Chatterjee K, Ports T. Immediate and sustained clinical improvement in chronic heart failure by an oral angiotensin converting enzyme inhibitor. Circulation 1980; 61:931–937.
35. Packer M. Vasodilator and inotropic drugs for the treatment of chronic heart failure: distinguishing hype from hope. J Am Coll Cardiol 1988; 12:1299–1317.
36. Colucci WS, Williams GH, Alexander RW, Braunwald E. Mechanisms and implications of vasodilator tolerance in the treatment of congestive heart failure. Am J Med 1981; 71:89–98.
37. Mettauer B, Rouleau JL, Bichet D, Kortas C, Manzini C, Tremblay G, Chatterjee K. Differential long-term intrarenal and neurohormonal effects of captropril and prazosin in patients with chronic congestive heart failure: importance of initial plasma renin activity. Circulation 1986; 73:492–502.
38. Ke Y, Manthey J, Dietz R, Leinberger H, Schomig A, Kubler W. Effects of hydralazine on sympathetic nervous activity in heart failure (abstr). Am J Cardiol 1982; 49:993.
39. Bayliss J, Norell MS, Canepa-Anson R, Reid C, Poole-Wilson P, Sutton G. Clinical importance of the renin-angiotensin system in chronic heart failure:

double blind comparison of captopril and prazosin. Br Med J 1985; 290:1861–1865.

40. Magorien RD, Unverferth DV, Leier CV. Hydralazine therapy in chronic congestive heart failure. Sustained central and regional hemodynamic responses. Am J Med 1984; 77:267–274.
41. Franciosa JA, Weber KT, Levine TB, Kinasewitz GT, Janicki JS, West J, Henis MMJ, Cohn JN. Hydralazine in the long-term treatment of chronic heart failure: lack of difference from placebo. Am Heart J 1982; 104:587–594.
42. Conradson TB, Ryden L, Ahlmark G, Saetre H, Person S, Nyquist O. Clinical efficacy of oral hydralazine in chronic heart failure. One year double-blind placebo controlled study. Am Heart J 1984; 108:1001–1006.
43. Franciosa JA, Jordan RA, Wilen MM, Leddy CL. Minoxidil in patients with left heart failure: contrasting hemodynamic and clinical effects in a controlled trial. Circulation 1984; 70:63–69.
44. Braunwald E, Colucci WS. Vasodilator therapy of heart failure. Has the promissory note been paid? N Engl J Med 1984; 310:459–461.
45. Cohn JN, Archibald DG, Ziesche S, Franciosa JA, Harston WE, Tristani FE, Dunkman WB, Jacobs W, Francis GS, Flohr KH, Goldman S, Cobb FR, Shah PM, Saunders R, Fletcher RD, Loeb HS, Hughes VC, Baker B. Effect of vasodilator therapy on mortality in chronic congestive heart failure. Results of a Veterans Administration Cooperative Study. N Engl J Med 1986; 314:1547–1552.
46. Wenting GJ, DeBrayn JHB, Man In't Veld AJ. Hemodynamic effects of captopril in essential hypertension and cardiac failure: correlations with short- and long-term effects on plasma renin. Am J Cardiol 1982; 49:1453–1459.
47. Fagard R, Amery A, Reybrouck T. Acute and chronic systemic and pulmonary hemodynamic effects of angiotensin converting enzyme inhibition with captopril in hypertensive patients. Am J Cardiol 1980; 46:295–305.
48. Fouad FM, Tarazi RC, Bravo EL, Hart NJ, Castle LW, Salcedo EE. Long-term control of congestive heart failure with captopril. Am J Cardiol 1982; 49:1489–1496.
49. Dunn FG, Oigman W, Ventura HO, Messerli FH, Kobrin I, Frohlich ED. Enalapril improves systemic and renal hemodynamics and allows regression of left ventricular mass in essential hypertension. Am J Cardiol 1984; 53:105–108.
50. Lund-Johansen P. Central hemodynamic effects of beta-blockers in hypertension. A comparison between atenolol, metoprolol, timolol, penbutolol, alprenolol, pindolol and bunitrolol. Eur Heart J 1983; 4(suppl):1–12.
51. Guazzi M, Polese A, Fiorentini C, Olivari MT, Magrini F. Cardiac performance and beta-adrenergic blockade in arterial hypertension. Am J Med Sci 1977; 273:63–69.
52. Tarazi RC, Dustan HP. Beta-adrenergic blockade in hypertension. Am J Cardiol 1972; 29:633–640.

53. Ferguson DW, Berg WJ, Sanders JS, Roach PJ, Kempf JS, Kienzle MG. Sympathoinhibitory responses to digitalis glycosides in heart failure patients. Direct evidence from sympathetic neural recordings. Circulation 1989; 80:65–77.
54. Swedberg K, Hjalmarson A, Waagstein F, Wallentin I. Beneficial effects of long-term beta-blockade in congestive cardiomyopathy. Br Heart J 1980; 44:117–133.
55. Swedberg K, Hjalmarson A, Waagstein F, Wallentin I. Adverse effects of beta-blockade withdrawal in patients with congestive cardiomyopathy. Br Heart J 1980; 44:134–142.
56. Weber KT, Likoff MJ, McCarthy D. Low-dose beta blockade in the treatment of chronic cardiac failure. Am Heart J 1982; 104:877–879.
57. Engelmeier RS, O'Connell JB, Walsh R, Rad N, Scanlon PJ, Gunnar RM: Improvement in symptoms and exercise tolerance by metoprolol in patients with dilated cardiomyopathy: a double-blind, randomized, placebo-controlled trial. Circulation 1985; 72:536–546.
58. Chadda K, Goldstein S. Byington R, Curb JD. Effect of propranolol after acute myocardial infarction in patients with congestive heart failure. Circulation 1986; 73:503–510.
59. Lambertz H, Meyer J, Erbel R. Long-term effects of prenalterol in patients with severe congestive heart failure. Circulation 1984: 69:298–305.
60. Roubin GS, Choong CY, Devenish-Meares S, Sadick NN, Fletcher PJ, Kelly DT, Harris PJ. β-adrenergic stimulation of the failing left ventricle: a double blind, randomized trial of sustained oral therapy with prenalterol. Circulation 1984; 69:955–962.
61. Weber KT, Andrews V, Janicki JS, Likoff M, Reichek N. Pirbuterol, an oral beta-adrenergic receptor agonist, in the treatment of chronic cardiac failure. Circulation 1982; 66:1262–1267.
62. Currie PJ, Kelly MJ, Middlebrook K, Federman J, Sainsbury E, Ashley J, Pitt A. Acute intravenous and sustained oral treatment with the $beta_1$ agonist prenalterol in patients with severe cardiac failure. Br Heart J 1984; 51:530–538.
63. Glover DR, Wather CG, Murray RG, Petch MC, Muir AL, Littler WA. Are the clinical benefits of oral prenalterol in ischemic heart failure due to beta blockade? A six month randomised double-blind comparison with placebo. Br Heart J 1985; 53:208–215.
64. Dahlstrom U, Areskog M, Wranne B, Karlsson E. Prenalterol as long-term therapy for chronic congestive heart failure: a randomized cross-over trial. Acta Med Scand 1984; 216:199–207.
65. Katz A. Potential deleterious effects of inotropic agents in the therapy of chronic heart failure. Circulation 1986; 73(suppl III):III-184–III-190.
66. The Xamoterol in Severe Heart Failure Study Group. Xamoterol in severe heart failure. Lancet 1990; 336:1–6.
67. Ikram H, Fitzpatrick D. Double blind trial of chronic oral beta blockade in congestive cardiomyopathy. Lancet 1981; 2:490–493.

68. Currie PJ, Kelly KJ, McKenzie A, Harper RW, Lim YL, Federman J, Anderson ST, Pitt A. Oral beta-adrenergic blockade with metoprolol in chronic severe dilated cardiomyopathy. J Am Coll Cardiol 1984; 3:203–209.
69. Feldman AM, Bristow MR. Adrenergic neuroeffector mechanisms in the failing human heart. In: Braunwald E, ed. Heart Disease (Update). A Textbook of Cardiovascular Medicine. 3rd ed. Philadelphia: W.B. Saunders, 1990.
70. Randall WC, ed. Nervous Control of Cardiovascular Function. New York: Oxford University Press, 1984.
71. Bristow MR, Hershberger RE, Port JD, Gilbert EM, Sandoval A, Rasmussen R, Cates AE, Feldman AM. β-adrenergic pathways in nonfailing and failing human ventricular myocardium. Circulation 1990; 82(suppl I):I-12–I-25.
72. Bristow MR, Kantrowitz NE, Ginsburg R, Fowler MB. β-adrenergic function in heart muscle disease and heart failure. J Mol Cell Cardiol 1985; 17:41–52.
73. Bristow MR, Sandoval AB, Gilbert EM, Deisher T, Minobe W, Rasmussen R. Myocardial α- and β-adrenergic receptors in heart failure: is cardiac-derived norepinephrine the regulatory signal? Eur Heart J 1988; 9(suppl H):35–40.
74. Bristow MR, Ginsburg R, Umans V, Fowler M, Minobe W, Rasmussen R, Zera P, Menlove R, Shah P, Jamieson S, Stinson EB. β_1- and β_2-adrenergic receptor subpopulations in nonfailing and failing human ventricular myocardium: coupling of both receptor subtypes to muscle contraction and selective β_1-receptor down-regulation in heart failure. Circ Res 1986; 59:297–309.
75. Stiles GL, Taylor S, Lefkowitz RJ. Human cardiac β-adrenergic receptors: subtype heterogeneity delineated by direct radioligand binding. Life Sci 1983; 33:467–473.
76. Frielle T, Collins S, Daniel KW, Caron MG, Lefkowitz RJ, Kobilda BK. Cloning of the cDNA for the human β_1-adrenergic receptor. Proc Natl Acad Sci USA 1987; 84:7920–7924.
77. Lands AM, Arnold A, McAuliff JP, Luduena FP, Brown TG. Differentiation of receptor systems activated by sympathomimetic amines. Nature 1967; 214:597–598.
78. Bristow MR, Minobe W, Rasmussen R, Hershberger RE, Hoffman BB. Alpha_1 adrenergic receptors in the nonfailing and failing human heart. J Pharmacol Exp Ther 1988; 247:1039–1045.
79. Rosendorf C. α-adrenoceptors in hypertension. J Cardiovasc Pharmacol 1986; 8(suppl 2):S3–S7.
80. McLeod AA, Brown JE, Kuhn C, Kitchell BB, Sedor FA, Williams RS, Shand DG. Differentiation of hemodynamic, humoral and metabolic responses to β_1- and β_2-adrenergic stimulation in man using atenolol and propranolol. Circulation 1983; 67:1076–1084.

81. Cody RJ, Laragh JH. The role of the renin-angiotensin-aldosterone system in the pathophysiology of chronic heart failure. In: Cohn JN, ed. Drug Treatment of Heart Failure. New York: Yorke Medical Books, 1983.
82. Curtiss C, Cohn JN, Vrobel T, Franciosa JA. Role of the renin-angiostensin system in the systemic vasoconstriction of chronic heart failure. Circulation 1978; 58:763–770.
83. Kluger J, Cody RJ, Laragh JH. The contributions of sympathetic tone and the renin-angiotensin system to severe chronic congestive heart failure: response to specific inhibitors (prazosin and captopril). Am J Cardiol 1982; 49:1667–1674.
84. Baker KM, Aceto JA. Characterization of avian angiotensin II cardiac receptors: coupling to mechanical activity and phosphoinositide metabolism. J Mol Cell Cardiol 1989; 21:375–382.
85. Baker KM, Campanile CP, Trachte GJ, Peach MJ. Identification and characterization of the rabbit angiotensin II myocardial receptor. Circ Res 1984; 54:286–293.
86. Aceto JF, Baker KM. [Sar^1] angiotensin II receptor-mediated stimulation of protein synthesis in chick heart cells. Am J Physiol 1990; 258:H806–H813.
87. Baker KM, Khosla MC. Cardiac and vascular actions of decapeptide angiotensin analogs. J Pharmacol Exp Ther 1986; 239:790–796.
88. Hughes J, Roth RH. Evidence that angiostensin enhances transmitter release during sympathetic nerve stimulation. Br J Pharmacol 1971; 41:239–255.
89. Zimmerman BG, Gomes SK, Liano JC. Action of angiotensin on vascular nerve adrenergic endings: facilitation of norepinephrine release. Fed Proc 1972; 31:1344–1350.
90. Roth RH. Action of angiotensin on adrenergic nerve endings: enhancement of norepinephrine biosynthesis. Fed Proc 1972; 31:1358–1364.
91. Tan LB, Jalil JE, Janicki JS, Weber KT, Clark WA. Cardiotoxic effects of angiotensin II (abstr). J Am Coll Cardiol 1989; 13(suppl A):2A.
92. Bristow MR, Port JD, Sandoval AB, Rasmussen R, Ginsburg R, Feldman AM: β-adrenergic receptor pathways in the failing human heart. Heart Failure 1989; 5:77–90.
93. Brown JH, Buxton IL, Brunton LL. α_1-adrenergic and muscarinic cholinergic stimulation of phosphoinositide hydrolysis in adult rat cardiomyocytes. Circ Res 1985; 57:532–537.
94. Williamson JR, Cooper RH, Joseph SK, Thomas AP. Inositol trisphosphate and diacylglycerol as intracellular second messengers in liver. Am J Physiol 1985; 248:C203–C216.
95. Nishizuka Y. The role of protein kinase C in cell surface signal transduction and tumour promotion. Nature 1984; 308:693–698.
96. Otani HM, Prasad R, Engelman RM, Otani H, Cordis GA, Das DK. Enhanced phosphodiesteratic breakdown and turnover of phosphoinositides during reperfusion of ischemic rat heart. Circ Res 1988; 63:930–936.

97. Steinberg SF, Kaplan LM, Inouye T, Zhang JF, Robinson RB. Alpha-1 adrenergic stimulation of 1,4,5-inositol trisphosphate formation in ventricular myocytes. J Pharmacol Exp Ther 1989; 250:1141–1148.
98. Otani H, Otani H, Das DK. α_1-adrenoceptor-mediated phosphoinositide breakdown and inotropic response in rat left ventricular papillary muscles. Circ Res 1988; 62:8–17.
99. Berridge MJ, Irvine RF. Inositol triphosphate, a novel second messenger in cellular signal transduction. Nature 1984; 312:315–321.
100. Schmitz W, Scholz H, Scholz J, Steinfath M. Increase in IP_3 prededes α-adrenoceptor-induced increase in force of contraction in cardiac muscle. Eur J Pharmacol 1987; 140:109–111.
101. Newman KB, Michael JR, Feldman AM. Activation of protein kinase C inhibits adenylate cyclase in endothelial cells via a pertussis toxin sensitive G protein (abstr). Circulation 1988; 78(suppl II):II-184.
102. Curiel R, Perez-Gonzalez J, Brito N, Zerpa R, Tellez D, Cabrera J, Curiel C, Cubeddu L. Positive inotropic effects mediated by α_1 adrenoceptors in intact human subjects. J Cardiovasc Pharmacol 1989; 14:603–615.
103. Arnold S, Williams R, Ports TA, Baughman RA, Benet LZ, Parmley WW, Chatterjee K. Attenuation of prazosin effect on cardiac output in chronic heart failure. Ann Intern Med 1979; 91:345–349.
104. Packer M, Meller J, Gorlin R, Herman MV. Hemodynamic and clinical tachyphylaxis to prazosin-mediated afterload reduction in severe chronic congestive heart failure. Circulation 1979; 59:531–539.
105. Franciosa JA, Schwartz DE. Acute hemodynamic effects of norepinephrine inhibition in patients with severe chronic congestive heart failure. J Am Coll Cardiol 1989; 14:624–630.
106. Vago T, Bevilacqua M, Norbiator G, Baldi G, Chebat E, Bertora P, Baroldi G, Accinni R. Identification of α_1-adrenergic receptors on sarcolemma from normal subjects and patients with idiopathic dilated cardiomyopathy: characteristics and linkage to GTP-binding protein. Circ Res 1989; 64:474–481.
107. Lee HR, Henderson SA, Reynolds R, Dunnmon P, Yuan D, Chien KR. α_1-adrenergic stimulation of cardiac gene transcription in neonatal myocardial cells. Effects on myosin light chain-2 gene expression. J Biol Chem 1988; 263:7352–7358.
108. Simpson P, McGrath A. Norepinephrine-stimulated hypertrophy of cultured rat myocardial cells is an alpha$_1$-adrenergic response. J Clin Invest 1983; 72:732–737.
109. Bristow MR, Port JD, Hershberger RE, Gilbert EM, Feldman AM. The β-adrenergic receptor-adenylate cyclase complex as a target for therapeutic intervention in heart failure. Eur Heart J 1989; 10(suppl B):45–54.
110. Murad F, Chi Y-M, Rall TW, Sutherland EW. Adenyl cyclase, III: the effect of catecholamines and choline esters on the formation of adenosine 3′,5′-phosphate by preparations from cardiac muscle and liver. J Biol Chem 1962; 237:1233–1238.

111. Gilman AG. G proteins and regulation of adenylyl cyclase. JAMA 1989; 262:1819–1825.
112. Casey PJ, Gilman AG. G protein involvement in receptor-effector coupling. J Biol Chem 1988; 263:2577–2580.
113. Yatani A, Brown AM. Rapid β-adrenergic modulation of cardiac calcium channel currents by a fast G protein pathway. Science 1989; 245:71–74.
114. Tada M, Katz A. Phosphorylation of the sarcoplasmic reticulum and sarcolemma. Ann Rev Physiol 1982; 44:401–423.
115. Winegrad S, McClellan G, Horowitz R, Tucker M, Lin LE, Weisberg A. Regulation of cardiac contractile proteins by phosphorylation. Fed Proc 1983; 42:39–44.
116. Greengard P. Phosphorylated proteins as physiological effectors. Science 1978; 199:146–152.
117. Kuo JF, Greengard JP. Cyclic nucleotide-dependent protein kinases. IV. Widespread occurrence of adenosine 3′,5′-monophosphate-dependent protein kinase in various tissues and phyla of the animal kingdom. Proc Natl Acad Sci USA 1969; 64:1349–1355.
118. Sperelakis N. Cyclic AMP and phosphorylation in regulation of Ca^{++} influx into myocardial cells and blockade by calcium antagonistic drugs. Am Heart J 1984; 107:347–357.
119. Kranias EG, Solaro J. Coordination of cardiac sarcoplasmic reticulum and myofibrillar function by protein phosphorylation. Fed Proc 1983; 42:33–38.
120. Lindemann JP, Jones LR, Hathaway DR, Henry BG, Watanabe AM. β-adrenergic stimulation of phospholamban phosphorylation and Ca^{2+}-ATPase activity in guinea pig ventricles. J Biol Chem 1983; 258:464–471.
121. Solaro RJ, Moir AJG, Perry SV. Phosphorylation of troponin I and the inotropic effect of adrenaline in the perfused rabbit heart. Nature 1976; 262:615–617.
122. Ezrailson EG, Potter JD, Michael L, Schwartz A. Positive inotropy induced by ouabain, by increased frequency, by X537A (RO2-2985), by calcium and by isoproterenol: the lack of correlation with phosphorylation of TnI. J Mol Cell Cardiol 1977; 9:693–698.
123. Chidsey CA, Braunwald E, Morrow AG. Catecholamine excretion and cardiac stores of norepinephrine in congestive heart failure. Am J Med 1965; 39:442–451.
124. Rose CP, Burgess JH, Cousineau D. Reduced aortocoronary sinus extraction of epinephrine in patients with left ventricular failure secondary to long-term pressure or volume overload. Circulation 1983; 68:241–244.
125. Swedberg K, Viquerat C, Rouleau JL, Roizen M, Atherton B, Parmley WW, Chatterjee K. Comparison of myocardial catecholamine balance in chronic congestive heart failure and in angina pectoris without failure. Am J Cardiol 1984; 54:783–786.
126. Sandoval AB, Gilbert EM, Rose CP, Bristow MR. Cardiac norepinephrine uptake and release is decreased in dilated cardiomyopathy (abstr). Circulation 1989; 80(suppl IV):393.

127. Spann JF, Sonnenblick EH, Cooper T, Chidsey CA, Willman VL, Braunwald E. Cardiac norepinephrine stores and the contractile state of heart muscle. Circ Res 1966; 19:317–325.
128. Bristow MR, Ginsburg R, Minobe W, Cubicciotti RS, Sageman WS, Lurie K, Billingham ME, Harrison DC, Stinson EB. Decreased catecholamine sensitivity and β-adrenergic receptor density in failing human hearts. N Engl J Med 1982; 307:205–211.
129. Fowler MB, Laser JA, Hopkins GL, Minobe W, Bristow MR. Assessment of the β-adrenergic receptor pathway in the intact failing human heart: progressive receptor down-regulation and subsensitivity to agonist response. Circulation 1986; 74:1290–1302.
130. Feldman Am, Cates AE, Veazey WB, Hershberger RE, Bristow MR, Baughman KL, Baumgartner WA, Van Dop C. Increase of the 40,000-mol wt pertussis toxin substrate (G protein) in the failing human heart. J Clin Invest 1988; 82:189–197.
131. Bohm M, Gierschik P, Jakobs KH, Schnabel P, Kemkes B, Erdmann E. Localization of a "postreceptor" defect in human dilated cardiomyopathy. Am J Cardiol 1989; 64:812–814.
132. Neumann J, Scholz H, Doring V, Schmitz W, von Meyerinck L, Kalmar P. Increase in myocardial G_i-proteins in heart failure. Lancet 1988; 2:936–937.
133. Feldman AM, Cates AE, Bristow MR, Van Dop C. Altered expression of α-subunits of G proteins in failing human hearts. J Mol Cell Cardiol 1989; 21:359–365.
134. Hammond HK, Ransnas LA, White FC, Bloor CM, Insel PA. Myocardial β-receptor number, pharmacological responsiveness, and G_s in volume overload hypertrophy in pigs (abstr). Circulation 1988; 78(suppl II):II-163.
135. Longabaugh JP, Vatner DE, Vatner SF, Homcy CJ. Decreased stimulatory guanosine triphosphate binding protein in dogs with pressure-overload left ventricular failure. J Clin Invest 1988; 81:420–424.
136. Vatner DE, Vatner SF, Nejima J, Uemura N, Susanni EE, Hintze TH, Homcy CJ. Chronic norepinephrine elicits desensitization by uncoupling the β-receptor. J Clin Invest 1989; 84:1741–1748.
137. Horn EM, Corwin SJ, Steinberg SF, Chow YK, Neuberg GW, Cannon PJ, Powers ER, Bilezilian JP. Reduced lymphocyte stimulatory guanine nucleotide regulatory protein and β-adrenergic receptors in congestive heart failure and reversal with angiotensin converting enzyme inhibitor therapy. Circulation 1988; 78:1373–1379.
138. Ransnas LA, Hjalmarson A, Insel PA. Dilated cardiomyopathy is associated with an impaired activation of the stimulatory G-protein, Gs, by GTP in heart membranes (abstr). Circulation 1988; 78(suppl II):II-178.
139. Feldman MD, Copelas L, Gwathmey JK, Phillips P, Warren SE, Schoen FJ, Grossman W, Morgan JP. Deficient production of cyclic AMP: pharmacologic evidence of an important cause of contractile dysfunction in patients with end-stage heart failure. Circulation 1987; 75:331–339.

140. Colucci WS, Leatherman GF, Ludmer PL, Gauthier DF. β-adrenergic inotropic responsiveness of patients with heart failure: studies with intracoronary dobutamine infusion. Circ Res 1987; 61(suppl I):I-82–I-86.
141. Heilbrunn SM, Shah P, Bristow MR, Valantine HA, Ginsberg R, Fowler MB. Increased β-receptor density and improved hemodynamic response to catecholamine stimulation during long-term metoprolol therapy in heart failure from dilated cardiomyopathy. Circulation 1989; 79:483–490.
142. Waagstein, F, Caidahl K, Wallentin I, Bergh C, Hjalmarson A. Long term β-blockade in dilated cardiomyopathy. Effects of short- and long-term metoprolol treatment followed by withdrawal and readministration of metoprolol. Circulation 1989; 80:551–563.
143. Eichhorn EJ, Bedotto JB, Malloy CR, Hatfield BA, Deitchman D, Brown M, Willard JE, Grayburn PA. Effect of beta-adrenergic blockade on myocardial function and energetics in congestive heart failure: improvements in hemodynamic, contractile, and diastolic performance with bucindolol. Circulation 1990; 82:473–483.
144. Gilbert EM, Anderson JL, Deitchman D, Yanowitz FG, O'Connell JB, Renlund DG, Bartholomew M, Mealey PC, Larrabee P, Bristow MR: Chronic β-blocker–vasodilator therapy improves cardiac function in idiopathic dilated cardiomyopathy: A double-blind, randomized study of bucindolol versus placebo. Am J Med 1990; 88:223–229.
145. O'Connor PC, Finch MJ, Harron DWG, Meredith PA, McDevitt DG, Shanks RG: Comparison of the hemodynamic effects of bucindolol, propranolol, and pindolol in healthy volunteers. Br J Clin Pharmacol 1985; 20:659–667.
146. Deitchman D, Perhach JL, Synder RW: β-adrenoceptor and cardiovascular effects of MJ 13105 (bucindolol) in anesthetized dogs and rats. Eur J Pharmacol 1980; 61:263–277.
147. Stanton HC, Dungan KW: In vitro effects of beta adrenoceptor agonists and antagonists on the rat ovarian suspensory ligament. J Pharmacol Exp Ther 1986; 239:591–596.
148. Hershberger RE, Wynn JR, Sundberg L, Bristow MR: Mechanism of action of bucindolol in human ventricular myocardium. J Cardiovasc Pharm 1990; 15:959–967.
149. Sweeney ME, Fletcher BJ, Fletcher GF. Exercise testing and training with β-adrenergic blockade: role of the drug washout period in "unmasking" a training effect. Am Heart J 1989; 118:941–946.
150. Kaiser P, Tesch PA, Thorsson A, Karlsson J, Kaijser L. Skeletal muscle glycolysis during submaximal exercise following acute β-adrenergic blockade in man. Acta Physiol Scand 1985; 123:285–291.
151. Vik-Mo H, Mjos OD. Influence of free fatty acids on myocardial oxygen consumption and ischemic injury. Am J Cardiol 1981; 48:361–365.
152. Mjos OD. Effect of inhibition of lipolysis on myocardial oxygen consumption in the presence of isoproterenol. J Clin Invest 1971; 50:1869–1873.

153. Bing RJ, Siegal A, Ungar J, Gilbert M. Metabolism of the human heart. II. Studies on fat, ketone and amino acid metabolism. Am J Med 1954; 16:504–515.
154. Kjekshus JK, Mjos OD. Effect on inhibition of lipolysis on myocardial oxygen consumption in the presence of isoproterenol. J Clin Invest 1972; 51:1767–1776.
155. Simonsen S, Kjekshus JK. The effect of free fatty acids on myocardial oxygen consumption during atrial pacing and catecholamine infusion in man. Circulation 1978; 58:484–491.
156. Bostrom M, Nie Z, Goertz G, Henriksson J, Wallberg-Henriksson H. Indirect effect of catecholamines on development of insulin resistance in skeletal muscle from diabetic rats. Diabetes 1989; 38:906–910.
157. Chiasson J-L, Shikama H, Chu DTW, Exton JH. Inhibitory effect of epinephrine on insulin-stimulated glucose uptake by rat skeletal muscle. J Clin Invest 1981; 68:706–713.
158. Neely J, Morgan H. Relationship between carbohydrate and lipod metabolism and energy balance of the heart. Ann Rev Physiol 1974; 36:413–459.
159. Waagstein F, Hjalmarson A, Swedberg K, Wallentin I. Beta-blockers in dilated cardiomyopathies: they work. Eur Heart J 1983; 4(suppl A):173–178.
160. Eichhorn EJ, McGhie AI, Bedotto JB, Corbett JR, Malloy CR, Hatfield BA, Deitchman D, Willard JE, Grayburn PA. Effects of bucindolol on neurohormonal activation in congestive heart failure. Am J Cardiol 1991; 67:67–73.
161. Henderson EB, Kahn JK, Corbett JR, Jansen DE, Pippin JJ, Kulkarni P, Ugolini V, Akers MS, Hansen C, Buja LM, Parkey RW, Willerson JT. Abnormal I-123 metaiodobenzylguanidine myocardial washout and distribution may reflect myocardial adrenergic derangement in patients with congestive heart failure. Circulation 1988; 78:1192–1199.
162. Hirakata H, Fouad-Tarazi FM, Bumpus M, Khosla M, Healy B, Husain A, Urata H, Kumagai H. Angiotensins and the failing heart. Enhanced positive inotropic response to angiotensin I in cardiomyopathic hamster heart in the presence of captopril. Circ Res 1990; 66:891–899.
163. Binkley PF, Lewe R, Lima J, Unverferth DV, Leier CV. Neurohormonal profile in congestive heart failure: response to β-blockade. J Lab Clin Med 1988; 111:393–398.
164. Rona G, Chappel CI, Balazs T, Gaudry R: An infarct-like myocardial lesion and other toxic manifestations produced by isoproterenol in the rat. Arch Pathol 1958; 67:443–455.
165. Reichenbach DD, Benditt EP: Catecholamines and cardiomyopathy: The pathogenesis and potential importance of myofibrillar degeneration. Hum Pathol 1970; 1:125–149.
166. Haft JI: Cardiovascular injury induced by sympathetic catecholamines. Prog Cardiovasc Dis 1974; 17:73–85.

167. Packer M. Pathophysiological mechanisms underlying the effects of β-adrenergic agonists and antagonists on functional capacity and survival in chronic heart failure. Circulation 1990; 82(suppl I):I-77–I-88.
168. Alderman J, Grossman W. Are β-adrenergic-blocking drugs useful in the treatment of dilated cardiomyopathy? Circulation 1985; 71:854–857.
169. Fowler MB, Bristow MR. Rationale for beta-adrenergic blocking drugs in cardiomyopathy. Am J Cardiol 1985; 55(suppl D):120D–124D.
170. Yusuf S, Peto R, Lewis J, Collins R, Sleight P. Beta blockade during and after myocardial infarction: an overview of the randomized trials. Prog Cardiovasc Dis 1985; 27:335–371.
171. Norwegian Multicenter Study Group. Timolol-induced reduction in mortality and reinfarction in patients surviving acute myocardial infarction. N Engl J Med 1981; 304:801–807.
172. ISIS-1 Collaborative Group. Randomized trial of intravenous atenolol among 16,027 cases of suspected acute myocardial infarction. Lancet 1986; 2:57–69.
173. Prichard BNC, Tomlinson B. Progress in antihypertensive therapy with multiple-action drug. Drugs 1988; 36(suppl 6):20–25.
174. DasGupta P, Broadhurst PA, Lahiri A. Improvement in congestive heart failure following chronic therapy with a new vasodilating beta-blocker: carvedilol (abstr). Circulation 1989; 80(suppl II):II-117.
175. Pouleur H, Etienne J, Van Mechelen H, Gurné O, Rousseau MF. Effects of the β_1-adrenergic receptor partial agonist xamoterol on left ventricular diastolic function. An evaluation after 1–6 years of oral therapy. Circulation 1990; 81(suppl III):III-87–III-92.
176. Marlow HF. Review of clinical experience with xamoterol. Effects on exercise capacity and symptoms in heart failure. Circulation 1990; 81(suppl III):III-93–III-98.
177. The German and Austrian Xamoterol Group. Double-blind placebo-controlled comparison of digoxin and xamoterol in chronic heart failure. Lancet 1988; 1:489–493.
178. Pouleur H, Rosseau MF, Mengeot P, Veriter C, Vincent MF, Brasseur LA. Improvement of global and regional left ventricular function in patients with previous myocardial infarction by a new β_1 adrenoceptor partial agonist, ICI 118,587. Eur Heart J 1982; 3(suppl D):123–127.
179. Hall JA, Kaufmann AJ, Brown MJ. Selective β_1-adrenoceptor blockade enhances positive inotropic responses to endogenous catecholamines mediated through β_2-adrenoceptors in human atrial myocardium. Circ Res 1990; 66:1610–1623.
180. Schubert B, Van Dongen AMJ, Kirsch GE, Brown AM. β-adrenergic inhibition of cardiac sodium channels by dual G-protein pathways. Science 1989; 245:516–519.
181. Swedberg K. Is neurohormonal activation deleterious to the long-term outcome of patients with congestive heart failure? II. Protagonist's viewpoint. J Am Coll Cardiol 1988; 12:550–554.

182. Woodley SL, Gilbert EM, Anderson JL, O'Connell JB, Deitchman D, Yanowitz FG, Mealey PC, Volkman K, Renlund DG, Bristow MR. β-blockade with bucindolol in heart failure due to ischemic vs idiopathic dilated cardiomyopathy. Circulation 1991; 84:2426–2441.
183. Cohn JN, Johnson G, Ziesche S, Cobb F, Francis G, Tristani F, Smith R, Dunkman WB, Loeb H, Wong M, Bhat G, Goldman S, Fletcher RD, Doherty J, Hughes CV, Carson P, Cintron G, Shabetai R, Haakenson C. A comparison of enalapril with hydralazine-isosorbide dinitrate in the treatment of chronic congestive heart failure. N Engl J Med 1991; 325:303–10.

13

Dopamine Receptor Agonists in Heart Failure

Cesare Casagrande
Zambon Research, Cormano, Milan, Italy

INTRODUCTION

It is commonly recognized that therapy for heart failure has progressed much faster in the past decade than at any previous time (1–4). This development was initiated by the proposal to use vasodilators (5) and was substantiated by the availability of angiotensin converting enzyme (ACE) inhibitors. Clinical investigations of this class of drugs have opened a debate on the therapeutic relevance not only of direct hemodynamic reduction of afterload but also on the reversal of neurohumoral activation (6). Progress in understanding the pathophysiological mechanisms underlying heart failure has been accompanied by advances in the design of controlled clinical trials, considering various end points, such as mortality, morbidity, quality of life, hemodynamics, and neurohumoral status, as well as the interrelation between such points, or lack of it (7). The initial expectations from new positive inotropic agents acting by phosphodiesterase inhibition ended in disappointment but created one (8) of several occasions on which controversy over the clinical efficacy of digitalis saw points being scored in favor of this classical drug. The search for safe and effective positive inotropic agents based on new mechanisms of action continues. The general consensus is that knowledge of heart failure and how to treat it is moving quickly, and also that further progress, including new therapeutic approaches, is needed, since the disease is becoming more prevalent as the age of the population increases (1,9).

Interest in dopamine receptor agonists, initiated by the pioneering work of L. I. Goldberg in the 1960s, led to the established use of dopamine (DA) in acute heart failure and shock in the following decade. Only a few investigators made contributions in this field, since progress was hindered by the lack of orally absorbed drugs. The "state of the art" at the time was recapitulated in a review by Goldberg and Kohli (10) that drew attention to the potential usefulness of peripherally acting dopaminergic agents in cardiovascular disease. In the last decade various other groups joined the field, contributing basic knowledge and experimental drugs. The purpose of this review is to examine the present state of the art and provide a perspective on the potential of dopamine receptor agonists as a new therapeutic approach in chronic congestive heart failure (CHF).

In the first clinical study of intravenous infusion of DA in CHF patients, Goldberg and his associates (11) observed a marked diuretic and natriuretic effect. Shortly afterward, in a second study (12), they were able to demonstrate that not only was sodium (Na^+) excretion increased, but also renal plasma flow (RPF) and glomerular filtration rate (GFR). These studies were the starting point of three interrelated avenues of research: (1) identification and classification of specific receptors mediating the effect of DA in the periphery; (2) exploration of the physiological role of DA in the cardiovascular and renal system; and (3) investigation of the therapeutic application of DA and, later on, of new dopaminergic drugs, not only in CHF, but also in hypertension, renal diseases, and other clinical conditions.

DOPAMINE RECEPTORS IN THE CARDIOVASCULAR AND RENAL SYSTEM

The pharmacology of peripheral dopamine receptors has recorded important progress (13,14) and has generated ideas, methodologies, and experimental drugs that are also important in exploring the physiological role of the amine. The investigations were developed by comparing the newly discovered receptors with the central nervous system (CNS) receptors subserving the central neurotransmitter function of DA, in terms of agonist and antagonist affinity, pharmacological response, and signal transduction mechanism. The use of the DA_1 and DA_2 denominations (15) arose from the need to analyze the two subtypes of peripheral receptors as being potentially distinct from the central D_1 and D_2 receptors.

The distribution of dopamine receptors is schematically shown in Figure 1. The existence of DA_1 receptors located on smooth muscle cells in the arterial bed, and their prevalence in the renal district, and also in the mes-

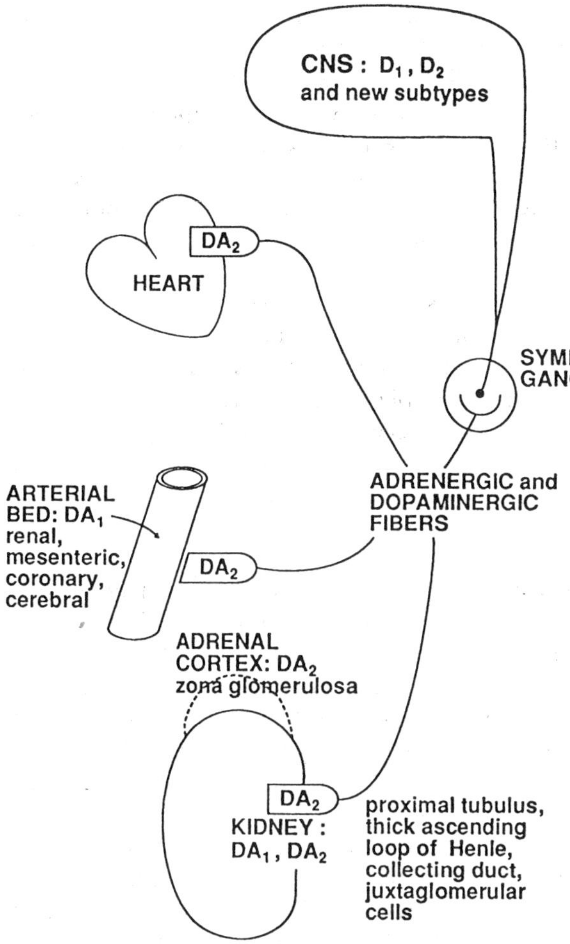

Figure 1 Dopamine receptors acting on the cardiovascular and renal system.

enteric, coronary, and cerebral bed, provided the main focus for the research of Goldberg and his group (13). The function of these receptors is to produce arterial vasodilation directly via stimulation of adenylate cyclase and increased availability of cAMP.

Receptors of the DA_2 subtype (16) are located in sympathetic fibers afferent to blood vessels, the kidney, and the heart. They decrease sympathetic transmission and norepinephrine (NE) release, thus buffering the influence of sympathetic activation of either central or peripheral origin on cardiac, vascular, and renal functions. DA_2 receptors in sympathetic ganglia similarly contribute to the control of sympathetic tone.

There are also a number of indications that activation of central D_2 receptors decreases sympathetic nerve activity in the periphery (17), but it was recently reported that quinpirole, a D_2 receptor agonist, induced a centrally mediated increase in sympathetic tone and in vasopressin release (18); further investigations are required in order to clarify whether these effects are actually mediated by dopamine receptors of either the D_2 or other subtypes.

An important physiological role is exerted by DA_2 receptors in the adrenal cortex, having a tonic inhibitory control on aldosterone secretion. The administration of dopamine receptor antagonists, such as metoclopramide, induces a marked increase in plasma aldosterone levels (19,20). In addition to prejunctional receptors, receptors of the DA_2 subtype have recently been reported to be present in postjunctional locations in blood vessels, as detected by biochemical (21) and autoradiographic techniques (22). It is still unclear whether these postjunctional receptors play any function role.

DA_2 receptors appear to be associated with various effector mechanisms, including inhibition of adenylate cyclase, inhibition of phosphatidyl inositol turnover, and increased potassium channel activity (20,21,23). An intriguing discussion of the possibility that the differences in potency observed with various agonist and antagonists may be related to the presence of different populations of both DA_1 and DA_2 receptors in the cardiovascular system was started a few years ago (24) but is still far from any conclusion (25).

Recently, there has been an impressive acceleration in research on central dopamine receptors, resulting from the use of molecular biology methodology. New receptors have been cloned and denominated D_3, D_4, and D_5 (26–28); D_3 and D_4 receptors have shown properties similar but not identical to D_2, while D_5 receptors appear to display properties similar but not identical to D_1. In addition to their difference in structure and affinity for agonist and antagonist, the distribution of D_3, D_4, and D_5 in various areas of the brain also appears to differ from that of the D_1 and D_2 receptors. This progress has opened new avenues in the search for new drugs for Parkinson's disease, schizophrenia, depression, and possibly other conditions. Transferring this knowledge to the analysis of peripheral receptors will most probably contribute to the understanding of the major issues still unresolved.

This is of particular importance for kidney receptors, which have been discovered in several locations, partially overcoming methodological problems in identifying pharmacological responses dependent on vascular receptors, prejunctional neuronal receptors, and receptors located in the elements of the nephron. Recent results have confirmed that receptors exist in the proximal convoluted tubule that inhibit Na^+ reabsorption by a twofold mechanism, involving both inhibition of the Na^+, H^+-exchanger at the brush-border membrane (29) and inhibition of Na^+, K^+-ATPase at the basolateral membrane. While the luminal-side receptor fits the previous hypothesis of a DA_1 subtype (action mediated by cAMP), the nature of the interstitial-side receptor is under discussion, propositions being advanced that this is either a DA_1-modulated DA_2 receptor, using diacylglycerol as a second messenger (30), or a new type of DA_1 receptor, mediating phospholipase activation (31). In addition, DAARP-32 (dopamine- and cAMP-regulated phosphoprotein), a phosphatase inhibitor previously identified in brain regions rich in dopaminergic innervation, has been shown to be involved in DA_1-mediated inhibition of Na^+, K^+-ATPase in the medullary thick ascending limb of Henle (32).

Very recently, the finding that there are dense ^{3}H-spiperone binding sites in the inner medulla led to the identification of a new receptor denominated DA_{2K} in cells of the collecting duct, i.e., the principal site of prostaglandin E_2 (PGE_2) production in the kidney (33). Cultured cells were shown to enhance production of PGE_2 under stimulation with DA or bromocriptine, a D_2 and DA_2 agonist, and the effect was counteracted by the DA_2 antagonist domperidone. These findings point to the possibility that the vasodilator and diuretic effects of DA may in part be mediated by PGE_2. However, an investigation of gludopa, a prodrug of DA endowed with selective renal effects, had failed to reveal any interference by indomethacin in the effects of the drug on healthy volunteers (34). On the other hand, DA infusion has been shown to increase urinary excretion of prostacyclin metabolites (35).

Previous findings of DA_2 receptors located in glomeruli in the rat kidney (36) have not been confirmed by recent studies using autoradiographic techniques (37). It is still hard to interpret the renal effects of selective DA_2 agonists and the involvement of intrarenal receptors (29,30,38–40), in part owing to the simultaneous activation of prejunctional DA_2 receptors on renal innervation.

The influence of DA on the release of renin has not been investigated in depth. Studies with DA itself, and particularly infusion in humans at various rates, were complicated by the α- and β-adrenergic effects of the amine. However, the presence of DA_1 receptors mediating renin release in the juxtaglomerular cells has been demonstrated both in vitro and in vivo (41,42). On the other hand, the observation that DA_2 stimulation

(43,44) decreases renin release requires further investigation in order to clarify whether this depends directly on a local receptor or whether it is mediated by neuronal DA_2 receptors affecting NE release.

Several dopamine agonists and antagonists have been used as experimental tools in analyzing peripheral dopaminergic receptors. In the original work of Goldberg and Kohli (13), DA and its *N,N*-dipropyl derivative, which prevailingly affect DA_1 and DA_2 receptors, respectively, were used to separate the functional responses. Later on, progress in the analysis of the DA_1 receptor was promoted by the availability of two structurally related benzazepine derivatives, i.e., fenoldopam, a selective agonist also used in clinical investigations, and SCH 23390, a selective antagonist. (S)-sulpiride and domperidone have been used as DA_2 antagonists, the latter providing both selectivity and peripheral distribution and allowing peripheral and central responses to be separated. Ergoline derivatives and congeners have also served as DA_2 agonists (45).

THE ORIGIN AND PHYSIOLOGICAL ROLE OF DOPAMINE IN THE CARDIOVASCULAR AND RENAL SYSTEM

Free DA is present in plasma in small amounts (40–50 pg/ml), versus a large amount (2500–5000 pg/ml) of DA conjugates. Free DA is almost 10 times less abundant than free NE, but conjugated DA represents approximately 50% of the total plasma catecholamine pool. In humans DA is sulfoconjugated, mostly as dopamine 3-O-sulfate. Circulating DA is basically derived from peripheral sources, since centrally generated catecholamines are almost completely metabolized within the CNS. A substantial portion of DA originates from noradrenergic neurons and the adrenal medulla, where it is synthesized as a precursor of NE and epinephrine. Maneuvers that induce strong sympathetic activation also increase circulating DA.

The existence and function of peripheral dopaminergic neurons have been debated for many years. They were finalistically postulated by associating the demonstrated neurotransmitter role of dopamine in the CNS and the presence of dopamine receptors mediating pharmacologically significant responses in various peripheral organs. Substantial evidence of dopaminergic innervation in the kidney has been provided by Bell (46) from biochemical and histochemical studies in the dog. Dopaminergic fiber terminals were found in proximity to tubular elements, juxtaglomerular cells, and the glomerular vascular pole. It was also shown that denervation decreased venous DA outflow, whereas renal nerve stimulation increased it. Significant, albeit more limited, information is available on the dopaminergic innervation of the human kidney and liver (47).

Investigating the functional role of dopaminergic nerves is made difficult by the predominance of noradrenergic terminals. Pharmacological results showing that DA_2 receptor blockade with domperidone increases dopamine release in the kidneys of normotensive and hypertensive subjects (48) provide indirect evidence suggesting the presence on dopaminergic neurons of "autoreceptors" controlling the release of DA by a feedback mechanism.

DA of neural origin therefore appears to be released in the kidney and possibly to contribute to circulating plasma levels. It is now recognized, however, that most renal DA, as well as urinary DA, is of nonneural origin, being produced from the decarboxylation of plasmatic L-dopa by dopa decarboxylase in the tubular epithelium. L-dopa is present in larger amounts in plasma than NE itself. The renal synthesis of DA was initially suggested by Ball and Lee (49) and has now been confirmed by extensive evidence (46,50,51), supporting a paracrine hormonal role of the amine, mediated by the various dopamine receptors in the kidney. Renal DA is partially circulated but largely excreted in urine, where it appears in amounts about 10 times greater than those of NE. Dopamine excretion is significantly increased (e.g., from 1.2 to 1.8 μmol/24 h) by a high-sodium diet. On the other hand, no correlation has been found between levels of endogenous DA in plasma and Na^+ excretion. Plasma concentrations of DA following intravenous administration of the drug in the doses required to induce natriuresis have proved to be much higher than the physiological levels (52).

Interestingly, along similar lines, it has recently been shown that DA in the adrenal cortex is also synthesized from plasma L-dopa (53) but not from tyrosine, which increases DA synthesis only in the medulla. These findings support a local link between endogenous production of DA and the DA_2 receptor controlling aldosterone release.

The hypothesis that a significant fraction of renal and urinary DA might be derived from the large amounts of sulfoconjugated DA present in plasma by sulfatase deconjugation (54) is no longer supported.

The presence of endogenous DA in organs provided with a variety of dopamine receptors suggested that it may elicit physiological control of kidney function, vascular resistance, and extracellular fluid volume and has promoted various investigations on the role of endogenous DA in essential hypertension (55). Alterations in both central and peripheral dopaminergic mechanisms are thought to be involved in the development of hypertension in various animal models and in humans (56). Recently, the idea has been put forward that dopaminergic mechanisms may be physiologically activated to counteract the increase in blood pressure in the early phases of the disease, but thereafter fail during its progression (57). Lee investigated the increase in renal synthesis and exertion of DA in response to salt loading in laboratory animals and humans and suggested that DA is released to act as an intrarenal natriuretic hormone. According to his hypothesis, the inability to mobilize kidney DA adequately under salt loading represents the fault of an essential natriuretic mechanism. This fault is peculiar to salt-sensitive hypertensives and is more common in West Africans and in their descendants on the American continent (58). It deserves thorough investigation as a causative factor in essential hypertension. The same, or a similar, fault was shown to be present in a group of patients with hypertension consequent to chronic glomerulonephritis. While this hypothesis awaits confirmation, pharmacological research directed to the treatment of hypertension with dopaminergic agents is certainly warranted.

Investigations on the role of endogenous DA in CHF have been more limited than those on hypertension. The ratio of DA to NE in cardiac tissues is known to increase in CHF, as a consequence of depressed dopamine β-hydroxylase activity (59). While any relevance of this increase to cardiac function is unknown, it appears improbable that it can contribute to a significant extent to the circulating pool of free DA.

Mercuro et al. have shown a threefold increase in the circulating level of dihydroxyphenylacetic acid (DOPAC), the main metabolite of DA, in a group of CHF patients, probably as a consequence of peripheral sympathetic hyperactivity. Whether this increased synthesis and metabolism represents the expression of metabolic waste, or an expression of increased availability of active DA in dopaminergic terminals, is at present unknown (60). Contrary to a previous report (61), plasma levels of DA were not increased in this group of patients. It is interesting, however, to note that plasma DOPAC was reduced when the overt symptoms of these patients regressed during hospitalization and treatment.

An interesting observation by Lang and Kaufmann (62) on the urinary excretion of DA in CHF patients of New York Heart Association (NYHA) classes II, III, and IV suggests a possible compensatory role of DA in mild heart failure, the efficiency of which could be decreased in patients with severe CHF. The urinary excretion of DA was increased in symptomatic conditions to 1900, 1400, and 1000 μg/d in class II, III, and IV, respectively, and went back to the normal range (400–800 μg/d) when the conditions of the patients were normalized by an efficacious treatment. A similar normalization of DA excretion following treatment of a group of class III and IV patients (2450 μg/d decreased to 529 μg/d after treatment) has recently been reported by another group (63). These results warrant further investigations on kidney DA synthesis CHF. Investigations in idiopathic edema have indicated that urinary DA excretion may be impaired in this condition (64,65).

Recently, two cases of severe orthostatic hypertension caused by congenital deficiency of dopamine β-hydroxylase have been reported (66). Plasma NE was absent, while free DA amounted to 250–300 pg/ml, i.e., five to six times normal values. Na^+ excretion was abnormally high. Intravenous treatment with metoclopramide or domperidone raised the pressure for 30 to 60 min, suggesting that not only the lack of NE, but also excessive DA, was part of the etiology of this syndrome. Treatment with DL-dihydroxyphenylserine, a precursor of NE bypassing the dopamine β-hydroxylase step, at 500 mg b.i.d. brought the patients back to normal conditions for over one year.

DOPAMINE AND ATRIAL NATRIURETIC FACTOR

Dopamine and atrial natriuretic factor (ANF) share a number of pharmacological effects, e.g., increasing renal blood flow (RBF), increasing diuresis and Na^+ excretion, and depressing aldosterone release. Human studies of applications of lower body positive pressure or water immersion suggest that endogenous DA is also involved in mediating natriuretic response in these conditions. This response was abolished by domperidone and metoclopramide treatment (67,68). A number of laboratory and clinical studies have dealt with the possible interrelation of ANF and DA effects. The mutual potentiation of receptorial effects has been investigated, as have the induction of ANF release by DA and the stimulation of DA synthesis in the kidney by ANF.

Differing points of view were recently summarized by Kurokawa and colleagues (69) and by Murphy and Bass (70), who considered, respectively, a multiplicity of studies either indicating that kidney DA plays a role as a necessary permissive factor in the natriuretic effect of ANF at a postreceptorial level, or denying it. Murphy and Bass analyzed a number of experimental studies and challenged the physiological meaning of results obtained by blockade of DA_1 receptor by SCH 23390 in the rat, in view of negative results in dogs, monkeys, and humans. They also pointed out the contrasting results obtained, using inhibition by carbidopa, on the requirement of active DA synthesis for the natriuretic effects of ANF. Other authors (71) substantially supported Kurokawa and colleagues' views (69) and even pointed out that ANF is able to displace competitively ^3H-SCH 23390, a DA_1 receptor ligand, in renal medulla preparations, but not in renal cortex preparations.

The picture is further complicated by results showing modifications of ANF effects by DA_2 receptor agonists, when recent information on intrarenal DA_2 receptors is considered. It has also been shown that ANF not only attenuates aldosterone response to angiotensin II, but also inhibits the release of aldosterone resulting from the withdrawal of dopaminergic control when the DA_2 antagonist metoclopramide is administered to healthy volunteers (72).

The natriuretic effects of dopamine appear not to be dependent on ANF release, as was shown by the induction of diuresis and natriuresis in healthy subjects by a DA infusion of 4 μg/kg/min without causing any change in plasma ANF levels (73). On the other hand, one would expect infusion of DA to modify ANF levels. Release of ANF may be stimulated when DA increases venous return and cardiac contractility, either directly or by releasing NE. On the contrary, elevated ANF plasma levels in CHF patients may decrease when cardiac preload is reduced by DA or related agents (74,75).

DOPAMINE AND DOPAMINE RECEPTOR AGONISTS IN THE TREATMENT OF HEART FAILURE

The clinical use of DA is based on the modulation of its multiple receptor interactions by progressively recruiting dopamine receptors, β-adrenoceptors, and α-adrenoceptors at increasing rates of infusion (76). Indeed, DA can represent three different medications, depending on whether the first class, or the first and second, or all three classes of receptors are activated. The combined positive inotropic and vasodilator effects elicited at intermediate rates of infusion, on the order of 5 μg/kg/min, recently led Opie to describe DA, as well as ibopamine, as a member of the therapeutic class of "inodilators" (77). In this class, however, DA and dopamine-like agents may represent a special category, since they can elicit a complex action that is not limited to inotropic stimulation and direct vasodilator effects. The multiplicity of dopaminergic mechanisms that are potentially amenable to therapeutic exploitation in CHF is outlined in Figure 2. Dopamine at low rates of infusion, on the order of 1–2 μg/kg/min, as well as dopamine receptor agonists endowed with DA_1 and DA_2 activity and devoid of β-receptor activity, can produce useful pharmacological effects promoting Na^+ excretion, reducing afterload, and counteracting sympathetic and renin-angiotensin-aldosterone stimulation. It is difficult to separate and analyze the therapeutic relevance of each of these effects; it may depend upon the drug used, as well as the clinical condition of the patient and concomitant therapy.

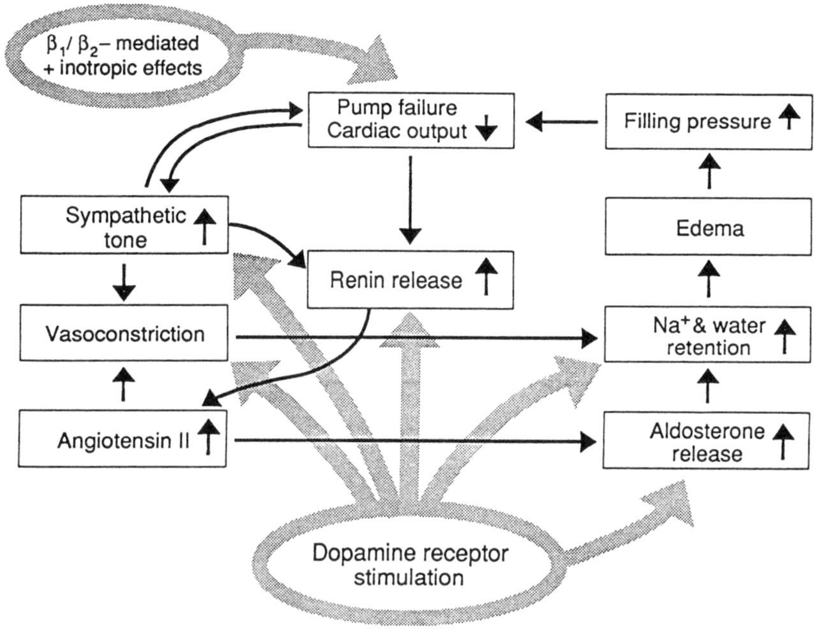

Figure 2 Components of the therapeutic action of dopamine receptor agonists in congestive heart failure.

Dopamine is not active by oral administration, and its effects, even on intravenous administration, are short-lived and can be sustained only by continuous infusion. In order to extend its potential therapeutic benefit in the chronic treatment of CHF, orally active dopamine-like drugs were desirable and were searched for by various investigators. The formulas of the drugs discussed in this paper are shown in Figure 3.

Some investigators were attracted by the possibility of developing agonists selective for the newly discovered dopamine receptors, and particularly for the DA_1 subtype held to be responsible for renal vasodilator and natriuretic effects. Their efforts led to the discovery of fenoldopam and dopexamine. Goldberg's group devoted attention to levodopa as an orally bioavailable precursor of DA. Other groups, including our own, started investigations on prodrugs of DA, and of dopamine analogues, suitably designed to overcome first-pass inactivation and prolong the duration of action. This work on dopaminergic prodrugs has recently been reviewed (78). The clinical application of ibopamine and some preliminary studies concerning docarpamine document the usefulness of this approach. An

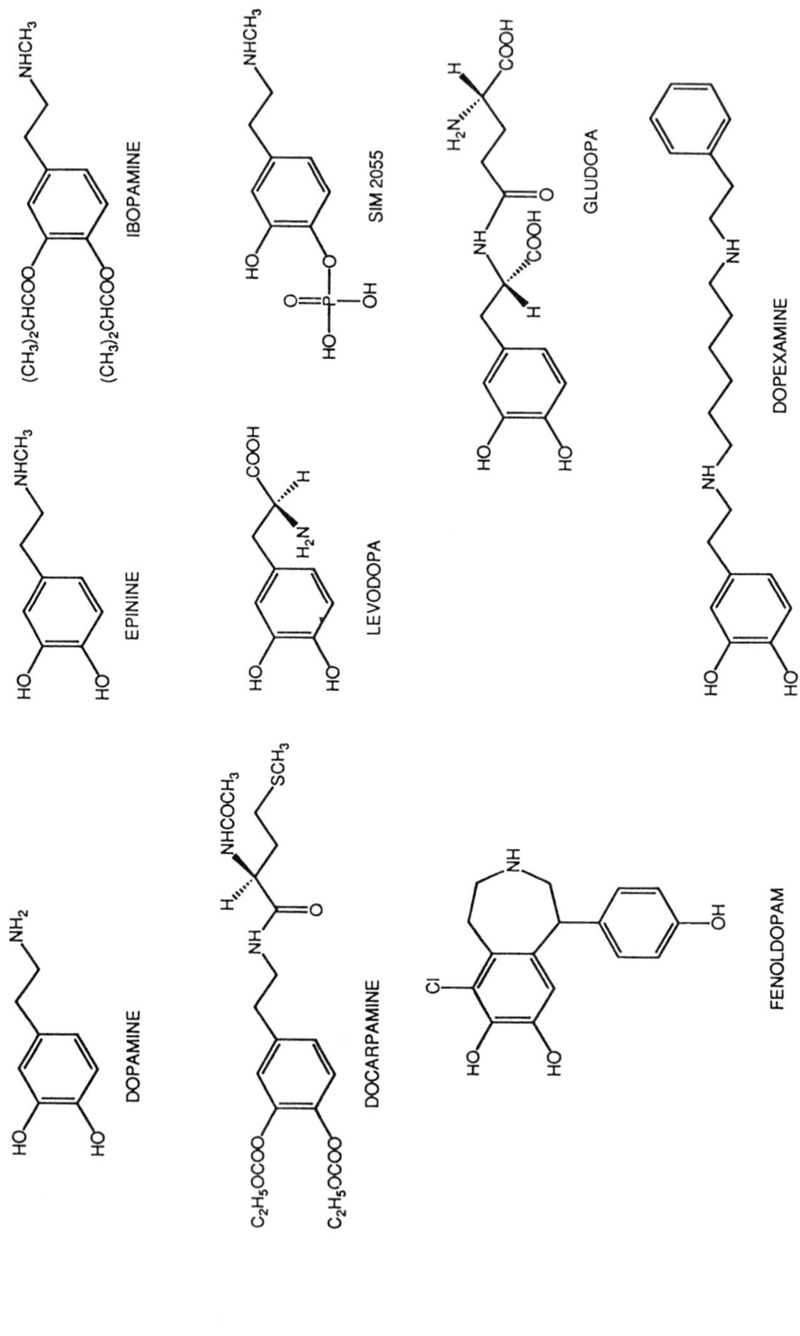

Figure 3 Dopamine receptor agonists and prodrugs.

additional possibility in the design of a prodrug is to use molecular moieties that metabolically determine selective delivery to a target organ; a notable example is gludopa, which achieves a good degree of renal selectivity. Gludopa, which is not orally active, has been used as a tool in the investigation of renal dopaminergic mechanisms in man (58). Recently, we have succeeded in producing a prodrug, Sim 2055 (*N*-methyldopamine 4-O-phosphate), showing oral activity and renal selectivity in laboratory studies.

Dopamine Infusion

The clinical use of DA, ranging from low ("renal") doses of 0.5–2 μg/kg/min to the intermediate doses of 4–5 μg/kg/min and up to the high rate of infusion used to induce pressor effects by stimulation of α-adrenoceptors, was reviewed by Goldberg in one of his last papers (76).

Some recent studies, providing additional information on its optimal use, either in comparison with or in combination with other sympathomimetic amines, are considered here. When a pressor effect is desired, as in the treatment of shock, the advantage of DA in comparison with NE is its superior effect on diuresis and cardiac output (CO). A combination of the two amines has been investigated as a way of optimally combining positive inotropic and pressor effects with the requirement of improving renal perfusion and diuresis (79).

A recent investigation on the action of DA on renal function, which was designed to explore the effects on ANF release, yielded several interesting observations (74). The study compared 10 normal subjects and 10 CHF patients in NYHA classes III and IV. With an infusion at 1.5 μg/kg/min, diuresis, natriuresis, and GFR were markedly and similarly increased in both groups, albeit starting from different basal levels. Plasma levels of NE, renin activity, and aldosterone were significantly reduced from their abnormally high values in patients, but were unchanged in normal subjects, except for NE, which doubled its value after 1 h of infusion. Atrial natriuretic factor was reduced (from 30 to 35 pg/ml) and augmented (from 9 to 17 pg/ml) in patients and normal subjects, respectively. In both groups a clear statistical correlation was shown between ANF and NE levels.

The contribution of vasodilator dopaminergic mechanisms, in addition to natriuresis, to the action of low-rate (2 μg/kg/min) DA has been described in a detailed analysis of the hemodynamic response (80). Cardiac output was increased and systemic vascular resistance (SVR) decreased. Left ventricular end-systolic wall stress also declined significantly, while the velocity of ventricular fiber shortening was scarcely modified, showing that afterload reduction was the main determinant of the effect, unlike that of dobutamine, which showed direct cardiac effects when tested at the same rate of infusion. The same group (81) has recently shown that myocardial oxygen consumption was significantly decreased by this dose of DA, whereas it was significantly increased at 6 μg/kg/min.

In order to exploit the beneficial action of the low doses, DA at 2.5 μg/kg/min was combined with dobutamine (approximately 7 μg/kg/min) in patients with heart failure following acute myocardial infarction, resulting in doubling of urine flow, as well as enhancement of the positive inotropic support of dobutamine (82). It was considered that the combination with dobutamine provides a greater increase in CO and avoids the α-adrenergic effect of high doses of DA.

A pharmacological investigation in dogs has revealed that differences between dobutamine and DA relate not only to stimulation of α_1-adrenoceptors in the arterial bed at high doses of DA, but also to an α_2-adrenergic component contributing prejunctionally to the control of heart rate (HR) and postjunctionally to venoconstriction. The latter mechanism may explain the inability of DA to decrease left ventricular filling pressure (LVFP) as effectively as dobutamine (83).

Dopamine, at increasing rates of infusion, and a bolus IV dose of enalaprilat, a potent ACE inhibitor, were compared in nine patients with severe CHF for their respective effects on RBF, measured by a local thermodilution technique, as well as on CO (84). Dopamine increased RBF by 99% at an average rate of 2.1 μg/kg/min, concomitantly with a lesser rise in CO, thus increasing the ratio of RBF to CO from 17% to 27%. At higher rates an additional increase in CO, but not in RBF, occurred. Enalaprilat increased with a parallel time course both CO and RBF, the latter to a maximum of 35%, representing 23% of CO. Both drugs thus increased RBF relative to CO, but DA was markedly more effective and selective. In view of the incidence of deterioration of renal function in patients treated with ACE inhibitors, these results suggest that dopaminergic drugs, or their combination with ACE inhibitors, may be indicated in the chronic treatment of those patients (particularly elderly subjects with normal or low blood pressure and partially impaired renal function) in whom the preservation of renal perfusion and GFR appears to be of major therapeutic importance.

Levodopa

Being available for clinical use in Parkinson's disease, levodopa afforded the first opportunity of investigating an orally active dopamine-like drug in the chronic treatment of CHF.

Starting from a preliminary observation of increased RPF and Na^+ excretion in parkinsonian patients treated with levodopa (85,86), two specific studies on CHF were conducted by Rajfer et al. (87,88).

In the first investigation (87), the acute effects of levodopa were assessed in ten patients in NYHA classes III and IV undergoing Swan-Ganz catheterization. Before the study, the patients were gradually introduced to the drug, starting with 250 mg every 6 h and gradually increasing to a total daily dose of 4 to 6 g, in order to reduce emetic effects. The drug was then withheld for 24 to 36 h before the hemodynamic investigation. An oral dose of 1.5 to 2 g of levodopa induced significant increases in cardiac index (CI) and decreases in SVR from 30 min to 4 h after administration. Blood pressure (BP) and HR were unchanged, and LVFP remained elevated. Of these patients, five continued on levodopa (1.5 to 2 g four times a day with 50 mg/d of pyridoxine hydrochloride, a cofactor of dopa-decarboxylase) in addition to their standard therapy of digitalis and diuretics for 3 to 12 months, showing an improvement in symptoms. These patients where then submitted to a second hemodynamic investigation, showing that the response to levodopa had been maintained and was similar to that of the first treatment. Heart rate was lower after the prolonged treatment.

In the second study (88), which included 14 CHF patients mostly in NYHA classes III and IV, the protocol for acute and chronic treatment was similar to that of the first study. Chronic treatment was continued for 12 weeks, after which 12 patients underwent a second hemodynamic evaluation. The clinical and hemodynamic observations were similar to those of the first study, confirming the lack of tolerance to the drug treatment, as well as a lowering of HR. In contrast to the observation on LVFP in the first study, pulmonary capillary wedge pressure (PCWP) was acutely lowered in the first hemodynamic evaluation of the second study.

A hemodynamic study (89) on levodopa (1500 mg), captopril, and their combination showed a moderate increase (2.03 to 2.40 L/min/m^2, $p < 0.05$) in CI. In combination with captopril, mean BP and PCWP significantly decreased, in a manner similar to the effects of captopril alone, and the increase in CI was maintained. Coronary blood flow (CBF) and myocardial oxygen consumption were practically unchanged. The successful replacement of DA infusion with oral levodopa (500 mg every 6 h) has been reported in one clinical case (90).

Following an investigation of eight patients treated for 4 weeks with 4000 mg daily, Hasenfuss et al. (91), notwithstanding the initial increase in fractional shortening assessed by echocardiography and an improvement in the clinical status of five patients, cast doubt on the persistence of improved hemodynamic and renal function, since no change was observed after the drug had been withdrawn for 2 weeks or more.

Plasma levels of NE were not decreased during levodopa administration. The hemodynamic effects were attributed to arterial vasodilation via DA_1 stimulation and to β_1-dependent inotropic stimulation, without any apparent contribution of effects mediated by prejunctional DA_2 receptors.

More extensive and controlled investigations would be required to assess the clinical efficacy of levodopa, but the use of the drug is hindered by its side effects (dyskinesia, nausea, and vomiting) (76,92).

Fenoldopam

Fenoldopam was discovered in a program of structural modification of SK&F 38393, the first example of a selective D_1 and DA_1 agonist, having both central and peripheral activity. Fenoldopam does not cross the blood–brain barrier and has served as an essential pharmacological tool in exploring the function of the DA_1 receptor not only in the laboratory, but also in clinical investigations (93,94). It is highly potent (about ten times more so than dopamine) and selective, showing α_2-adrenergic inhibitory properties only at doses that are not considered to be relevant to its clinical effect (95). Fenoldopam is proposed as a vasodilator in hypertensive emergencies by intravenous infusion; its effect after oral administration was shown to last about 2 h.

Oral fenoldopam was initially proposed for the chronic treatment of CHF, but its clinical development to treat this condition has been discontinued. Available reports of studies in CHF patients include six studies on intravenous administration (96–101); four studies on oral administration of single or repeated doses (100,102–104); and preliminary information on two placebo-controlled therapeutic trials (105,106), giving conflicting indications as to the ability of fenoldopam to increase exercise tolerance.

Intravenous administration at 0.36 μg/kg/min in 16 patients induced a significant increase in CO and a decrease in mean SVR from 1981 to 1212 dyne/s/cm^{-5} but these effects were lost after 22 h of infusion (97). An infusion of 0.75 μg/kg/min (100) in six patients increased CO and decreased MAP, but did not modify renal function; plasma renin activity (PRA) was significantly increased. In a third study (99) the infusion was titrated (mean rate 0.6 μg/kg/min) to induce a 25% increase in CI and then maintained for 24 h. The effects were rapid in onset, reaching peak values of +27% in CI and −37% in SVR, but gradually attenuated from the second hour; at 16 to 20 h the residual effect was +14% in CI and −13% in SVR. A comparison of intravenous fenoldopam and nitroprusside was conducted at mean rates of 1.45 and 2.99 μg/kg/min respectively (101); the effects on

MAP, CI, and SVR were similar, whereas only nitroprusside appeared to be able to reduce right atrial pressure, indicating the prevailing character of fenoldopam as an arteriolar vasodilator. Plasma levels of NE tended to increase with fenoldopam.

In a comparative study (96) of oral doses of 100 mg of fenoldopam and 30 mg (mean dose) of captopril, similar effects on MAP, CI, and SVR were observed with both treatments, but only captopril was able to decrease mean pulmonary arterial pressure and pulmonary vascular resistance.

The effects of single doses of 50, 100, and 200 mg in 10 patients were shown to be dose-related, and statistically significant for the 100- and 200-mg dose at 30 min to 1 h after administration. At 200 mg MAP decreased from 96 to 83 mm Hg, SVR decreased from 1987 to 1191 dyne/s/cm^{-5}, and CI increased from 2.2 to 3.1 L/min/m^2, returning to baseline values in 3 to 4 h (104).

Francis et al. (102) investigated hemodynamics and renal function in eight patients after a single dose of 100 mg and then after repeated doses of 100 mg q.i.d. for 3 days. The hemodynamic modifications observed after the first dose were similar to those reported in the previous studies, but it was shown that RBF was reduced after the first and last dose, while urine volume and Na^+ excretion remained unchanged over the 3-day treatment. An increase in PRA was observed after the first and the last dose, leading to the suggestion that activation of the renin-angiotensin system might be responsible for lack of the expected renal effects.

In a 3-day administration of 100 mg t.i.d. (98) to 17 patients, hemodynamic effects were regularly observed at the first dose, after 1 day, and after 3 days, returning to basal value within 3 h after each dose. The treatment was prolonged (103) to 4 to 12 weeks in 14 patients in order to investigate the effects on Na^+ excretion. No overall modifications were observed in the group. A subgroup of eight patients showing reduced Na^+ excretion was also shown to have increased PRA and decreased renal perfusion pressure and creatinine clearance.

Reflex activation of the sympathetic nervous system and the renin-angiotensin system thus appears to obliterate the effects of fenoldopam (102). Direct activation of renin release by stimulation of DA_1 receptors (41,42) is probably involved. A recent evaluation of the therapeutic potential of DA_1 agonists in hypertension (94) indicated that the combination of moderate DA_2 receptor stimulant activity with DA_1 agonistic activity may result in an ideal pharmacological profile for a dopaminergic antihypertensive drug, counteracting any reflex-mediated increase in HR, vasoconstrictor tone, and renin secretion. The same conclusion may well apply to congestive heart failure.

Dopexamine

Dopexamine, an *N*-substituted dopamine congener, has been investigated in a number of studies in heart failure as an acute intravenous infusion in doses ranging from 1 to 6 μg/kg/min (107,108); it is not active by the oral route. It has recently been approved in the United Kingdom for acute treatment of low cardiac output states, including heart failure and post-surgical conditions. With respect to DA, the pharmacological profile of dopexamine has the potential advantage of the absence of α-adrenergic activity, allowing an upward titration of the rate of infusion until an optimal vasodilator effect is achieved. The latter is dependent on DA_1 and β_2-receptor stimulation, since dopexamine is almost as active as dopamine at DA_1 receptors, but is markedly more potent on β_2-adrenoceptors, while it is devoid of any direct activity on the β_1 subtype. It is moderately active on DA_2 receptors. In addition, dopexamine inhibits the neuronal uptake of NE, thus exerting an indirect sympathomimetic action resulting in a positive inotropic and chronotropic effect that is possibly potentiated by direct effects of cardiac β_2-adrenoceptors.

In patients with acute heart failure following myocardial infarction and in CHF, dopexamine produced a marked reduction in afterload and increase in CO. Heart rate was generally increased, while BP was practically unchanged. Studies on CHF patients did not altogether produce conclusive evidence of redistribution of blood flow to the kidney and of diuretic effects, whereas evidence of increased RPF has been provided in healthy subjects (109) and hypertensive patients (110). The analysis of renal effects of dopexamine in therapeutic studies in CHF may be complicated by the attenuation, or loss, of effect when the infusion is prolonged to 12 h or more (107,111). This could result from increased sympathetic stimulation and circulating NE, and increased PRA.

Ibopamine

Ibopamine has hitherto been the only dopaminergic drug to be extensively investigated in the chronic treatment of CHF. Broad clinical experience has been achieved with ibopamine in acute, medium-term, and long-term clinical trials in over 3000 patients. Controlled trials have been extended to 3 and 6 months' duration. Moreover, since ibopamine has been approved for the chronic treatment of CHF in Italy, 3700 patients have been followed up for a median time of 1 year in postmarketing surveillance programs. Comprehensive reports discussing the pharmacological profile, clinical efficacy, and safety of ibopamine are available (78,112). The dose of ibopamine usually advised is 100 mg t.i.d.; in clinical studies it ranged from 50 to 200 mg two or three times per day.

The experimental approach used in the development of ibopamine has been simply directed at improving the oral bioavailability of DA and its duration of action. For this purpose, a number of ester prodrugs of DA and its *N*-substituted analogues were tested to assess their ability to overcome first-pass metabolism, which is responsible for inactivating orally administered DA, and to produce hemodynamic and renal effects comparable with those of infused DA in various animal models.

Among these prodrugs, ibopamine, i.e., the 3,4,-*O*-diisobutyric ester of *N*-methyldopamine, or epinine, showed a sequential activation of dopaminergic, β-adrenergic, and α-adrenergic receptors when administered to dogs in a series of intraduodenal doses ranging from 0.8 to 24 mg/kg, similarly to IV DA at increasing rates of infusion. Ibopamine selectively increased RBF and decreased RVR at doses of 0.8–2 mg/kg. These effects increased dose-proportionally up to 24 mg/kg. Cardiac contractility was stimulated, and CO was increased, starting from 8 mg/kg, with a simultaneous but less marked increase in MAP. Systemic vascular resistance was unchanged at 8–12 mg/kg and reduced at 24 mg/kg. Heart rate was slightly decreased, except at the highest dose. Cardiac relaxation was improved, and oxygen demand appeared to be met by adequate supply. These effects lasted 1 to 3 h, depending on the dose and the parameters considered. Since the intensity and mutual balance of dopaminergic and adrenergic effects of DA show considerable differences among species, the effects of ibopamine on DA_1 dopaminergic receptors were also investigated in the rabbit. In this species oral ibopamine did not elicit any pressor effects up to 50 mg/kg, suggesting a predominance of vasodilator effects. Intravenous bolus doses of ibopamine, or epinine, ranging from 1 to 100 nmol/kg slightly reduced MAP and significantly increased RBF and decreased RVR at doses 3 to 10 times lower than those of DA (113).

The diuretic and natriuretic action of ibopamine were investigated in rats under various experimental conditions. In normal, conscious rats the effects of oral doses of 25–100 mg/kg of ibopamine matched those of DA administered intraperitoneally at 0.5–4 mg/kg. The diuretic effect of ibopamine in anesthetized rats was neatly antagonized by d-sulpiride, a partially selective DA_1 antagonist. Ibopamine, like DA but unlike levodopa, appeared to be devoid of CNS effects when it was administered peripherally in various laboratory models of central dopaminergic activity. Essentially, ibopamine is well absorbed on oral administration and rapidly hydrolyzed by esterases in plasma and in peripheral tissues, generating a pharmacologically useful amount of epinine. Epinine shows the spectrum of dopaminergic and adrenergic activity of dopamine, but it is significantly more active on DA_1 receptors and on prejunctional DA_2 and α_2 receptors. It is also more active than dopamine on β_2- and α_1-adrenoceptors. Its indirect sympathomimetic activity is less than that of DA (78).

Several studies investigating the hemodynamic effects of ibopamine in CHF patients by right-heart catheterization have been reviewed (114) and discussed in comparison with the hemodynamic effects of DA. Some investigators established a direct comparison and considered an infusion of 2–4 μg/kg/min of DA as equivalent to 100 mg (115), 200 mg (116), or 300 mg of ibopamine (117). As an example, the modification of various hemodynamic parameters after 200 mg of ibopamine was found to parallel that occurring with an infusion of dopamine, individually adjusted for each patient in the range of 4–6 μg/kg/min (118). Ibopamine and dopamine, respectively, increased CI by 34.6% and 33.3%, increased stroke volume index by 36.7% and 32.3%, decreased SVR by 29.3% and 24.7%, and decreased PCWP by 10.5% and 13.8%, while BP and HR were virtually unchanged. The effect of ibopamine in these hemodynamic studies lasted 4 to 5 h. Since BP and HR were generally not modified, beneficial effects on CO and vascular resistance appeared to be achieved without any increase in cardiac workload and a constant organ perfusion pressure. The modest echocardiographic changes in systolic time intervals and inotropic indexes, in comparison with the relatively more marked effects on vascular resistance and cardiac output, led Ren et al. (117) to conclude that ibopamine exerts its effects mainly by reduction of afterload dependent on arteriolar vasodilation, rather than by direct cardiac stimulation. The α_1-adrenergic component of the pharmacological profile of epinine was not overtly manifested, since BP was not increased over a large range of doses, reaching 1500 mg as a single dose in healthy subjects, thus showing that the vasodilator components of the pharmacological spectrum of epinine compensate for any α-adrenergic effect in this respect. On the other hand, an effect on α_2-postsynaptic receptors, similarly to what has been reported for DA (83,119), is probably manifested in a transient increase in PCWP, which was observed in studies at doses of 200 mg or higher. This effect appeared shortly after administration (15–30 min), in correspondence with the peak plasma levels of epinine, and returned to basal, or lower than basal, values at the maximum hemodynamic effect (1–1.5 h).

The peripheral vasodilation induced by ibopamine was shown to be mediated by dopaminergic stimulation, since it was antagonized by racemic sulpiride, a mixed DA_1 and DA_2 antagonist (120).

Moderate diuretic effects were observed in normal subjects. The time-course of the effects was followed in three periods of 80 min after the administration of a 50-mg dose (121). Urine volume, Na^+ excretion, and

GFR were increased by 142%, 170%, and 42%, respectively, in the first period. The increase in urine volume and sodium excretion, but not in GFR, was still significant in the second and third period. These effects of ibopamine were not dose-dependently increased at high doses. The diuretic effect was maintained in 5-day administration at 50 mg b.i.d. (122). More marked and clinically significant effects were reported in a 7-day treatment of CHF patients (123). Twenty-four-hour urine and Na^+ excretion was gradually increased, reaching a plateau of +95% and +50%, respectively, at the end of the treatment. Creatinine clearance was also significantly increased, rising by 39%.

Neurohumoral modifications dependent on the stimulation of DA_2 receptors were investigated as a clinically important component of the effect of ibopamine in CHF patients.

A reduction in plasma levels of aldosterone (124–126), PRA (121,125–127), and NE (119,126,127) has been reported in both short- and long-term treatment, showing the ability of ibopamine to buffer activation of the sympathetic nervous system and the renin-angiotensin-aldosterone system, thereby resetting cardiovascular-renal homeostasis toward normal values.

The results of these clinical pharmacology studies underline the importance of the combined actions of ibopamine on DA_1 and DA_2 receptors, although a possible contribution of effects mediated by prejunctional α_2-adrenoceptors, particularly on NE release, should not be excluded.

Ibopamine has been investigated in chronic-therapy trials in all degrees of severity of CHF. These trials have been reviewed (78,128). The efficacy of ibopamine as single-drug therapy in mild heart failure has been investigated by Kleber et al. (129,130) in two multicenter trials, indicating the usefulness of a dopamine-like drug beyond the scope of its use as an addition to multiple-drug therapy for severe CHF, which was predictable from the experience with DA infusion. The first study was conducted with three parallel treatments of 4-week duration, using ibopamine, 200 mg b.i.d., versus placebo in double-blind conditions and versus digoxin as an open group. The second study, of 8-week duration, used a double-blind design of four groups of patients, in which ibopamine was compared at the same dose with placebo and hydrochlorothiazide, as well as a combination of ibopamine and hydrochlorothiazide. In both studies, ibopamine was consistently better than the placebo in terms of signs and symptoms, edema, and body weight, and also in the number of patients withdrawn for lack of efficacy, which was significantly higher in the placebo groups. The active treatments were considered similarly effective. Even so, some differences were noted, e.g., in a questionnaire score by which ibopamine showed advantage in terms of functional capacity in comparison with digoxin, or in a greater improvement in edema and body weight with the combination of ibopamine and hydrochlorothiazide than with the diuretic alone. Furthermore, ibopamine did not cause hypokalemia.

In another multicenter study of patients with mild CHF, ibopamine 100 mg t.i.d. for 6 weeks was compared with placebo, and a variable dose of diuretics was allowed according to need during a 6-week double-blind treatment (131). Both the number of patients withdrawn from the study owing to clinical deterioration and the dose of diuretics used in the patients completing the trial showed a significant difference in favor of ibopamine.

The effect of ibopamine 100 mg t.i.d. in elderly patients with mild CHF (NYHA class II) having a mean age of 70 years was investigated in another controlled study (132). In this study, treatment with diuretics was allowed when needed. After 3 months of treatment, the patients in the ibopamine group showed a significant improvement in exercise tolerance, as assessed by a bicycle ergometer test, and also showed a lesser degree of fatigue in a daily-life model of effort based on a 6-min walking test, notwithstanding the earlier use and higher consumption of diuretics in the placebo group (361 mg) in comparison with the ibopamine group (250 mg).

Ibopamine, given at a dosage of 100 t.i.d. for 3 months to NYHA class III patients receiving standard therapy with digoxin and diuretics, was investigated in a multicenter, placebo-controlled trial (133). A markedly improved effort capacity was shown by an ergometric bicycle test at the first month, which was sustained and further increased at the second and the third month of treatment. Cardiothoracic ratio was significantly lowered, as was end-systolic wall stress, assessed by echocardiography. New York Heart Association class and symptom scoring also improved. Exercise tolerance was also shown to be improved in a 6-month multicenter, placebo-controlled study (134), as was NYHA class, as a result of administering ibopamine 200 mg t.i.d. and concomitant treatment with digitalis and diuretics.

The hemodynamic response to ibopamine, which had been shown to be preserved in long-term open treatments of up to 1 year, was investigated in an "ad hoc" study (135), by a double-blind, crossover invasive investigation against placebo, both at the beginning and at the end of 3-month open treatment with ibopamine. In both hemodynamic sessions, a significant response to 100 mg of ibopamine in comparison with placebo was apparent in CI and SVR.

The safety of ibopamine was investigated in 1-year treatment in 847 patients in two open studies (136,137), and also in postmarketing surveillance studies in which three cohorts of patients receiving ibopamine (N = 2169), ibopamine and digoxin (N = 1540), or digoxin (N = 628), and additional treatment as needed, were followed up for a median time of 1 year (138,139). The general conclusion of the detailed analyses provided with these studies indicates that ibopamine has an excellent safety profile in terms both of mortality and of serious adverse effects, notably in its lack of untoward effects on cardiac rhythm. Observations of the latter effects were relatively rare, and their causal relationship to the drug was generally questionable. A specific electrophysiological investigation (140), including atrial and ventricular electrical stimulation, was performed on seven patients before and after they were given 200 mg of ibopamine. The electrophysiological parameters were not modified, and the frequency of serial responses following atrial or ventricular electrical stimulation was not augmented. In addition, no increase in spontaneous arrhythmias was detected by Holter monitoring of these patients for 24 h.

The lack of arrhythmogenic potential was confirmed by a double-blind, crossover study conducted on 97 patients, in whom 48-h Holter monitoring failed to reveal any difference between ibopamine and placebo in effect on heart rate, ectopic supraventricular beats, couples of runs, and ventricular ectopic beats (141). In a second study with a single-blind design, a 48-h Holter recording was used in three consecutive 1-week periods, on placebo, 100 mg of ibopamine t.i.d., and 200 mg of ibopamine t.i.d. The safety of ibopamine was confirmed, and a significant reduction in rhythm disturbances was observed. These favorable results were considered to be possibly related to either the improvement of hemodynamic conditions or the activation of the cardiac presynaptic dopaminergic receptors, or both (142). These authors extended their observations to a 6-month open treatment, with similar results (142).

A controlled study of the influence of ibopamine on survival is not yet available. A meta-analysis of controlled trials did not generate any hint of increased mortality in ibopamine-treated groups versus active-treatment or placebo comparison groups. On the contrary, the analysis of the incidence of mortality in long-term trials of ibopamine in historical comparison with active treatment and the placebo groups in reported survival studies led Taylor to infer that the drug may have a beneficial effect on life span, suggesting that a formal prospective study is warranted (143).

The ability of ibopamine to replace DA infusion has been investigated. Orally administered ibopamine, in divided doses of 100 mg 6 to 8 times a day, acutely and chronically supported hemodynamic function in 15 critically ill, dopamine-dependent patients, allowing a survival rate of 61% at 1 year (144).

Docarpamine

Docarpamine is a prodrug derived from dopamine by esterification of the catechol group and acylation of the amino group with *N*-acetylmethionine. Intraduodenal administration at doses ranging from 3.3 to 35 mg/kg in dogs indicated a pharmacological profile comparable to that of intravenous DA (145,146).

A single dose of 1200 mg was administered to 12 CHF patients in NYHA classes III and IV (147). M-mode echocardiography showed a significant decrease in left ventricular end-systolic volume. The mean velocity of circumferential fiber shortening and fractional shortening improved, while end-diastolic volume did not change. Mean arterial pressure and HR were unchanged. Renal function was monitored for 3 h after the administration, showing significant modifications. Renal plasma flow was increased from 216 to 384 ml/min, GFR from 67 to 119 ml/min, urine volume from 99 to 158 ml/h, and Na^+ excretion from 9.9 to 21.8 mEq/h.

A more complete description of the hemodynamic effects could be provided by cardiac catheterization studies. Information on the clinical efficacy of the drug is expected from controlled clinical trials, which are reported to be in progress with a 750 mg q.i.d. dose schedule.

Kidney-Selective Dopaminergic Prodrugs

The results obtained with ibopamine and docarpamine demonstrate that DA or its near-analogue epinine can be converted into orally active prodrugs, mimicking all the cardiovascular and renal effects of the parent compounds. The therapeutic potential of the action of DA in the kidney has stimulated research aimed at obtaining prodrugs that not only overcome the first-pass metabolic inactivation, as in the case of ibopamine and docarpamine, but also may be able to deliver the parent compound selectively to the kidney.

Various efforts in this field have been reviewed (78). The most interesting compound to emerge has been gludopa, an *N*-γ-glutamyl derivative of L-dopa that is cleaved with a good degree of selectivity to give L-dopa, and thereafter dopamine, in the proximal tubular cells, owing to the high local concentration of γ-glutamyl transpeptidase. These properties have been exploited by intravenous infusion in clinical pharmacological studies aimed at investigating the role of defective renal dopaminergic mechanisms in hypertension (58). Unfortunately, gludopa is not active orally, and the search for a therapeutically useful compound must thus be continued. We have recently reported (148,149) that a new prodrug of epinine, Sim 2055, i.e., epinine 4-*O*-phosphate, induced marked renal vasodilation in dogs starting from oral doses of 0.625 mg/kg. Sim 2055 shows a high degree of renal selectivity in comparison with ibopamine, possibly owing to local activation by alkaline phosphatases in the brush-border membrane of proximal tubular cells. Clinical pharmacological investigations are now awaited to provide information on the renal effects of this prodrug in humans.

CONCLUSIONS

This overview has analyzed in sequence the composite pattern of distribution and action of dopamine receptors, the possible physiological role of endogenous dopamine in the cardiovascular and renal system, and the results of clinical investigations on dopamine receptor agonists in congestive heart failure. Speculation on the compensatory role of endogenous dopamine in maintaining renal and circulatory homeostasis, and its relevance in cardiovascular disease, has mainly been based on pharmacological evidence, considered in combination with the local availability of the amine in organs, such as the kidney, that are richly endowed with dopamine receptors. Clinical pharmacology studies have produced important contributions to our knowledge of the function of dopamine receptors in humans, particularly by using drugs provided with receptor subtype selectivity, such as fenoldopam, or organ selectivity, such as gludopa.

From a therapeutic point of view, however, it has been the use of a nonselective, dopamine-like drug such as ibopamine that has led to the most significant progress, confirming in the chronic treatment of both mild and severe heart failure the perception of clinical benefit previously derived from the intravenous use of dopamine. Although it is clear that dopamine DA_1 and DA_2 receptor stimulation plays a prominent role in the clinical effects of ibopamine, and of low doses of dopamine as well, it remains to be established which of the various pharmacological mechanisms are most important in determining the clinical benefit.

What are the future prospects? The definition of the structure and function of new subtypes of peripheral dopamine receptors will open the way to the design of more advanced drugs, and to better understanding of their clinical action. It may well also provide some answers to the unsolved questions about the pathophysiological role of dopamine.

In the meantime, available clinical results highlight the peculiar characteristics of dopamine-like agents, in which the simulation of various dopamine receptors, currently encompassed in the DA_1/DA_2 classification, contribute to the pharmacological profile of the drug. If we consider the following features of these agents:

1. Hemodynamic properties allowing afterload to be reduced without lowering the perfusion pressure of critical organs, such as the heart, brain, and kidney
2. Ability to improve renal function, which, together with the preservation, or improvement, of renal perfusion, suggests use in patients, particularly elderly ones, who cannot tolerate ACE inhibitors, owing to hypotension or deterioration of renal function

3. Usefulness in mild heart failure, in particular by allowing diuretic intake to be lowered, thus reducing the hypokalemia and neurohumoral activation linked to intensive diuretic therapy
4. Favorable neurohumoral effects, involving a combined action on sympathetic tone and the renin-angiotensin-aldosterone system

It may be concluded that these dopamine receptor agonists constitute a novel and useful addition to the range of drugs used to treat congestive heart failure, and warrant further clinical investigation and application to establish their optimal use.

REFERENCES

1. Francis GS. Heart failure in 1991. Cardiology 1991; 78:81–94.
2. Katz MA. Changing strategies in the management of heart failure. J Am Coll Cardiol 1989; 13:513–523.
3. Cohn JN. Current therapy of the failing heart. Circulation 1988; 78:1099–1107.
4. Packer M. Symposium on the therapeutic challenge of congestive heart failure. Foreword. J Am Coll Cardiol 1988; 12:262–264.
5. Cohn J, Franciosa JA. Vasodilation therapy of heart failure. N Engl J Med 1977; 297:24–31, 254–257.
6. Swedberg K, Eneroth P, Kjekshus J, Whilhelmesel. Hormones regulating cardiovascular function in patients with severe congestive heart failure and their relation to mortality. Circulation 1990; 82:1730–1736.
7. Packer M. How should we judge the efficacy of drug therapy in patients with congestive heart failure? The insights of six blind men. J Am Coll Cardiol 1987; 9:433–438.
8. Di Bianco R, Shabetai R, Kostak W, Moran J, Schlant RC, Wright R. A comparison of oral milrinone, digoxin and their combination in the treatment of patients with chronic heart failure. N Engl J Med 1989; 320:677–683.
9. Williams JF Jr. Evolving concepts in congestive heart failure. Mod Con Cardiovasc Dis 1990; 59:43–53.
10. Goldberg LI, Kohli JD. Agonist and antagonist of peripheral pre- and post-synaptic dopamine receptors: clinical implications. In: Gessa GL, Corsini GU, eds: Apomorphine and Other Dopaminomimetics. New York: Raven Press, 1981:273–284.
11. Goldberg LI, McDonald RH Jr, Zimmerman AM. Sodium diuresis produced by dopamine in patients with congestive heart failure. N Engl J Med 1963; 269:1060–1064.
12. McDonald KH Jr, Goldberg LI, McNay JL, Tuttle EP. Effects of dopamine in man: augmentation of sodium excretion, glomerular filtration rate, and renal plasma flow. Clin Invest 1964; 43:1116–1124.

13. Goldberg LI, Kohli JD. Differentiation of dopamine receptors in the periphery. In: Kaiser C, Kebabian JW, eds. Dopamine, Receptors. Symposium Series No. 224. Washington, D.C.: American Chemical Society, 1983:101–113.
14. Lokhandwala MF, Barrett JF. Cardiovascular dopamine receptors: physiological, pharmacological and therapeutic implications. J Autonom Pharmacol 1982; 3:189–215.
15. Goldberg LI, Kohli JD. Peripheral pre- and post-synaptic dopamine receptors: are they different from dopamine receptors in the central nervous system? Commun Psychopharmacol 1979; 3:447–456.
16. Langer SZ. Presynaptic regulation of the release of catecholamines. Pharmacol Rev 1980; 32:337–358.
17. Mok JSL, Hutchinson JS, Sim MK. Effects of dopamine on blood pressure and heart rate after microinjection in the hypothalamus of spontaneously hypertensive and normotensive Wistar-Kyoto rats. Clin Exp Hypertension Theory Pract A12 15–36.
18. Damase-Michel C, Montrastruc JL, Gharib C, Geelen G, de Saint G, Tran MA. Effect of quinpirole, a specific dopamine DA, receptor agonist, on the sympathoadrenal system in dogs. J Pharmacol Exp Ther 1990; 252:770–777.
19. Carey RM, Drake CR. Effects of metoclopramide and bromocriptine on the renin-angiotensin-aldosterone system in man: dopaminergic control of aldosterone. J Clin Invest 1979; 63:727–735.
20. Missale C, Liberini P, Memo M, Carruba MO, Spano PF. Characterization of dopamine receptors associated with aldosterone secretion in rat adrenal glomerulosa. Endocrinology 1986; 119:2227–2232.
21. Missale C, Castelletti L, Memo M, Carruba MO, Spano PF. Identification and characterization of postsynaptic D_1- and D_2-dopamine receptors in the cardiovascular system. J Cardiovasc Pharmacol 1988; 11:643–650.
22. Ricci A, Amenta F. Autoradiographic localization of dopamine DA_2-receptor site in the rat mesenteric vascular tree. J Pharmacol Exp Ther 1990; 254:750–755.
23. Memo M, Pizzi M, Missale C, Carruba MO, Spano PF. Pharmacological and functional basis of dopamine D-2 receptor diversity (abstr). Pharmacol Res 1990; 22(suppl) 324.
24. Hilditch A, Drew GM. Peripheral dopamine receptor subtypes: a closer look. Trends Pharmacol Sci 1985; 6:396–400.
25. Andersen PH, Gingrich JA, Bates, MD, Dearry A, Falardeau P, Senogles SE, Caron MG. Dopamine receptors subtypes: beyond the D_1/D_2 classification. Trends Pharmacol Sci 1990; 11:231–236.
26. Sokoloff P, Giros B, Martres MP, Bouthenet ML, Schwartz JC. Molecular cloning and characterization of a novel dopamine receptor (D_3) as a target for neuroleptics. Nature 1990; 347:146–151.
27. Van Tol HHM, Bunzow JR, Guan HC, Sunahara RK, Seeman P, Niznik HG, Cive O. Cloning of the gene for a human dopamine D_4 receptor with high affinity for the antipsychotic clozapine. Nature 1991; 350:610–614.

28. Sunahara RK, Guan HC, O'Dowd BF, Seeman P, Laurier LG, Gordon N, George SR, Torchia J, Van Tol HHM, Niznik HB. Cloning of the gene for a human dopamine D_5 receptor with higher affinity for dopamine than D_1. Nature 1991; 350:614–619.
29. Felder CC, Campbell T, Albrecht F, Jose PA. Dopamine inhibits Na^+-H^+ exchanger activity in renal brush-border membrane vesicles. Am J Physiol, 1990; 259:F297–F303.
30. Bertorello A, Aperia A. Short-term regulation of Na^+, K^+-ATPase activity by dopamine. Am J Hypertension 1990; 3:51S–54S.
31. Felder CC, McKelvey AM, Gitler MS, Eisner GM, Jose PA. Dopamine receptor subtypes in renal brush-border and basolateral membranes. Kidney Int. 1989; 36:183–189.
32. Aperia AA, Hökfelt T, Meister B, Bertorello A, Frycksted J, Holtbäck U, Seri I. The significance of L-amino acid decarboxylase and DARPP-32 in the kidney. Am J Hypertension 1990; 3:11S–13S.
33. Huo T, Ye MQ, Healy DP. Characterization of a dopamine receptor DA_{2K} in the kidney inner medulla. Proc Natl Acad Sci USA 1990; 88:3170–3174.
34. Jeffrey RF, MacDonald TM, Marwick K, and Lee MR. The effect of carbidopa and indomethacin on the renal response to γ-glutamyl-L-dopa in normal man. Br J Clin Pharmacol 1988; 25:195–201.
35. Manoogian C, Nadler J, Ehrlich L, Horton R. The renal vasodilating effect of dopamine is mediated by calcium flux and prostacyclin release in man. J Clin Endocrinol Metab 1988; 66:678–683.
36. Felder RA, Belcher AM, Eisner GM, Jose PA. Cortical tubular and glomerular dopamine receptors in the rat kidney. Am J Physiol 1984; 247:F557–F568.
37. Amenta F. Density and distribution of dopamine receptors in the cardiovascular system and in the kidney. J Autonom Pharmacol 1990; 10(suppl 1):1–18.
38. Carey RM, Siragy HM, Ragsdale NV, Howell NL, Felder RA, Peach MJ, Chevalier R. Dopamine-1 and dopamine-2 mechanisms in the control of renal function. Am J Hypertension 1990; 3:59S–63S.
39. Seri I. Dopamine and natriuresis. Mechanism of action and developmental aspects. Am J Hypertension, 1990; 3:82S–86S.
40. Watkins HO, Eutmnu P, Hedge SS, Lokhandwala MF. Renal effects of the dopamine-2 receptor agonist bromocryptine in dogs (abstr). FASEB J 1990; 4:A607.
41. Kurtz A, Della Bruna R, Pratz J, Cavero I. Rat juxtaglomerular cells are endowed with DA_1 dopamine receptors mediating renin release. J Cardiovasc Pharmacol 1988; 12:658–663.
42. Montier F, Katchadourian P, Pratz J, Cavero I. The increase in plasma renin activity evoked by fenoldopam in dogs in directly mediated by dopamine-1 receptor stimulation. J Cardiovasc Pharmacol 1989; 13:739–747.

43. Worth DP, Harvey JN, Brown J, Worral A, Lee MR. Domperidone treatment in man inhibits the fall in plasma renin activity induced by intravenous gamma-L-glutamyl-L-Dopa. Br J Clin Pharmacol 1986; 21:497–502.
44. Sowers JR, Sharp B, McCallum RW. Dopaminergic modulation of renin release. Clin Exp Hypertension 1981; 3:15–21.
45. Struyker-Boudier HAJ. Cardiovascular and renal effects of dopamine agonists. In: Van Zwieten PA, Man in't Veld AJ, Lie KI, eds. Heart Failure in Perspective: Focus on Ibopamine. London: Royal Society of Medical Services, 1990:43–52.
46. Bell C. Dopamine and the kidney, In: Amenta F, ed. Peripheral Dopamine pathophysiology. Boca Raton, FL: CRC Press, 1990:87–98.
47. Bell C, Mann R. Identification of dopaminergic nerves in humans. Am J Hypertension 1990; 3:4S–6S.
48. Salvetti A, Lucarini AR, Bernini GP, Simonini H. Dopaminergic (DA_2) receptors and renal circulation in normotensive subjects and in patients with essential hypertension. J Cardiovasc Pharmacol 1987; 10(suppl 5):S19–S23.
49. Ball SG, Lee MR. The effect of carbidopa administration on urinary sodium excretion in man. Is dopamine an intrarenal natriuretic hormone? Br J Clin Pharmacol 1977; 4:115–119.
50. Lee MR. Dopamine and the kidney. Clin Sci 1982; 62:439–448.
51. Zimlichman R, Levinson PD, Kelly G, Stull R, Keiser HR, Goldstein D. Derivation of urinary dopamine from plasma dopa. Clin Sci 1988; 75:515–520.
52. Levinson PD, Goldstein DS, Munson PJ, Gill JR, Kaiser HR. Endocrine, renal and hemodynamic responses to graded dopamine infusion in normal men. J Clin Endocrinol Metab 1985; 60:821–826.
53. Buu NG, Lussier C. Origin of dopamine in the adrenal cortex. Am J Physiol 1990; 258:F287–291.
54. Unger T, Buu NT, Kuchel O. Sulphoconjugated catecholamines, nutrition and hypertension. Can J Physiol Pharmacol 1980; 58:22–27.
55. Smit AJ. Renal effects of exogenous and endogenous dopamine. Studies on the renal haemodynamic and natriuretic effects of dopamine in man, Thesis, University of Groningen, the Netherlands, 1988.
56. Sowers JR, Golub MS, Berger ME, Whitfield L. Dopaminergic modulation of pressor and hormonal responses in essential hypertension. Hypertension 1982; 4:424–430.
57. Kuchel O. Peripheral dopamine in essential hypertension: an early defense against hypertension failing during its progression? Am J Hypertension 1990; 3:104–107.
58. Lee MR. Salt, renal dopamine and essential hypertension. Triangle 1987; 26:11–21.
59. Pierpont GL, Francis GS, De Master EG, Levin B, Bolman RM, Cohn JN. Elevated left ventricular myocardial dopamine in preterminal idiopathic cardiomyopathy. Am J Cardiol 1983; 52:1033–1035.

60. Mercuro G, Rossetti Z, Rivano C, Ruscazio M, Tocco L, Sau F, Lai L, Gessa GL, Cherchi A. Marked increase of peripheral dopamine metabolism in congestive heart failure in man. J Appl Cardiol 1988; 3:19–27.
61. Viquerat CE, Daly P, Swedberg K, Evers C, Curran D, Parmley WW, Chatterjee K. Endogenous catecholamine levels in chronic heart failure: relation to the severity of hemodynamic abnormalities. Am J Med 1988; 78:455–460.
62. Lang R, Kaufmann W. Zur Rolle der sympathischen Aktivität bei chronischer Herzinsuffizienz. Therapie Woche 1984; 34:132–142.
63. Asakura S, Tabei K, Muto S, Asano Y, Hosoda S. The role of endogenous dopamine in congestive heart failure. Jpn Heart J 1989; 30:115–127.
64. Kuchel O, Buu NT, Racz K, Gutkowska J. Hormonal correlates of the inadequate natriuretic response to salt loading in idiopathic edema. Clin Invest Med 1987; 10(2):71–77.
65. Sowers JR. Altered dopaminergic modulation of sodium homeostasis in idiopathic edema. In: Amenta F, ed. Peripheral Dopamine Pathophysiology. Boca Raton, FL: CRC Press, 1990:211–217.
66. Man in't Veld AJ. Congenital dopamine β-hydroxylase deficiency: an exercise in catecholamine pathophysiology. In: Casagrande C, ed. Experimental Cardiology: Linking Laboratory and Clinical Investigations. Milan: CNM, 1993:223–228.
67. Bennett ED, Tighe D, Wegg W. Abolition by dopamine blockade of the natriuretic response produced by lower body positive pressure. Clin Sci 1982; 63:361–366.
68. Coruzzi P, Musiari L, Biggi A, Ravanetti C, Novarini A. Dopamine blockade abolishes the exaggerated natriuretic response of essential hypertension. J Hypertension 1987; 5:587–591.
69. Kurokawa K, Sophasan S, Katoh T. Dopamine and renal action of atrial natriuretic peptide. In: Brenne MM, Laragh JH, eds. Progress in Atrial Peptide Research. American Society of Hypertension Symposium Series, Vol. 3. New York: Raven Press, 1989:89–94.
70. Murphy MB, Bass AS. Dopamine, its receptors, and atrial natriuretic peptide. Am J Hypertension 1990; 3:55S–58S.
71. Hedge SS, Ricci A, Vega J, Amenta F, Lokhandwala MF. Evidence for the role of the endogenous renal dopamine and DA_1-receptors in the renal effects of atrial natriuretic factor. XI International Congress of Pharmacology, IUPHAR, Amsterdam, July 1–6, 1990.
72. Lang CC, Rahman AR, Coutil WJR, Balfour DJK, Struthers AD. Atrial natriuretic factor inhibits metoclopramide-stimulated aldosterone release in humans. Br J Clin Pharmacol 1990; 29:606P–607P.
73. Shenker Y, Weder AB, Grekin RJ. Atrial natriuretic hormone is not elevated during dopamine induced natriuresis. Life Science 1987; 40:1965–1970.
74. Fontana F, Ruffini M, Cappelli M, Bernardi P. Effetti della infusione della dopamina sulla liberazione del fattore natriuretico atriale. Giorn It Cardiol 1990; 20:227–237.

75. Stangl K, Baumann G, Weil J, Gerzer R, Kersher M, Blömer H. Akute Senkung erhöhter Spiegel des atrialen natriuretische Peptids (ANP) und des Zyklischen Guanosinmonophosphat (cGMP) by Patienten mit chronischer Herzinsuffizienz durch beta-adrenerge Stimulation mit Dopexamin-Hydrochlorid. Z Kardiol 1990; 79:417–423.
76. Goldberg LI. The role of dopamine receptors in the treatment of congestive heart failure. J Cardiovasc Pharmacol 1989; 14(suppl 5):S19–S27.
77. Opie LH. Pharmacological profile of ibopamine and related dopamine-like inodilators. Cardiovasc Drugs Ther 1989; 3:1041–1054.
78. Casagrande C, Santangelo F. Dopaminergic prodrugs. In: Amenta F, ed. Peripheral Dopamine Pathophysiology. Boca Raton, FL: CRC Press, 1990:308–343.
79. Shaer GL, Fink MP, Parrillo JE. Norepinephrine alone versus norepinephrine plus low-dose dopamine enhanced renal blood flow with combination pressor therapy. Crit Care Med 1985; 13:492–496.
80. Rajfer SI, Borow KB, Lang RM, Neumann A, Carroll JD. Effects of dopamine on left ventricular afterload and contractile state in heart failure: relation to the activation of β_1-adrenoceptors and dopamine receptors. J Am Coll Cardiol 1988; 12:498–506.
81. Borow KM, Lang RM, Neumann A, Weinert L, Marcus R, Sareli P. Effects of dopamine on left ventricular mechanics and energetics: importance of differential receptor activation (abstr). J Am Coll Cardiol 1990; 15:210A.
82. El Allaf D, Cremers S, D'Orio V, Carlier J. Combined hemodynamic effects of low doses of dopamine and dobutamine in patients with acute infarction and cardiac failure. Arch Int Physiol Biochem 1984; 92:S49–S55.
83. Lang RM, Carroll JD, Nakamura S, Itoh H, Rajfer S. Role of adrenoceptors and dopamine receptors in modulating left ventricular diastolic function. Circulation Res 1988; 63:126–134.
84. Maskin CS, Ocken S, Chadwig B, LeJemtel T. Comparative systemic and renal effects of dopamine and angiotensin-converting enzyme inhibition with enalaprilat in patients with heart failure. Circulation 1985; 72:846–852.
85. Finlay GD, Whitesett TL, Cucinell EA, Goldberg LI. Augmentation of sodium and potassium excretion, glomerular filtration rate and renal plasma flow by levodopa. N Engl J Med 1971; 284:865–870.
86. Whitsett TL, Goldberg LI. Effects of levodopa in systolic pre-ejection period, blood pressure, and heart rate during acute and chronic treatment of Parkinson's disease. Circulation 1972; 45:97–106.
87. Rajfer SI, Anton AH, Rossen JD, Goldberg LI. Beneficial hemodynamic effects of oral levodopa in heart failure. N Engl J Med 1984; 310:1357–1362.
88. Rajfer SI, Rossen JD, Nemanich JW. Sustained hemodynamic improvement during long-term therapy with levodopa in heart failure: role of plasma catecholamines. J Am Coll Cardiol 1987; 10:1286–1293.
89. Daly PA, Curran D, and Cahtterjee K. Effects of L-DOPA and captopril on resting hemodynamic and coronary blood flow (abstr). Circulation 1985; 72:III–406.

90. Maddox RW, Arnold WS, Sliger VO. Beneficial hemodynamic effects of oral levodopa in a patient with cardiomyopathy. Clin Pharm 1982; 4:502.
91. Hasenfuss G, Kasper W, Meinertz T, Busch W, Hofman T, Krause T, Holubarsch C, Lehmann M, Just H. Does long term oral levodopa therapy improve cardiac function in congestive heart failure? Circulation 1985; 72:III–303.
92. Hasenfuss G, Just H. Clinical relevance of long-term therapy with levodopa and orally active dopamine analogues in patients with chronic congestive heart failure. Basic Res Cardiol 1989; 84(suppl 1):191–196.
93. Beck TR, Clancy A, Creegen R. Clinical effects of fenoldopam, a potent dopamine (DA_1) agonist. In: Hieble JP, ed. Cardiovascular Function of Peripheral Dopamine Receptors. New York: Marcel Dekker, 1990:331–344.
94. Clark BJ. Postjunctional dopamine receptor stimulants. In: Amenta F, ed. Peripheral Dopamine Pathophysiology. Boca Raton, FL: CRC Press, 1990:307–343.
95. Kohli JD, Glock D, Goldberg LI. Relative DA_1-dopamine-receptor agonist and α-adrenoceptor antagonist activity of fenoldopam in the anesthetized dog. J Cardiovasc Pharmacol 1988; 11:213–216.
96. Green J, Nara A, Jarvis MD, Pospisil R, Kasmer R, Beek T. Invasive hemodynamic comparison of fenoldopam and captopril in heart failure (abstr). Clin Pharmacol Ther 1987, 41:242.
97. Kimmelstiel CD, Benotti JR, McCue JE. Acute hemodynamic effect of fenoldopam in patients with advanced congestive heart failure (abstr). Circulation 1988;78(suppl II):II-624.
98. Kukin ML, Gottlieb SS, Medina N, Yushak M, Packer M. Oral fenoldopam produces favorable but short-lived hemodynamic effects in heart failure (abstr). Circulation 1988; 78(suppl II):II-618.
99. Munger MA, Benotti JR, Jeffrey AG, Jarvis RC, Nara AR, McCue JE, Pospisil RA, Kasmer RJ. Assessment of hemodynamic tolerance from a 24-hour intravenous infusion of fenoldopam mesylate in congestive heart failure. Am J Cardiol 1990; 65:206–210.
100. Uretsky BF, Murali S, Betschart A, Tokarsky T, Kolesar JA. The dopamine receptor agonist fenoldopam improves hemodynamics without improving urine flow or sodium excretion (abstr). Circulation 1989; 80(suppl II):630.
101. Young JB, Leon CA, Pratt CM, Kyngry C, Taylor AA, Roberts R. Intravenous fenoldopam in heart failure: comparing the hemodynamic effects of $dopamine_1$ agonism with nitroprusside. Am Heart J 1988; 115:378–384.
102. Francis GS, Wilson BC, Rector TS. Hemodynamic, renal and neurohumoral effects of a selective oral DA_1 receptor agonist (fenoldopam) in patients with congestive heart failure. Am Heart J 1988; 116:473–479.
103. Kukin ML, Packer M, Neuberg GW, Medina N, Yushak M. Changes in renal perfusion pressure limit the natriuretic response to dopamine receptor stimulation in human heart failure (abstr). Circulation 1989; 80(suppl II):493.

104. Young JB, Leon CA, Pratt CM, Suarez JM, Aronoff RD, Roberts R. Hemodynamic effects of an oral dopamine receptor agonist (fenoldopam) in patients with congestive heart failure. J Am Coll Cardiol 1985; 6:792–796.
105. King BD, Beck TR, Snyder MM, Musser TK. Efficacy of fenoldopam (SK&F 82526) in chronic congestive heart failure (abstr). Circulation 1987; 76(suppl IV):71.
106. MacDonald TM, Jeffrey RF, Muir AL, Lee MR. A preliminary study of fenoldopam in the treatment of chronic left ventricular failure due to ischaemic heart disease. Br J Clin Pharmacol 1988; 27(suppl I):662P–663P.
107. Fitton A, Benfield P. Dopexamine hydrochloride. A review of its pharmacodynamic and pharmacokinetic properties and therapeutic potential in acute cardiac insufficiency. Drugs 1990; 39:308–330.
108. Meinertz T, Drexler H, Just H. Dopexamine in heart failure: how does the pharmacological situation translate into the clinical situation? Basic Res Cardiol 1990; 84(suppl 1):177–186.
109. Mousdale S, Ceyburn PA, Mackie AM, Groves ND, Rosen M. Comparison of the effect of dopamine, dobutamine, and dopexamine upon renal blood flow: a study in normal healthy subjects. Br. J Pharmacol 1988; 25:555–560.
110. Magrini FR, Foulds R, Roberts N, Macchi G, Mondadori C, Zanchetti A. Renal hemodynamic effects of dopexamine. Am J Cardiol 1988; 62:53C–56C.
111. Böhm M, Reuschel-Janetschek E, Erdmann E. Lack of sustained hemodynamic effect of the beta$_2$-adrenoceptor agonist dopexamine in end-stage congestive heart failure. Am J Cardiol 1990; 65:395–396.
112. Godfraind T, Spano PF, Carruba MO, Casagrande C, eds. Inodilators: a new strategy in the therapy of heart failure. J Cardiovasc Pharmacol 1990; 14(suppl 8):S1–S132.
113. Miragoli G, Ferlenga P, Semeraro C. Renal and systemic vasodilator effects of ibopamine in awake rabbits (abstr). J Autonom Pharmacol 1990; 10(suppl 1):132.
114. Lopez-Sendon J. Hemodynamic and neurohumoral effects of ibopamine in patients with chronic congestive heart failure. Cardiology 1990; 77(suppl 5):9–21.
115. Sannia L, Ibba GV, Castellaccio M, Dore L. Comparison of the acute hemodynamic effects of ibopamine and dopamine in chronic congestive heart failure. Arzneim Forsch 1986; 46:355–359.
116. Ciampani N, Berrettini U, Caruso L. Effetti emodinamici acuti dell'ibopamina nei pazienti con insufficienza cardiaca congestizia (abstr). X Congr. Cardiol. Nazionale. IN-RCA, Ancona Italy, October, 1986:113.
117. Ren JH, Unverferth DV, Leier CV. The dopamine congener, ibopamine, in congestive heart failure. J Cardiovasc Pharmacol 1984; 6:748–755.
118. De Vita C, Triulzi E, Devizzi S, Colombo G, Palvarini M, Pocchiari F, Pataccini R. Evaluation of acute hemodynamic effects and pharmacokinetic behaviour of ibopamine in patients with severe heart failure. Arzneim Forsch 1986; 36:349–354.

119. Rajfer SI, Rossen JD, Douglas FL, Goldberg LI, Karrison T. Effects of long-term therapy with oral ibopamine on resting hemodynamics and exercise capacity in patients with heart failure: relationship to the generation of *N*-methyl-dopamine and to plasma norpinephrine levels. Circulation 1986; 73:740–748.
120. Longhini C, Ansani L, Musacci FG, Aggio S, Baracca F, Toselli T, Ghirardi P. Peripheral hemodynamic effects of ibopamine in patients with congestive heart failure. A placebo-controlled, double-blind study. Cardiovasc Drugs Ther 1989; 3:199–202.
121. Incerti PL, Badalamenti S, Lorenzano E, Graziani G, Morganti A, Salerno F, Ghirardi P. Humoral and renal effects of ibopamine in normal subjects. Arzneim Forsch 1986; 36:405–407.
122. Melloni GF, Minoja GM, Scarazzati S, Bauer R, Brusoni B, Ghirardi P. Renal effects of SB 7505: A double-blind study. Eur J Clin Pharmacol 1981; 19:177–180.
123. Dei Cas L, Manca C, Bernardini B, Vasini G, Visioli O. Non-invasive evaluation on the effects of oral ibopamine (SB 7505) on cardiac and renal function in patients with congestive heart failure. J Cardiovasc Pharmacol 1982; 4:436–440.
124. Rolandi E, Marchetti G, Franceschinis R, Cicchetti V, Gianrossi R, Cantoni V, Barreca T. Inhibition of prolactin and aldosterone secretion by the dopamine derivative, ibopamine. Eur J Clin Pharmacol 1986; 29:629–630.
125. Missale C, Metra M, Sigala S, Memo M, Dei Cas L, Spano PF. Inhibition of aldosterone secretion by dopamine, ibopamine and dihydroergotoxine in patients with congestive heart failure. J Cardiovasc Pharmacol 1989; 14(suppl 8):S72–S76.
126. Caponnetto S, Terrachini V, Canale C, Bruzzone F, Masperone MA, Pastorino L, Licciardello L, Marchetti GV. Long-term treatment of congestive heart failure with oral ibopamine. Effects on rhythm disorders and neurohumoral alterations. Cardiology 1990; 77(suppl 5):43–48.
127. Nakano T, Morimoto Y, Kakuta Y, Konishi T, Kodera T, Kanamaru M, Takezawa H. Acute effects of ibopamine hydrochloride on hemodynamics, plasma catecholamine levels, renin activity, aldosterone, metabolism and blood gas in patients with severe congestive heart failure. Arzneim Forsch 1986; 36:1829–1834.
128. Taylor SH, Cicchetti V. Efficacy of ibopamine in the treatment of heart failure. Am Heart J 1990; 120:1583–1590.
129. Kleber FX, Thyroff-Friesinger U. Treatment of mild congestive heart failure with ibopamine, hydrochlorothiazide, ibopamine plus hydrochlorothiazide, or placebo. A double-blind comparative study. Cardiology 1990; 77(suppl 5):67–74.
130. Kleber FX, Thyroff-Friesinger U. Ibopamine versus digoxin in the treatment of mild congestive heart failure. A double-blind randomized, placebo-controlled trial. Cardiology 1990; 77(suppl 5):75–80.

131. Dalla Volta S, Razzolini R, Roshan-Ali Y. Clinical efficacy of ibopamine in heart failure. Results of a double-blind clinical study. Am J Noninvas Cardiol 1991; 5(suppl 1):15–17.
132. Pizzorni C, Barabino A, Di Benedetto G, Musso N, Vergassola C, Azzollini A, Lotti G. Neurohumoral evaluation and long-term treatment of mild congestive heart failure in elderly patients with ibopamine: a double-blind, placebo controlled study. Am J Noninvas Cardiol 1991; 5(suppl 1):23–31.
133. Condorelli M, Mattioli G, Caponnetto S, Varricchio M, Colonna L, Guiducci U, Paciaroni E, Gavazzi A, Cucchini F, Canale C, Terrachini V, Montemartini C, Bonaduce A, Montemurro A, Cappello C, Cacciapuoti F, De Luca I, Brandi L, Gigli L. The long-term efficacy of ibopamine in treating patients with severe heart failure: a multicenter investigation. J Cardiovasc Pharmacol 1989; 14(suppl 8):S83–S92.
134. Kayanakis JG, and The European Ibopamine Study Group. Six months treatment of congestive heart failure with ibopamine: a double-blind randomized, placebo-controlled multicenter trial. Am J Noninvas Cardiol 1991; 5(suppl 1):32–38.
135. Reffo GC, Gabellini A, Forattini C, Fracalossi C, Ziacchi V, Lomanto B, Cantoni V, Ghirardi PE, Licciardello L. Double-blind, acute hemodynamic invasive evaluation in congestive heart failure before and after open sustained treatment with ibopamine. Curr Ther Res 1988; 44:723–730.
136. Rolandi E, Sabino F, Cantoni V, Ghirardi P, Marchetti GV, Cicchetti V. Long-term therapy of chronic congestive heart failure with ibopamine: a multicenter trial. J Cardiovasc Pharmacol 1989; 14(suppl 8):S93–S103.
137. Riva E, Cavalli A, Abbondati G, Cedrini MC, Schleman M, Fuccella LM, and the Italian Working Group. Ibopamine: long-term safety study in patients with congestive heart failure. Int J Clin Pharmacol Res 1989; 9:21–28.
138. Sher D, Ferrari V. Ibopamine post-marketing surveillance. Arzneim Forsch 1987; 37:869–902.
139. Sher D, Licciardello L, Ferrari V, Sirtori F, Cesana B. Safety of ibopamine in congestive heart failure. Ibopamine cohort study: baseline and 1-year results. Arzneim Forsch 1991; 41:402–409.
140. Ciampani N, Massacci C, Capestro F, Brescia Fratadocchi G, Moccheggiani R, Ruga O, Purcano A. The diisobutyryl ester of *N*-methyldopamine, ibopamine: evaluation of electrophysiological properties and arrhythmogenicity studies. Arzneim Forsch 1986; 366:363–366.
141. Furlanello F. Influence of ibopamine on heart rate and arrhythmic pattern in patients with congestive heart failure. G It Cardiol 1989; 19:71–80.
142. Caponnetto S, Terrachini V, Canale C, Bruzzone F, Licciardello F, Marchetti GV. Absence of proarrhythmic effects of ibopamine on patients with congestive heart failure. J Cardiovasc Pharmacol 1989; 14:S104–S110.
143. Taylor SH. Ibopamine and lifespan. Cardiovasc Drugs Ther 1989; 3:1059–1063.

144. Dei Cas L, Metra M, Nodari S, Visioli O. Efficacy of ibopamine treatment in patients with advanced heart failure: purpose of a new therapeutic scheme with multiple daily administrations. J Cardiovasc Pharmacol 1989; 14(suppl 8):S111–S117.
145. Yamaguchi I, Nishiyama S, Akimoto Y, Yoshikawa M, Nakajima H. A novel orally active dopamine prodrug TA-870. I. Renal and cardiovascular effects and plasma levels of free dopamine in dogs and in rats. J Cardiovasc Pharmacol 1989; 13:879–886.
146. Nishiyama S, Yamaguchi I, Akimoto Y, Yoshikawa M, Nakajima H. A novel orally active dopamine prodrug TA-870. III. Positive inotropic effects and cardiorenal selectivity in anesthetized dogs. J Cardiovasc Pharmacol 1990; 15:283–290.
147. Kubota J, Kubo S, Nishimura H, Ueyama M, Kino M, Nakayama A, Hara K, Kawamura K. Cardiorenal effects of an orally active dopamine prodrug (TA 870) in patients with congestive heart failure. J Cardiovasc Pharmacol 1989; 14:53–57.
148. Casagrande C, Merlo L, Ferrini R, Miragoli G, Semeraro C. Cardiovascular and renal action of dopaminergic prodrugs. J Cardiovasc Pharmacol 1989; 14(suppl 8):S40–S59.
149. Casagrande C, Merlo L, La Regina A. Development of dopaminergic drugs for the chronic treatment of congestive heart failure. J Autonom Pharmacol 1990; 10(suppl 1):S85–S93.

14

Calcium Entry Blockers in Congestive Heart Failure and in Asymptomatic Left Ventricular Dysfunction

Hubert Pouleur
University of Louvain, Brussels, Belgium

INTRODUCTION

Calcium entry blockers, also called calcium antagonists and slow calcium channel blockers, have become a widely accepted therapy for hypertension and angina pectoris (1,2), and evidence has accumulated that some of them might have additional therapeutic potential in subarachnoid hemorrhage, in head injury, and perhaps even in stroke (3–6).

When these agents were introduced on a large scale, 10 to 15 years ago, there was also hope that they might become used as first-line therapy for heart failure. Most were, indeed, powerful vasodilators, and afterload reduction remained a desirable goal in heart failure. Their beneficial effects on the balance between myocardial oxygen supply and demand and, for some of them, clear effects on myocardial perfusion even during oral therapy (7) suggested a place in therapy for ischemic heart failure. There was also a large body of experimental evidence indicating that calcium overload played a role in the progression of myocardial dysfunction (8), and many authors reported beneficial effects of calcium entry blockers in isolated heart preparations and in animal survival studies. The prognosis of the alcoholic hamster and of the Syrian hamster with hereditary cardiomyopathy appeared brighter than ever (9,10), and clinical trials were optimistically undertaken on the above rationale. Simultaneously, and despite the lack of firm clinical evidence, thousands of heart failure patients worldwide received calcium antagonists for their routine management, nifedipine and diltiazem probably being the most widely prescribed. The magnitude of this use in academic hospitals is well illustrated by the fact that approximately 38% of heart failure patients enrolled between 1986 and 1990 in the large multicenter, multinational trial Studies of Left Ventricular Dysfunction (SOLVD) still received a calcium antagonist (11).

Recently, however, there has been a growing concern that calcium antagonists might worsen symptoms of heart failure or might precipitate the development of heart failure in previously asymptomatic patients with left ventricular dysfunction (12–16). The hopes that they could be useful in unstable angina pectoris or in acute myocardial infarction have also been seriously undermined (17,18).

So what? Are all calcium antagonists contraindicated in all forms of heart failure? Where do we stand in 1993? The purpose of this chapter is to try to answer these questions, at least partially, by reviewing the pharmacology of these agents in the perspective of the progress made during the last decade in our understanding of the pathophysiology of heart failure.

PHARMACOLOGY OF THE CALCIUM ANTAGONISTS

Negative Inotropic Action

Basically, all slow calcium channel blockers reduce calcium influx in vascular smooth muscle, thereby causing vasodilation. This vasodilation can be produced in normotensive as well as in hypertensive subjects, and, provided that the doses are adapted, an identical result can be achieved on resistance vessels by practically all calcium entry blockers (2) (Fig. 1). However, these agents also impair calcium entry in the myocardial cell, thereby depressing cardiac function. The opening of a voltage-dependent calcium channel and the resultant intracellular calcium influx play an important role in the depolarization of the sinus node, in the propagation of the impulse, particularly at the atrioventricular node, and in the regulation of the mechanical performance of the myocytes. Thus, all calcium channel blockers have the potential to depress both mechanical and electrophysiologic performance, to the point that at high concentrations, cardiac standstill can occur. The failing heart, which already suffers from an impairment in its excitation-contraction relaxation coupling mechanisms (19), is in this respect more sensitive than the normal heart (20,21) to the depressant action of calcium antagonists.

As schematized in Figure 2, the negative inotropic effect of a calcium antagonist is dose-dependent. In contrast, most beta-blockers are devoid

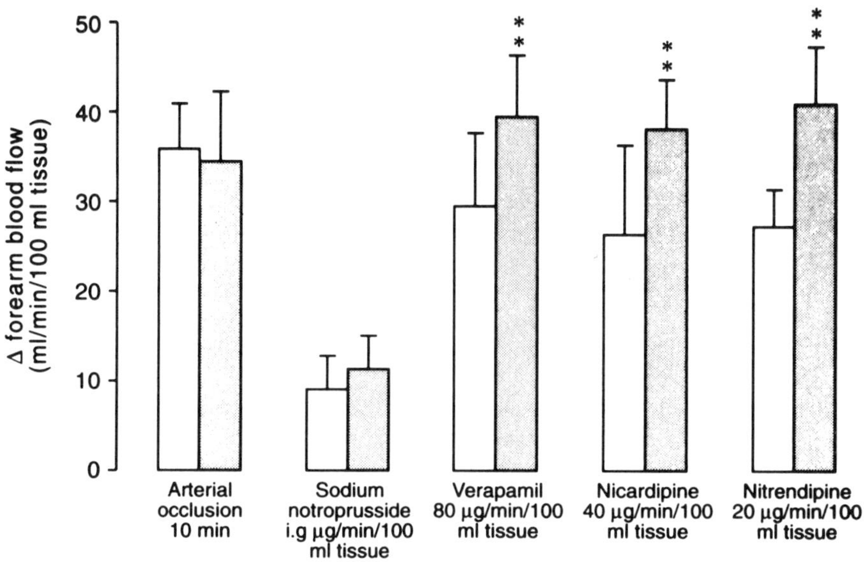

Figure 1 Increases in forearm blood flow during intra-arterial infusions of calcium antagonists verapamil, nicardipine, and nitrendipine, during "non-specific" vasodilation by sodium nitroprusside, and during reperfusion after 10 min of ischemia. Means ± SD; shaded bars, hypertensive subjects; open bars, age-matched normotensive controls. In comparison with the corresponding value for normotensive control subjects, $**p < 0.01$. (From Ref. 2.)

of direct effects on the membrane and will not lower the inotropic state below the level of "zero sympathetic drive," leaving intact the other mechanisms of regulation of myocardial performance, such as the Frank-Starling mechanism.

To minimize these drawbacks, calcium antagonists have been synthesized that have a much greater affinity for smooth muscle than for the myocardium. Nicardipine and nisoldipine (20,21) are good examples of this category: at a therapeutic dose (plasma concentration below 0.5 µM) it may not be possible to detect a reduction in contractility with these compounds (22–24), although in patients with severe congestive heart failure some negative inotropism can be evidenced during intravenous infusion (25). In contrast, agents such as verapamil, diltiazem, and nifedipine already depress the contractile function of a normal heart at therapeutic doses (26,27).

Until recently, it was not clearly established that this depression might be of any clinical significance. However, Packer et al. have shown that in patients with severe congestive heart failure a single oral dose of 20 mg of nifedipine could produce a serious, and in some cases life-threatening,

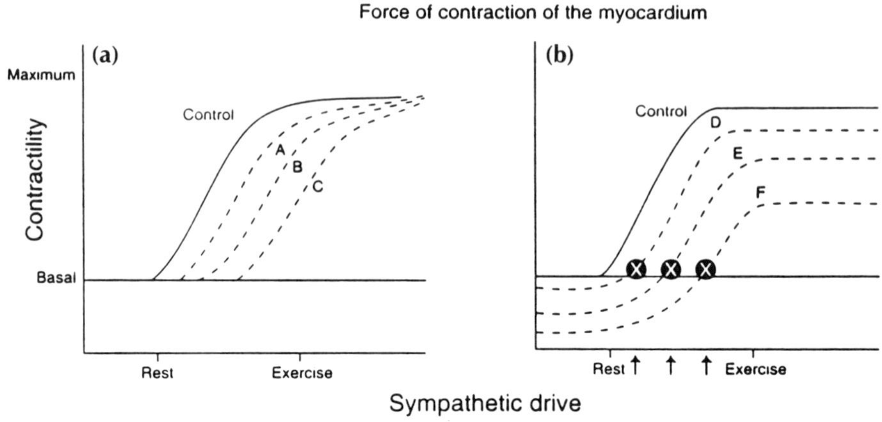

Figure 2 (a) Schematic representation of the effects of three increasing doses (A, B, and C) of a pure β_1-antagonist on myocardial performance at rest and at peak exercise. (b) Schematic representation of the effects of three increasing doses (D, E, and F) of a slow calcium channel blocker on myocardial performance at rest and at peak exercise. In contrast to beta-blockers, calcium channel blockers depress contractility at rest and during exercise. To maintain cardiac performance, sympathetic drive must be increased at rest (arrows) as a compensatory mechanism.

hemodynamic deterioration (28). This hemodynamic deterioration was characterized by a marked decrease in arterial pressure and in right and left ventricular stroke work indexes (Fig. 3). As the changes in systemic vascular resistance were comparable in the patients who tolerated nifedipine well and in the patients who deteriorated (Fig. 3), this dramatic hemodynamic situation was clearly caused by a pronounced depressant effect of nifedipine on the myocardium rather than by more intense vasodilation. These data therefore point out a major problem with the use of this agent in heart failure, namely a dose-related myocardial depression.

Neurohumoral Activation

In an important trial using nifedipine in unstable angina (17,29), a detrimental effect of nifedipine on mortality was detected. Interestingly, the excess in mortality was no longer present when nifedipine was associated with metoprolol. Thus, the detrimental effect of nifedipine in unstable angina may not necessarily be related to its negative inotropic effects but rather to other factors susceptible to attenuation by metoprolol, such as a neurohumoral activation (Fig. 4). Indeed, the intense systemic vasodilation

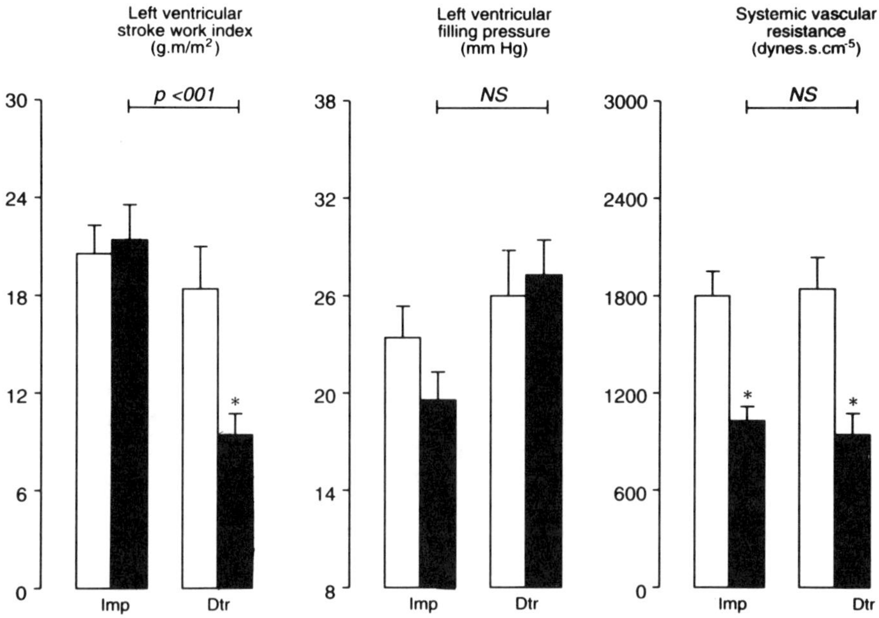

Figure 3 Left ventricular stroke work index, left ventricular filling pressure, and systemic vascular resistance before (open bars) and after (filled bars) the administration of nifedipine in patients with severe congestive heart failure who either tolerated nifedipine well and showed improvement (Imp) or deteriorated under nifedipine (Dtr). In comparison with the corresponding value for the before-treatment condition, $*p < 0.001$. (From Ref. 28.)

induced by the calcium antagonists activates compensatory mechanisms such as sympathetic drive and the renin-angiotensin system (13,30). Acutely, the reflex increase in sympathetic tone may mask or compensate for the depression in contractility, but in clinical settings such as unstable angina or acute myocardial infarction, it can be expected to be detrimental. It is also possible that calcium entry blockade could trigger a direct release of renin as a result of a direct action on the juxtaglomerular apparatus (30), or that it could affect neurohumoral postural responses by a sensitization of cardiopulmonary and arterial baroreceptors (31).

Furthermore, during prolonged administration to patients with heart failure, this neurohumoral activation may create a circle leading to a worsening of their clinical status (13). In a recent randomized, crossover study to compare the safety of nifedipine and isosorbide in patients with mild to moderate heart failure, episodes of hospitalization and increases in diuretic

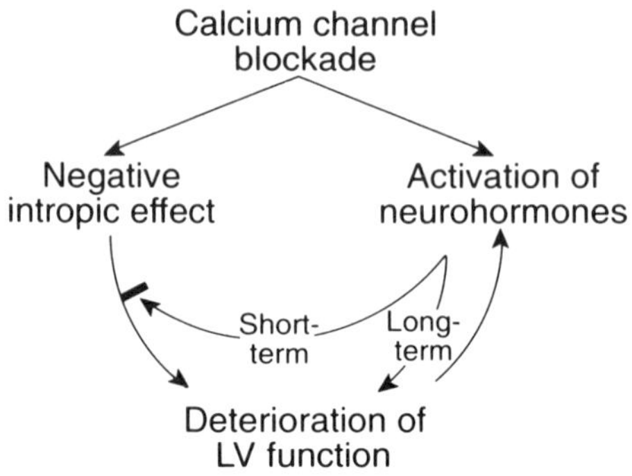

Figure 4 Potential mechanisms by which calcium channel blockers may exert deleterious effects on left ventricular (LV) function. Short-term hemodynamic and clinical deterioration is most likely to be related to negative inotropic effects; adverse effects during long-term therapy appear to be related to prolonged activation of neurohormonal systems, although such activation may help to counterbalance the negative inotropic effects occurring during short-term therapy. (From Ref. 13.)

dosages for worsening of heart failure were significantly more frequent when the patients were receiving nifedipine (15). In an elegant study, Barjon et al. made similar observations with nisoldipine and were able to show that this effect was at least partially related to an alteration in renal clearance of water (32) (Fig. 5) and to alterations in the response in plasma renin activity, vasopressin, aldosterone, and norepinephrine during a water load. Finally, it has also been observed that prolonged administration of diltiazem to patients with left ventricular dysfunction significantly increased the incidence of new congestive heart failure (16). In this last trial, it was also observed that the patients receiving beta-blockers were not at increased risk of heart failure, once again emphasizing the differing nature of the myocardial depression induced by beta-blockade or direct calcium entry blockade. In the presence of a limited cardiac reserve, however, there was a trend toward exacerbation of heart failure and atrioventricular conduction disturbances when beta-blockers were associated with calcium entry blockers (16).

Moreover, when patients with transmural infarction were given diltiazem, a significant increase in mortality was observed among those with pulmonary congestion (14). Other trials in unstable angina or acute myocardial infarction with verapamil or nifedipine administered during the acute phase have been unable to demonstrate a clinical benefit, in contrast to beta-blockers (18).

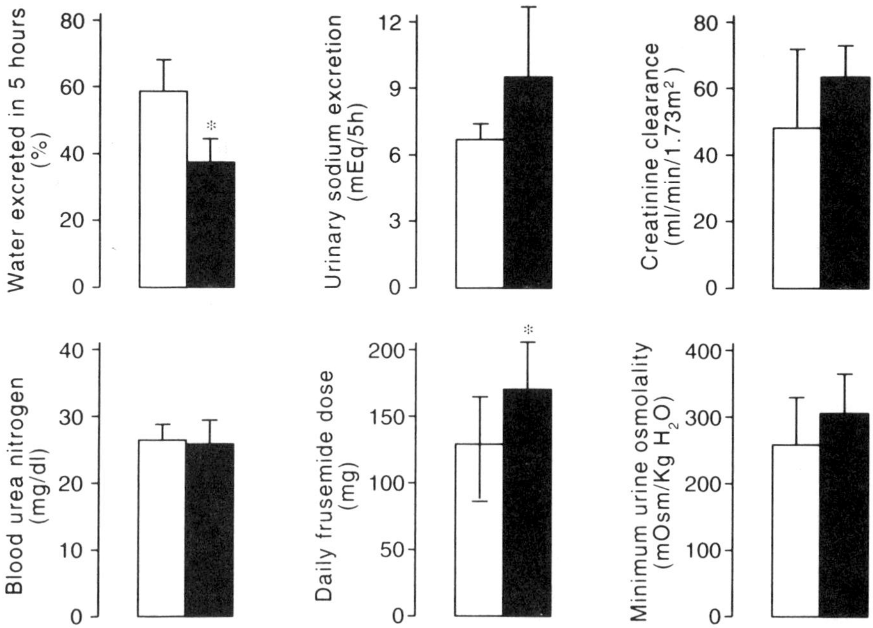

Figure 5 Chronic renal effects of nisoldipine, which was found to decrease water excretion and to increase daily furosemide requirements, as well as tending to increase urinary sodium excreted and minimum urinary osmolality. Means ± SD; filled bars, nisoldipine; open bars; controls; in comparison with the corresponding value for control subjects, $^*p < 0.05$. (From Ref. 32.)

It is clear, therefore, that the negative inotropic effect and the neurohumoral activation caused by some calcium antagonists put patients with heart failure at higher risk. Exhaustive reviews of these distressing observations have been made by Packer (12,13,30). Most data so far suggest that these effects are primarily a "class effect," although this hypothesis may require further testing, as we will discuss later.

Effects on Calcium Overload, Myocardial Perfusion, and Other Potentially Useful Properties of Calcium Blockers in Heart Failure

Despite the negative findings, it may be premature to reject, once and for all, the therapeutic possibilities provided by this class of drugs in heart failure or cardiac dysfunction. Direct monitoring of intracellular calcium concentration in human papillary muscle has revealed the presence, in most forms of heart failure, of abnormally high calcium concentrations during diastole (33). An increased level of free cytoplasamic calcium not only causes delayed or incomplete relaxation of the contractile proteins but may also activate detrimental biochemical processes (8,34). Such abnormalities in calcium handling are particularly severe in pressure-overload hypertrophy and in idiopathic hypertrophic cardiomyopathy (33,34). Thus, when heart failure develops in idiopathic hypertrophic cardiomyopathy, left ventricular systolic function is generally preserved and the patient's symptoms appear primarily related to an impaired diastolic distensibility caused by a reduced rate of calcium sequestration. In this setting, the administration of verapamil or nifedipine improves the diastolic properties of the left ventricle and the patient's functional status (35,36). In another trial studying patients with heart failure and a normal ejection fraction, a greater improvement in exercise tolerance and symptomatology was also observed with verapamil than with placebo (37).

Although long-term prognostic information is still lacking, there is therefore at least one subset of heart failure patients who may benefit clinically from a reduction in myocardial calcium influx. These patients, as a rule, have a normal left ventricular ejection fraction and symptoms of pulmonary congestion or impaired exercise tolerance caused by severe diastolic dysfunction.

Another area in which calcium entry blockade might prove useful is that of the progression of left ventricular dysfunction. Despite the negative effects of diltiazem and nifedipine evidenced in some trials, it may indeed be worthwhile to identify a subset of patients in whom a calcium antagonist might possibly slow down the relentless process of ventricular enlargement.

Although many different mechanical stimuli (including systolic wall stress and diastolic wall stress) and neurohumoral stimuli (angiotensin II, norepinephrine, aldosterone) are responsible for the complex process of myocardial hypertrophy, reorganization of the collagen matrix, and remodeling of the ventricular cavity, intracellular calcium is frequently involved as a second messenger. Calcium overload, as already said, or subendocardial ischemia (34,35), related to fibrosis, impaired relaxation, or microvascular spasms (39,40), may also play a role in preventing hypertrophy from fully compensating for the cardiac overload.

In theory, therefore, calcium entry blockers might reduce the rate of progression of ventricular remodeling by several mechanisms: reduction in wall stress, prevention of vascular spasms, effects on the fibroblasts, perhaps even effects on calcium overload. Experimental data in several models of heart failure or hypertension support this hypothesis and indicate that calcium antagonists may reduce myocardial hypertrophy as well as prevent or correct changes in the collagen network (41). Furthermore, in hypertensive patients with ventricular hypertrophy, the regression of hypertrophy appears comparable to that achieved with angiotensin converting enzyme (ACE) inhibitors. In patients with ischemic left ventricular dysfunction, the calcium antagonist nisoldipine appeared able to selectively improve shortening and relaxation in chronically ischemic areas (hibernating myocardium) and to delay the progression of left ventricular dysfunction (42,43). Which group of patients and which calcium antagonists should then be considered to test these hypotheses on a prospective basis?

A first interesting subgroup might be that of patients with aortic or mitral regurgitation who do not yet require valvular surgery. Prolonged afterload reduction with hydralazine has been shown to be useful in these patients (44). Calcium antagonists have a better side effect profile and a better overall tolerance than hydralazine. Delaying valvular surgery without compromising left ventricular function might undoubtedly be useful, particularly in young patients, and a controlled clinical trial comparing a calcium antagonist with placebo, and perhaps with an ACE inhibitor in a third arm, might therefore be worth considering in this clinical setting.

The most important group to study remains, however, patients with chronic ischemic heart disease or idiopathic dilated cardiomyopathy and severely depressed pump function (ejection fraction $< 40\%$). These patients might be in New York Heart Association functional class I, II, or III. It is precisely in this type of heart failure that detrimental effects have been reported with diltiazem, nifedipine, or nisoldipine. However, more encouraging results have been reported in other studies using nicardipine, amlodipine, or felodipine (45–47). In subsets of patients with dilated cardiomyopathy, favorable effects have also been reported with diltiazem (48). Moreover, in most of these studies ACE inhibitors, which are now becoming standard therapy for all degrees of heart failure (11), were not yet used. It is quite possible that the use of ACE inhibitors will be able to reduce the consequences of neurohumoral activation while preserving other beneficial properties of the calcium blockers, particularly the additional afterload reduction and the coronary vasodilation. This hypothesis is supported by the SOLVD results, in which the benefit of the ACE inhibitor enalapril on mortality and prevention of heart failure was comparable in patients who were and who were not receiving calcium antagonists (mainly nifedipine and diltiazem). This rules out a significant detrimental effect of these calcium blockers in the presence of an ACE inhibitor.

Thus, it may be worthwhile to reconsider the potential of calcium blockers in heart failure, but this time with the protective umbrella of an ACE inhibitor. Such a trial is currently planned by the Veterans Administration (VHeFT 3). Which type of calcium antagonist should be preferred in this setting? Although the answer is unknown, we may try to define the profile desirable for this purpose. In contrast to patients with hypertrophic cardiomyopathy, who easily tolerate the negative inotropic effect of verapamil or nifedipine, any further depression in performance should preferably be avoided in patients with heart failure. Preference should be given to compounds with a high selectivity for smooth muscle. Furthermore, because of their nonlinear first-pass metabolism, many of these compounds had to be given at relatively high doses, causing high peak plasma levels and low trough levels. These high peaks are not only likely to activate reflex mechanisms more strongly but may also be sufficient to depress contractility in a failing heart. New slow-release formulations or long-acting compounds are now available in the dihydropyridine family. With these formulations, the steady-state plasma levels obtained are more suitable to achieve a constant afterload reduction with minimal side effects.

Finally, the long-term effects on neurohormones and renal function appear to differ between compounds, for reasons still unclear. For example, the water retention and the incidence of worsening of congestive heart failure seen with nisoldipine have not been reported with nicardipine or felodipine, and decreases in plasma catecholamines have been reported in small studies during treatment of heart failure patients with felodipine or amlodipine (45–47). It is too early to suggest that the absence of catecholamine rise with some compounds will result in clinically different benefit, particularly in the presence of an ACE inhibitor. Although some direct effect of the compound on hormone release may exist (30), it remains to be determined if this is true in humans. Some of the apparent differences between compounds may simply be related to differences in pharmacokinetics and might be reduced by use of sustained-release formulations. Finally, one must also remember how variable are the neurohumoral values in heart failure patients. The real end points will be survival, exercise tolerance, and patients' well-being.

A last subset of patients in whom long-term effects of calcium antagonists could be worth examining is hypertensive patients with coronary artery disease. Two placebo-controlled and randomized trials using nifedipine or nicardipine (49,50) have shown that these agents, albeit unable to influence the progression of established stenoses, significantly reduced the progression of minimal lesions or the development of new lesions (49,50). The magnitude of the beneficial effects of nifedipine and of nicardipine appeared remarkably similar and could be related to the ability of calcium channel blockers to enhance cholesteryl ester hydrolysis and to reduce cholesterol accumulation in human vascular tissue (51). The relationship between hypertension and coronary artery disease was discovered many years ago; in contrast to the incidence of stroke, it has been notoriously difficult to reduce the incidence of coronary events in this population. Further studies are obviously necessary to confirm that the angiographic findings of the INTACT study (49) and of Waters et al. (50) have clinical implications. Still, in a disease for which treatment may span many years and start at an early age, reduction in the progression of coronary atherosclerosis is highly desirable. In this respect, dihydropyridine derivatives might therefore have an "edge" over other therapies.

In conclusion, despite the wide use of these compounds in the early 1990s, the prescription of a calcium-antagonist to treat heart failure is justified by clinical data only in a small subset of patients with normal systolic function and impaired diastolic filling. Even in this group, controlled clinical trials of the size necessary to obtain regulatory approval for the indication are still lacking.

In most other forms of heart failure and in an acute myocardial infarction, there is currently more evidence of detrimental effects than of clinical benefit. Even in patients with heart failure and angina pectoris, objective evidence is lacking that physical capacity is significantly improved by the addition of a calcium blocker. Nevertheless, there are still enough experimental and positive clinical observations to justify controlled clinical trials in heart failure, particularly with dihydropyridine derivatives of the second generation and in patients already receiving an ACE inhibitor.

ACKNOWLEDGMENT

The authors thank Ms. Isabelle Mottard for her careful secretarial assistance.

REFERENCES

1. Cohn PF, Braunwald E. Chronic ischemic heart disease. In: Braunwald E, ed. Heart Disease. A Textbook of Cardiovascular Medicine. Philadelphia: W. B. Saunders, 1984:1334–1383.
2. Kiowski W, Bolli P, Erne P, Müller FB, Hulthen UL, Bühler FR. Mechanisms of action and clinical use of calcium antagonists in hypertension. Circulation 1989; 80:IV-136–144.
3. Flamm ES. The potential use of nicardipine in cerebrovascular disease. Am Heart J 1989; 117:236–242.
4. Flamm ES, Adams HP, Beck DW, Pinto RS, Marler JR, Walker MD, Godersky JC, Loftus CM, Biller J, Boarini DJ, O'Dell C, Banwart K, Kongable G. Dose-escalation study of intravenous nicardipine in patients with aneurysmal subarachnoid hemorrhage. J Neurosurg 1988; 68:393–400.
5. Handa J, Matsuda M, Nakasu Y, Nakasu S, Kidooka M, Watanabe K. Early operation of aneurysmal subarachnoid hemorrhage—use of nicardipine, a calcium channel blocker. Arch Jpn Chir 1984; 53:619–630.
6. Neil-Dwyer G, Mee E, Dottance D, Lowe D. Early intervention with nimodipine in subarachnoid hemorrhage. Eur Heart J 1987; 8:11–47.

7. Rousseau MF, Hanet C, Desager JP, Pouleur H. Effects of long-term therapy with the association of nisoldipine and a β-blocker on exercise tolerance and coronary hemodynamics in patients with stable angina: a comparison with monotherapy. In: Hugenholtz PG, Meyer J, eds. Nisoldipine 1987. Berlin: Springer-Verlag, 1987:213–222.
8. Wrogemann K, Nylen EG. Mitochondrial calcium overloading in cardiomyopathic hamsters. J Mol Cell Cardiol 1978; 10:185–195.
9. Wu S, White R, Wikman-Coffelt J, Sievers R, Wendland M, Garrett J, Higgins CB, James T, Parmley WW. The preventive effect of verapamil on ethanol-induced cardiac depression: phosphorus-31 nuclear magnetic resonance and high-pressure liquid chromatographic studies of hamsters. Circulation 1987; 75:
10. Rouleau JL, Chuck LHS, Hollosi G, Kidd P, Sievers RE, Wikman-Coffelt J, Parmley WW. Verapamil preserves myocardial contractility in the hereditary cardiomyopathy of the syrian hamster. Circ Res 1982; 50:405–412.
11. The SOLVD Investigators. Effect of enalapril on survival in patients with reduced left ventricular ejection fractions and congestive heart failure. N Engl J Med 1991; 325:293–302.
12. Packer M, Kessler PD, Lee WH. Calcium-channel blockade in the management of severe congestive heart failure: a bridge too far. Circulation 1987; 75:V-56–V-64.
13. Packer M. Pathophysiological mechanisms underlying the adverse effects of calcium channel-blocking drugs in patients with chronic heart failure. Circulation 1989; 80:IV-59–67.
14. The Multicenter Diltiazem Postinfarction Trial Research Group. The effect of diltiazem on mortality and reinfarction after myocardial infarction. N Engl J Med 1988; 319:385–392.
15. Elkayam U, Amin J, Mehra A, Vasquez J, Weber L, Rahimtoola SH. A prospective, randomized, double-blind, crossover study to compare the efficacy and safety of chronic nifedipine therapy with that of isosorbide dinitrate and their combination in the treatment of chronic congestive heart failure. Circulation 1990; 82:1954–1961.
16. Goldstein RD, Boccuzzi SJ, Cruess D, Nattel S, the Adverse Experience Committee, and the Multicenter Diltiazem Postinfarction Research Group. Diltiazem increases late-onset congestive heart failure in postinfarction patients with early reduction in ejection fraction. Circulation 1991; 83:52–60.
17. Holland University Nifedipine/Metoprolol Trial (HINT) Research Group. Early treatment of unstable angina in the coronary care unit. A randomized double-blind, placebo controlled comparison of recurrent ischemia in patients treated with nifedipine or metoprolol or both. Br Heart J 1986; 56:400–413.
18. Held PH, Yusuf S, Furberg CD: Calcium channel blockers in acute myocardial infarction and unstable angina: an overview. Br Med J 1989; 299:1187–1192.
19. Feldman MD, Copelas L, Gwathmey JK, Phillips P, Warren SE, Schoen FJ. Deficient production of cyclic AMP: pharmacologic evidence of an important cause of contractile dysfunction in patients with end-stage heart failure. Circulation 1987; 75:331–339.

20. Satoh K, Yanagisawa T, Taira N. Mechanisms underlying the cardiovascular action of a new dihydropyridine vasodilator, YC-93. Clin Exper Pharmacol Physiol 1980; 7:249–262.
21. Kazda S, Garthoff B, Meyer H, Schlobeta/mann K, Stoepel K, Towart R, Vater W, Wehinger E. Pharmacology of a new calcium antagonist compound, isobutyl methyl 1,4-Dihydro-2,6-dimethyl-4(2-nirophenyl)-3, 5-pyridinedicarboxylate (nisoldipine, Bay k 5552). Drug Res 1980; 30(II):2144–2162.
22. Lambert CR, Buss DD, Pepine CJ. Effects of nicardipine on myocardial function in vitro and in vivo. Circulation 1990; 81:III-139–147.
23. Rousseau MF, Vincent MF, Cheron P, Van Den Berghe G, Charlier AA, Pouleur H. Effects of nicardipine on coronary blood flow, left ventricular inotropic state and myocardial metabolism in patients with angina pectoris. B J Clin Pharmacol 1985; 20:147S–157S.
24. Rousseau MF, Etienne J, Van Mechelen H, Veriter C, Pouleur H. Hemodynamic and cardiac effects of nicardipine in patients with coronary artery disease. J Cardiovasc Pharmacol 1984; 6:833–839.
25. Aroney CN, Semigran MJ, Dec GW, Boucher CA, Fifer MA. Inotropic effect of nicardipine in patients with heart failure: assessment by left ventricular end-systolic pressure-volume analysis. J Am Coll Cardiol 1989; 14:1331–1338.
26. Walsh RA, Badke RF, O'Rourke RA. Differential effects of systemic and intracoronary calcium channel blocking agents on global and regional left ventricular dysfunction in conscious dogs. Am Heart J 1981; 102:341.
27. Rousseau MF, Vincent MF, Van Hoof F, Van den Berghe G, Charlier AA, Pouleur H. Effects of nicardipine and nisoldipine on myocardial metabolism, coronary blood flow and oxygen supply in angina pectoris. Am J Cardiol 1984; 54:1189–1194.
28. Packer M, Lee WH, Medina N, Yushak M, Berstein JL, Kessler PD: Prognostic importance of the immediate hemodynamic response to nifedipine in patients with severe left ventricular dysfunction. J Am Coll Cardiol 1987; 10:1303–1311.
29. Lubsen J. Medical management of unstable angina. What have we learned from the randomized trials? Circulation 1990; 82(II):82–87.
30. Francis GS: Calcium channel blockers and congestive heart failure. Circulation 1991; 83(1):336–338.
31. Kassis E, Amtorp O. Cardiovascular and neurohumoral postural responses and baroreceptor abnormalities during a course of adjunctive vasodilator therapy with felodipine for congestive heart failure. Circulation 1987; 75:1204–1213.
32. Barjon JN, Rouleau JL, Bichet D, Juneau C, De Champlain J: Chronic renal and neurohumoral effects of the calcium entry blocker nisoldipine in patients with congestive heart failure. J Am Coll Cardiol 1987; 9:622–630.
33. Morgan JP, Erny RE, Allen PD, Grossman W, Gwathmey JK. Abnormal intracellular calcium handling, a major cause of systolic and diastolic dysfunction in ventricular myocardium from patients with heart failure. Circulation 1990; 81-2:III21–III32.

34. Lorell BH, Grossman W: Cardiac hypertrophy: consequences for diastole. J Am Coll Cardiol 1987; 9:1189–1193.
35. Bonow RO, Rosing DR, Bacharach SL, Green MV, Kent KM, Lipson LC, Maron BJ, Leon MB, Epstein SE. Effects of verapamil on left ventricular systolic function and diastolic filling in patients with hypertrophic cardiomyopathy. Circulation 1981; 64:787–796.
36. Lorell BH, Paulus WJ, Grossman W, Wynne J, Cohn PF. Modification of abnormal left ventricular diastolic properties by nifedipine in patients with hypertrophic cardiomyopathy. Circulation 1982; 65:499–507.
37. Setaro JF, Schulman DS, Black HR, LaCroix M, Zaret BL, Soufer R: Congestive heart failure, intact systolic function, and abnormal diastolic filling: improvement with verapamil in a placebo-controlled trial. Circulation 1988; 78:II-204.
38. Hittinger L, Shannon RP, Bishop SP, Gelpi RJ, Vatner SF. Subendomyocardial exhaustion of blood flow reserve and increased fibrosis in conscious dogs with heart failure. Circ Res 1989; 65:971–980.
39. Factor SM, Sonnenblick EH: Hypothesis: is congestive cardiomyopathy caused by a hyperreactive myocardial microcirculation (microvascular spasm)? Am J Cardiol 1982; 50:1149–1152.
40. Factor SM, Minase T, Cho S, Dominitz R, Sonnenblick EH: Microvascular spasm in the cardiomyopathic Syrian hamster: a preventable cause of focal myocardial necrosis. Circulation 1982; 66:342–354.
41. Frishman WH, Skolnick AE, Strom JA: Effects of calcium entry blockade on hypertension-induced left ventricular hypertrophy. Circulation 1989; 80(IV):151–161.
42. Rousseau MF, Gurné O, Benedict CR, van Eyll C, Pouleur H: Effects of nisoldipine on the time-dependent changes in left ventricular function and neurohumoral status in patients with ischemic heart disease. In: Lichtlen PR, Krayenbühl HP, eds. Aspects of Nisoldipine (Symposium in Nice during XIth Congress of the European Society of Cardiology). Stuttgart: Schattauer, 1990:69–83.
43. Pouleur H, van Eyll C, Gurné O, Van Mechelen H, Rousseau MF. Contrasting effects of the calcium antagonist nisoldipine on the normal and hibernating myocardium. Circulation 1991; 84(4):II-515.
44. Greenberg B, Massie B, Bristow JS, Cheitlin M, Siemienczuk D, Topic N, Wilson RA, Szlachcic J, Thomas D. Long-term vasodilator therapy of chronic aortic insufficiency. A randomized double-blinded, placebo-controlled clinical trial. Circulation 1988; 78:92–103.
45. Lahiri A, Robinson CN, Kohli RS, Caruana MP, Raftery EB. Acute and chronic effects of nicardipine on systolic and diastolic left ventricular performance in patients with heart failure. A pilot study. Clin Cardiol 1986; 9:257–261.
46. Packer M: Calcium channel blockers in chronic heart failure. The risks of "physiologically rational" therapy. Circulation 1990; 82:2254–2257.
47. Kassis E, Amtorp O. Long-term clinical, hemodynamic, angiographic, and

neurohumoral responses to vasodilation with felodipine in patients with chronic congestive heart failure. Cardiovasc Pharmacol 1990; 15:347–352.
48. Figulla HR, Rechenberg JV, Wiegand V, Soballa R, Kreuzer H. Beneficial effects of long-term diltiazem treatment in dilated cardiomyopathy. J Am Coll Cardiol 1989; 13:653–658.
49. Lichtlen PR, Hugenholtz PG, Rafflenbeul W, Hecker H, Jost S, Deckers JW on behalf of the INTACT Group Investigators. Retardation of angiographic progression of coronary artery disease by nifedipine. Results of the International Nifedipine Trial on Antiatherosclerotic Therapy (INTACT). Lancet 1990; 335:1109–1113.
50. Waters D, Lespérance J, Francetich M, Causey D, Théroux P, Chiang Y, Hudon G, Lemarbre L, Reitman M, Joyal M, Gosselin G, Dyrda I, Macer J, Havel RJ. A controlled clinical trial to assess the effect of a calcium channel blocker on the progression of coronary atherosclerosis. Circulation 1990; 82:1940–1953.
51. Etingin OR, Hajjar DP. Calcium channel blockers enhance cholesteryl ester hydrolysis and decrease total cholesterol accumulation in human aortic tissue. Clin Res 1990; 66:185–190.

15

Phosphodiesterase Inhibitors, Calcium Sensitizers, and Ion Channel Active Agents

Wilson S. Colucci and Joel S. Landzberg
Brigham and Women's Hospital and Harvard Medical School, Boston, Massachusetts

INTRODUCTION

A long-standing goal in the treatment of congestive heart failure has been the development of an orally active positive inotropic agent (1). It has seemed logical that such an agent would be of clinical value by correcting, at least partially, the fundamental hemodynamic abnormality in the process of congestive heart failure, insufficient cardiac pump function. This thesis has been further supported by the demonstrated value of intravenously administered positive inotropic agents, such as dobutamine, to improve hemodynamic function and stabilize the clinical situation in patients. However, there has also been concern that the chronic administration of potent positive inotropic agents could be associated with adverse clinical effects related to inordinate energy requirements, the stimulation of arrhythmias, or impairment of diastolic myocardial relaxation (2,3). Furthermore, it remains to be proven that an improvement in pump function caused by a positive inotropic agent will translate into a clinically useful improvement in functional capacity, quality of life, or survival.

The last decade has witnessed an explosion of new therapeutic agents that exert a positive inotropic effect when administered orally. These agents utilize a variety of pharmacological mechanisms to increase myocardial contractility, and in some cases a single agent may exert a positive inotropic action by more than one mechanism (Table 1). In addition, many of these new agents exert significant vasodilatory effects that may contribute, to various degrees, to the clinical activity of the agent. Although many such compounds have been evaluated in various preclinical models, relatively few have undergone significant clinical testing in humans. In the discussion that follows, we will focus primarily on those agents that have undergone substantial clinical testing in patients with congestive heart failure.

REGULATION OF MYOCARDIAL CONTRACTILE FORCE

The generation of myocardial contractile force is due to the ATP-dependent interaction or "cross-bridging" of the contractile proteins, actin and myosin. This interaction is regulated by tropomyosin and troponin, proteins that in turn are regulated by the free cytosolic concentration of calcium. Calcium binds to the troponin-C subunit of troponin, thereby inducing a conformational change in troponin that favors an increase in cross-bridge formation.

Contraction and relaxation of the heart are due to cyclic increases and decreases in cytosolic free calcium concentration. The major source of this calcium is the sarcoplasmic reticulum, from which calcium release is triggered by the influx of a smaller amount of "trigger" calcium that enters the cell via voltage-dependent calcium channels of the L-type. These channels are cyclically activated by membrane depolarization, and in addition, their conductance of calcium is modulated by cAMP: An increase in cAMP promotes a greater influx of calcium for a given level of membrane de-

Table 1 Pharmacologic Mechanisms of Action of Several New Inotropic Agents

	Amrinone, milrinone, enoximone	Pimobendan	DPI 201-106	OPC-8212
Phosphodiesterase inhibition	+	+		+
Calcium sensitization		+	+	
Sodium current			+	+
Potassium current				+
Vasodilation	+[a]	+[a]	+[b]	

[a]Due to phosphodiesterase inhibition
[b]Due to calcium channel inhibition

polarization. A variety of calcium channel agonists are now available that can directly activate the L-type calcium channel in the absence of membrane depolarization. β-Adrenergic agonists (e.g., isoproterenol, dobutamine) and phosphodiesterase inhibitors (e.g., amrinone, milrinone, enoximone) increase the availability of cAMP, and thereby increase L-type channel flux indirectly.

Voltage-dependent calcium channel influx can also be increased by prolonging the time of depolarization, as may occur if outward potassium currents are inhibited. There is evidence that α_1-adrenergic receptor stimulation and some of the new inotropic agents (e.g., OPC-8212) may act, in part, by this mechanism (4,5).

Calcium may also enter the myocardial cell by way of Na^+-Ca^{2+} exchange, a process that is promoted by an increase in intracellular sodium concentration. Intracellular sodium concentration can be increased by inhibition of Na^+/K^+-ATPase (e.g., digitalis glycosides), or by increasing the inward conductance of sodium by "fast" sodium channels, as may occur with some of the new inotropic agents including DPI 201-106 and OPC-8212 (6,7).

The sensitivity of the contractile apparatus to calcium can be modulated, apparently by multiple mechanisms (8–10). Some hormones that act by stimulation of phospholipase-C to cause mobilization of intracellular calcium and activation of protein kinase-C (PK-C) (e.g., α-adrenergic receptor agonists, endothelin, angiotensin II) may increase the calcium sensitivity of the contractile apparatus. This action may be due to a PK-C-mediated increase in intracellular pH, but other mechanisms are also possible. Several pharmacological agents have now been identified which can increase calcium sensitivity (i.e., DPI 201-106, pimobendan). These agents apparently do not act by an effect on intracellular pH, since they exert this effect in permeabilized cells where the pH is fixed. It appears that some of these agents act by a direct effect on various components of the contractile apparatus, such as troponin-C.

PHOSPHODIESTERASE INHIBITORS

Several agents that inhibit phosphodiesterase have been evaluated clinically in patients with congestive heart failure, and at least three agents, amrinone, milrinone, and enoximone, are currently available in various countries for intravenous use in patients with refractory congestive heart failure. A number of new inotropic agents exert phosphodiesterase inhibitory activity in combination with at least one other action that may also exert a positive inotropic effect, such as calcium sensitization or sodium channel activation. These agents with multiple mechanisms of positive inotropic activity will be considered separately.

Phosphodiesterase inhibitors cause an increase in intracellular cAMP levels by inhibiting the enzyme responsible for degradation of cAMP. It is not surprising that the effects of phosphodiesterase inhibitors on the heart are quite similar to those caused by β-adrenergic agonists, which also act by increasing the availability of intracellular cAMP. Phosphodiesterase is a ubiquitous enzyme with several isoforms that exhibit a certain degree of tissue specificity. The predominant isoform in myocardium and vascular smooth muscle is referred to as F-III (11). Phosphodiesterase inhibitors differ in their selectivity for the various isoforms of phosphodiesterase. Increased selectivity for F-III should result in greater specificity for the cardiovascular system and reduced nonspecific activity in noncardiovascular tissues, such as the gastrointestinal tract. A characteristic of the new phosphodiesterase inhibitors is a relative selectivity for the F-III isoform, and as a consequence, a lower incidence of gastrointestinal intolerance, a common adverse effect seen with nonselective phosphodiesterase inhibitors such as aminophylline, particularly when used in concentrations that would significantly affect myocardial contractility. The phosphodiesterase inhibitors exert a positive inotropic effect in most animal species, although rats are a notable exception (12).

Since F-III phosphodiesterase is present in vascular smooth muscle, as well as in myocardium, it is not surprising that most of the phosphodiesterase inhibitors so far evaluated also exert a potent, direct vasodilator effect. This action is mediated by cAMP, and generally manifests as a balanced arterial and venous dilation, not unlike that caused by nitroprusside (13). The relative importance of the positive inotropic and vasodilator actions of the phosphodiesterase inhibitors is often difficult to determine, since both actions can result in marked hemodynamic improvement in patients with heart failure.

The positive inotropic response to phosphodiesterase inhibitors may be attenuated in patients with end-stage heart failure. In vitro studies with myocardium explanted from patients with end-stage heart failure at the time of cardiac transplantation show an attenuated positive inotropic response to these agents when compared with normal myocardium (14). The response is normalized if the tissue is first "primed" with forskolin, an agent that directly increases cAMP levels by stimulating the catalytic unit of adenylate cyclase. It is likely that myocardial cAMP levels are deficient in the severely failing heart, in part because of the attenuated function of the β-adrenergic receptor/adenylate cyclase pathway (15), and it would not be surprising, therefore, if the response to a phosphodiesterase inhibitor were likewise attenuated. It is also likely that assessment of the response to a phosphodiesterase inhibitor in vitro exaggerates the magnitude of this attenuation, since it creates a situation in which the myocardium is removed from its in situ milieu, which in a patient with severe heart failure often consists of a heightened level of sympathetic tone that may elevate the basal cAMP level.

Since β-adrenergic agonists and phosphodiesterase inhibitors increase cAMP levels by different mechanisms, it is predicted that the combination of these agents should result in a complementary effect on contractility. In patients with heart failure, the maximal positive inotropic response to the intracoronary infusion of a β-adrenergic agonist such as dobutamine is substantially attenuated because of altered β-adrenergic receptor pathway function (16). Prior intracoronary infusion of the phosphodiesterase inhibitor milrinone both exerts a direct positive inotropic effect and results in a significantly greater positive inotropic response to the subsequent administration of the same dose of dobutamine (16). Clinically, it has been shown that the combination of a β-adrenergic agonist (dobutamine) and a phosphodiesterase inhibitor (amrinone) causes a greater increase in +dP/dt and a substantially better hemodynamic response than either agent alone (17).

The relative contributions of the positive inotropic and direct vasodilator actions of the phosphodiesterase inhibitors to the overall improvement in hemodynamic performance is not clear (18). Early studies with amrinone suggested that a positive inotropic action might not contribute to the overall systemic effects of the drug (19). More recent studies that compared the effect of intracoronary infusion of milrinone with that of systemic administration of the drug have indicated that in therapeutic concentrations, this agent exerts a direct positive inotropic effect, even in patients with severe heart failure, and that this effect contributes significantly to the overall hemodynamic action of the drug (20). It is possible that the positive inotropic-to-vasodilator ratio varies from agent to agent, and even at different drug concentrations for the same agent.

Amrinone

Amrinone was the first of the phosphodiesterase inhibitors to undergo extensive clinical testing. The intravenous administration of amrinone to patients causes a marked increase in stroke volume, stroke work, and cardiac output, and substantial decreases in right atrial pressure, pulmonary capillary wedge pressure, and left ventricular end-diastolic pressure, generally associated with only a small increase in heart rate (19,21,22). Some (21,22), but not all (19), investigations found that intravenous administration of amrinone was associated with an increase in +dP/dt, suggesting a positive inotropic effect. The presence of a positive inotropic effect and its clinical relevance have been questioned (18,19).

The intravenous form of amrinone was approved in several countries, including the United States, for the treatment of refractory congestive heart failure. Intravenous amrinone has been useful in the acute hemodynamic stabilization of patients, particularly those who are not adequately responsive to β-adrenergic agonists. Amrinone may be used alone or in combination with a β-adrenergic agonist. Because of its potent vasodilator actions, amrinone should be avoided in patients who do not have elevation of cardiac filling pressures. Amrinone should also be used with caution in patients with depressed arterial pressure, although many such patients will tolerate the drug and may be benefited. The major dose-limiting side effects are tachycardia, an increase in supraventricular or ventricular arrhythmias, and hypotension. Thrombocytopenia occurs in a small percentage of patients but generally is not clinically significant and responds to withdrawal of the drug.

Clinical studies with the oral form of amrinone failed to demonstrate clinical efficacy with regard to exercise capacity or symptomatology, and its use was associated with an unacceptable level of adverse effects, predominantly involving gastrointestinal intolerance, and to a lesser extent thrombocytopenia (23).

Milrinone

Milrinone is an analogue of amrinone that is both more potent on a per-milligram basis and more selective for the F-III isoform of phosphodiesterase (24). The hemodynamic effects of intravenous milrinone are similar to those described for amrinone, although an increase in +dP/dt has been observed more consistently than with amrinone (12,18,25,26). Studies with direct intracoronary infusion of milrinone have demonstrated a positive inotropic effect that contributes to the overall hemodynamic actions of the intravenous agent (20). The hemodynamic responses to milrinone are maintained over prolonged periods of several days. Intravenous milrinone has been approved for use in several countries, including the United States. The dose-limiting toxicity of milrinone is similar to that of amrinone, except that thrombocytopenia rarely occurs.

In contrast to the experience with amrinone, the oral form of milrinone is not associated with gastrointestinal intolerance, and thus, the agent has received substantial scrutiny as a long-term therapy for patients. The largest of the long-term trials, reported by DiBianco et al. (27), compared milrinone, digitalis, and the combination of milrinone and digitalis with placebo in 230 patients with moderate congestive heart failure (Fig. 1). All

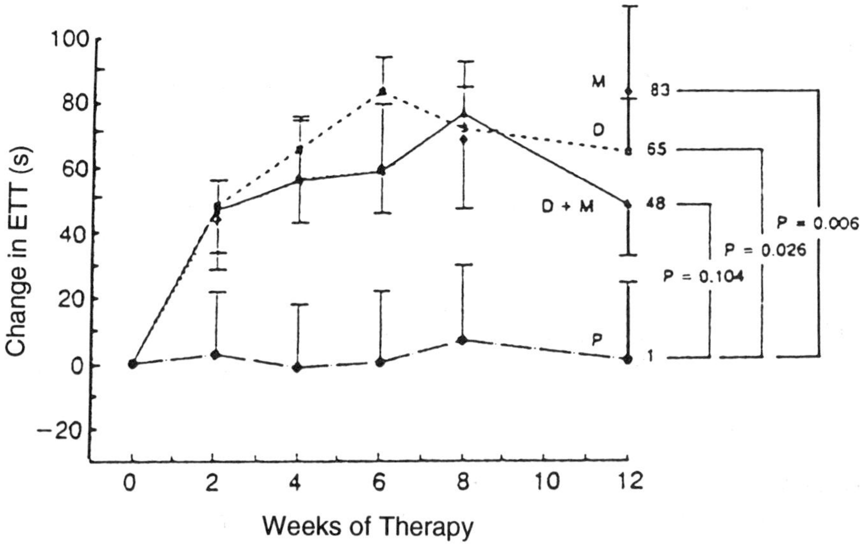

Figure 1 Change in exercise duration, relative to baseline, in patients treated with placebo (P), milrinone (M), digitalis (D), or the combination of digitalis and milrinone (D + M). (From Ref. 27.)

patients were in sinus rhythm and received maintenance therapy consisting of diuretics. In this study, converting enzyme inhibitors and other vasodilators were not allowed. Over the 12-week course of the study, it was found that both milrinone and digoxin, as well as the combination of the two agents, caused a significant increase in exercise capacity, although the combination caused no greater increase than either digitalis or milrinone alone. Both milrinone and digitalis decreased the incidence of clinical decompensation, although milrinone was less efficacious in this regard than digitalis. Milrinone treatment was associated with an increase in ventricular arrhythmias and a trend toward an increase in mortality, although much of this trend could be attributed to a significant imbalance in the randomization of high-risk patients with a low ejection fraction to the milrinone group.

The effect of milrinone on survival was specifically addressed by Packer et al. (28) in the PROMISE trial, a study that examined the effect of adjunctive milrinone therapy in New York Heart Association (NYHA) class III and IV patients already receiving optimal conventional therapy consisting of (in most cases) diuretics, digitalis, and converting enzyme inhibitors or other vasodilators. Patients (N = 1088) were randomized and followed for a median period of 6.1 months, at which time the trial was terminated because of a significant 28% increase in cardiovascular mortality in the milrinone-treatment group (Fig. 2). The increase in mortality was primarily in class IV (risk ratio = 1.53) versus class III (risk ratio = 1.03) patients, and was apparently related to a proarrhythmic effect and an increase in the incidence of sudden death (29). Further analysis has suggested that this adverse effect of milrinone may have been related to digoxin, since the increased incidence of sudden death with milrinone was largely among patients with a digoxin level greater than the median for the group (30). The PROMISE data suggest that arrhythmias leading to sudden death are a serious adverse effect with milrinone. Largely on the basis of this trial, the further development of oral milrinone was curtailed.

Enoximone

Enoximone and the related agent piroximone are F-III–selective phosphodiesterase inhibitors whose acute hemodynamic effects with intrave-

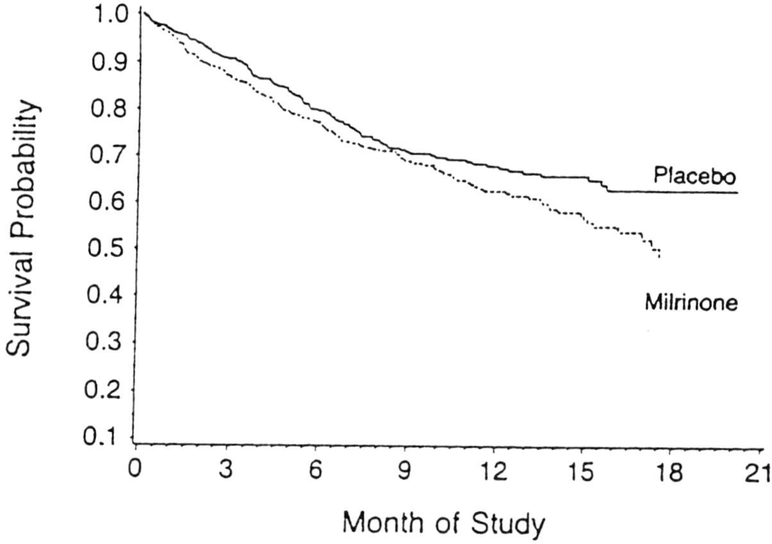

Placebo	527	375	270	185	137	77	21
Milrinone	561	395	284	184	132	74	14

Figure 2 Probability of survival in New York Heart Association class III and IV patients treated with maximal conventional therapy plus the addition of placebo or milrinone. The decreased survival with milrinone was statistically significant. (From Ref. 28.)

nous administration are similar to those already described for amrinone and milrinone (31,32). The hemodynamic actions of these agents are also due to a combination of positive inotropic and vasodilator effects (32). Intravenous enoximone has been approved for the management of severe myocardial failure in several countries. As with amrinone and milrinone, the major dose-limiting effects are related to tachycardia, arrhythmias, and hypotension.

Oral enoximone is well absorbed and appears to be hemodynamically efficacious for at least several months (33). A 12-patient randomized, controlled, crossover-design trial compared enoximone to placebo, with each treatment arm lasting for 6 weeks (34). All patients in this study received diuretics, and 8 of 12 patients received digoxin. Vasodilators and converting enzyme inhibitors were excluded. During the enoximone treatment arm, exercise duration increased significantly by 30% to 43%, symptoms of heart failure improved, and NYHA class decreased by at least one level in all patients.

The largest placebo-controlled trial of enoximone, however, failed to demonstrate clinical benefit of the agent. Uretsky et al. (35) evaluated 102 patients with NYHA functional class II–III congestive heart failure on long-term treatment with diuretics and digoxin. Vasodilators and converting enzyme inhibitors were excluded. Over the 16-week course of this study, enoximone caused no significant change in exercise duration. Dropouts due to a combination of worsening heart failure and adverse effects were more frequent in the enoximone group, as was the incidence of diarrhea. The incidence of death was significantly higher among patients receiving enoximone, with no deaths in the placebo group as compared with five deaths in the enoximone group (sudden death, 2; progressive heart failure, 2; myocardial infarction, 1).

In the study of Uretsky et al., enoximone was administered in a low dose for the first 4 weeks (50–75 mg t.i.d.), and subsequently the dose was increased to 100–150 mg t.i.d., if tolerated. It is of interest that in a subset of patients in whom metabolic gas analysis was performed, anaerobic threshold was significantly increased at 4 weeks, but not thereafter. This observation led the authors to speculate that a lower dose of enoximone might have been more efficacious clinically, and probably would have been tolerated better (35). This thesis appears to have been supported by recent data presented in abstract form (36).

CALCIUM SENSITIZING AGENTS

Several compounds have been identified that increase the sensitivity of the contractile apparatus to calcium. These agents cause a leftward/upward shift of the relationship between calcium and tension development. Although the exact site of action for these agents is not known, it may involve effects on troponin-C, the subunit of troponin that interacts with calcium. At least three agents that can be shown to sensitize myocardium to calcium in vitro have been evaluated clinically in patients with congestive heart failure—sumazole, DPI 201-106, and pimobendan. Of these agents, sumazole received only limited intravenous testing, and although DPI 201-106 was evaluated more extensively, it is no longer under investigation. Pimobendan is currently undergoing extensive clinical testing as an oral agent.

Pimobendan

Pimobendan (UDCG-115) exerts both positive inotropic and direct vasodilator activities. In skinned myocytes, it can be shown that pimobendan increases the sensitivity of the contractile apparatus to calcium (37,38). In addition, pimobendan inhibits phosphodiesterase at therapeutically relevant concentrations (39). The parent compound (UDCG-115) is metabolized to UDCG-212, which exerts a more potent positive inotropic effect than UDCG-115.

Acute intravenous administration of pimobendan to patients with congestive heart failure results in an increase in stroke volume and cardiac index, associated with decreases in left ventricular end-diastolic pressure, systemic vascular resistance, and mean arterial pressure, and a small increase in heart rate (40). Left ventricular peak +dP/dt is increased, which, in the presence of decreases in arterial and left ventricular end-diastolic pressures, is evidence of a positive inotropic effect. The improvement in hemodynamic function is associated with a decrease in myocardial oxygen demand coincident with a decrease in the left ventricular systolic stress-time interval (40).

The administration of a single oral dose of pimobendan to patients with heart failure is associated with hemodynamic effects similar to those observed with intravenous drug administration. Two randomized, placebo-controlled trials have evaluated the efficacy of oral pimobendan in patients. Katz et al. evaluated 52 patients with NYHA class III and IV congestive heart failure treated with diuretics (52/52), digoxin (47/52), converting enzyme inhibitors (40/52), and hydralazine/nitrates (4/52) (41). Patients were randomized to placebo or pimobendan, 5 or 10 mg/d for 4 weeks. When taken together, patients who received pimobendan showed a significant increase in exercise duration in comparison with placebo-treated patients.

Kubo et al. reported a larger, placebo-controlled trial that evaluated 198 patients randomized to placebo vesus 2.5, 5, or 10 mg/d of pimobendan for 12 weeks (42). Patients in this trial were primarily in NYHA class III, and most were receiving diuretics, digoxin, and a converting enzyme inhibitor or other non–converting enzyme inhibitor vasodilator. In this trial, patients who received 5 mg/d of pimobendan showed a significant increase in exercise duration, and those who received 10 mg/d showed a smaller but still significant increase (Fig. 3). This pattern of a greater improvement with the 5 mg/d dosage was likewise found with regard to quality of life scores, which increased significantly with the 5 mg/d dosage, and to a lesser extent with the 10 mg/d dosage. The 2.5 mg/d dosage did not signficantly improve exercise or quality of life in this trial.

SODIUM AND POTASSIUM CHANNEL ACTIVE AGENTS

Agents that affect sodium and potassium ion flux can exert a positive inotropic action by a variety of mechanisms, which in all cases culminate in the increased entry of extracellular calcium. By promoting greater so-

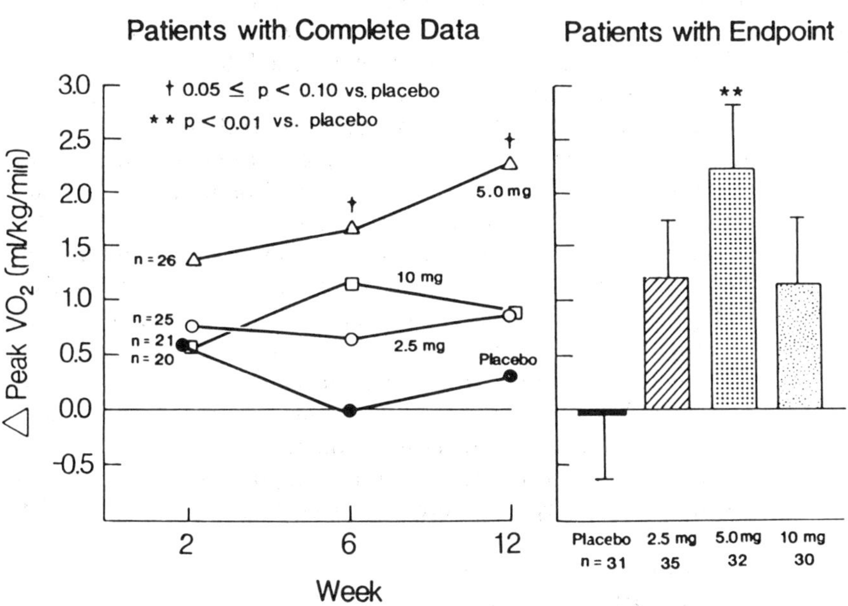

Figure 3 Changes in peak oxygen consumption during exercise in patients treated with placebo or three doses of pimobendan (2.5, 5, and 10 mg/d). (From Ref. 42.)

dium influx via fast sodium channels, sodium channel agonists such as DPI 201-106 and OPC-8212 make more intracellular sodium available for exchange with extracellular calcium via the Na^{+}-Ca^{2+} exchange mechanism. Alternatively, by interfering with outward rectifying K^{+} currents, agents such as OPC-8212 prolong the duration of depolarization and thereby increase the inward conductance of calcium via voltage-dependent calcium channels. Both DPI 201-106 and OPC-8212 have been evaluated in patients. Although DPI 201-106 is no longer under investigation, some of the observations made with this agent may be relevant to future agents. OPC-8212 is currently being evaluated as an oral agent.

DPI 201-106

DPI 201-106 has two actions that in theory may exert a positive inotropic effect. First, the agent prolongs the open time for the fast sodium channel, thus making more sodium available for exchange with extracellular calcium (6,43). In addition, there is evidence from experiments performed with skinned myocardial trabeculae that this agent may increase the sensitivity of the contractile apparatus to calcium (44). The relative importance of these two mechanisms is not clear. However, in several species including humans, the positive inotropic effect is blocked by tetrodotoxin, a specific inhibitor of fast sodium channels, removal of extracellular sodium, or prior depolarization, all maneuvers that would suggest that the major positive inotropic mechanism is increased conductance by fast sodium channels (45). However, there is evidence that this sensitizing effect may be more prominent in myopathic tissue as compared with normal tissue (44). DPI 201-106 may also exert a negative lusitropic effect (46), presumably related to altered calcium handling. In relevant concentrations, this agent has no effect on phosphodiesterase, but appears to exert a significant antagonistic action on voltage-dependent calcium channels, since it inhibits potassium-stimulated contraction and calcium uptake in rabbit aorta (46). This effect on voltage-dependent calcium channels may also contribute to slowing of heart rate, an effect that may occur with this agent. DPI 201-106 also exerts significant electrophysiological effects in myocardium, most prominently a concentration-dependent prolongation of action potential duration (47). This effect is antagonized by tetrodotoxin, suggesting that it is related to increased sodium influx.

When administered by intravenous infusion to patients with congestive heart failure, DPI 201-106 results in increases in cardiac index and +dP/dt, and decreases in systemic vascular resistance and left ventricular end-diastolic pressure (48). Heart rate may decrease as well. Oral administration of DPI 201-106 to patients with severe heart failure resulted in increases in cardiac index, stroke volume, and stroke work without significant changes in heart rate or systemic arterial pressure (47). The QT_c interval was increased and correlated with the plasma DPI 201-106 concentration, an observation that raised some concerns about potential arrhythmogenicity (47). This agent has not undergone further clinical evaluation.

OPC-8212

OPC-8212 is a quinolinone derivative with multiple mechanisms of action involving ion channels, some or all of which may contribute to a positive inotropic effect in myocardium. At least four activities have been identified: (1) inhibition of the outward delayed rectifying potassium current (5); (2) an increase in fast sodium inward current (7); (3) an increase in whole-cell calcium influx, probably due to inhibition of phosphodiesterase and elevated cAMP levels (49); and (4) a rate-dependent prolongation of the action potential duration (50). All of these actions would result in a greater influx of calcium. The relative importance of these mechanisms with regard to the inotropic effect of the agent is not clear, and it is possible that more than one mechanism contributes.

The acute oral administration of OPC-8212 to patients with congestive heart failure results in beneficial hemodynamic effects characterized by an increase in cardiac output and modest reductions in left and right heart filling pressures, generally with no increase or a small decrease in heart rate (51).

OPC-8212 has undergone substantial evaluation in patients with congestive heart failure, both in Japan and in the United States. This agent is currently approved for the treatment of heart failure in Japan and has been administered to several thousand patients there. Results of two double-blind, placebo-controlled trials are available. The first trial, conducted in Japan, evaluated 83 patients with moderate to severe congestive heart failure, cardiomegaly, and reduced left ventricular ejection fraction (mean ejection fraction 43%) (52). Patients were randomized to placebo or OPC-8212, 60 mg/d for a 3-month period. Most patients also received diuretics, digitalis, and vasodilators. Patients treated with OPC-8212 exhibited a reduction in clinical deterioration, improvement in quality of life as assessed by a questionnaire, and a significant increase in left ventricular ejection fraction associated with a reduced left ventricular end-systolic dimension. Exercise function was not evaluated.

Feldman et al. (53) reported a second controlled trial performed in the United States. This trial evaluated 76 patients with NYHA functional class II–IV congestive heart failure despite therapy with diuretics, digitalis, and converting enzyme inhibitors in most patients. The median ejection fraction in this study (24%) was substantially lower than in the Japanese study. Patients were randomized to placebo or OPC-8212 (60 mg/d) for a period of 12 weeks. OPC-8212 therapy was associated with an improvement in the quality of life, as assessed by the sickness impact profile questionnaire, and a significant reduction in the combined end points of major morbidity and mortality (Fig. 4). OPC-8212 treatment was associated with small improvements in exercise performance, and Holter monitoring revealed no significant change in the number of ventricular premature concentrations per hour. The major side effect of OPC-8212 is a small incidence (approximately 2% to 4%) of reversible agranulocytosis in Caucasian patients. The electrocardiographic QT interval is prolonged, as would be anticipated on the basis of the mechanism of action.

FUTURE ISSUES

It remains to be determined whether a positive inotropic agent can be developed that is both clinically efficacious and safe. A number of orally active positive inotropic agents have now been studied in patients with heart failure. From this early experience, several important realizations

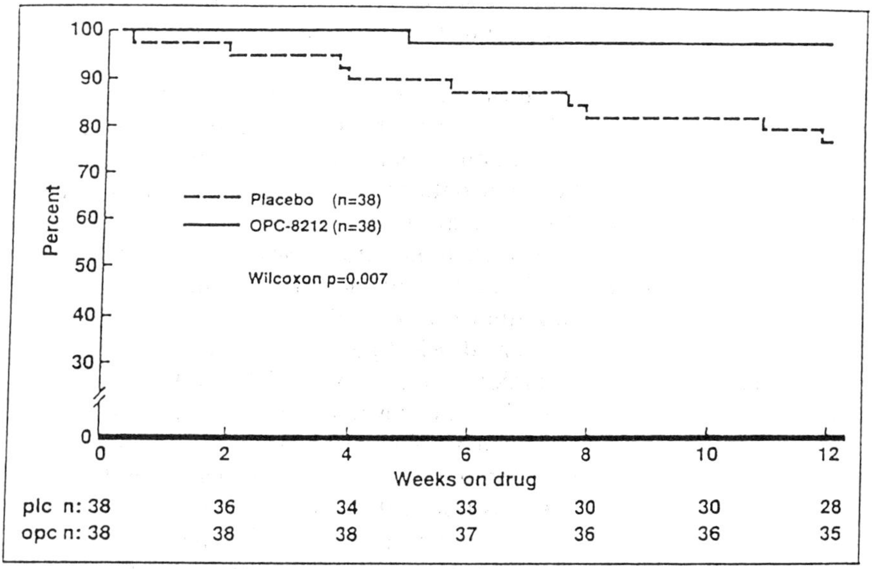

Figure 4 Percent of patients free of the combined end point of morbidity and mortality during treatment with placebo or OPC-8212. (From Ref. 53.)

have emerged, and more important, new issues have been raised for future attention. The pure phosphodiesterase inhibitors such as amrinone, milrinone, and enoximone may improve exercise capacity. However, the utility of these agents has been seriously hindered by adverse effects such as gastrointestinal intolerance, hypotension, and arrhythmias. In addition, serious questions have been raised regarding the safety of both enoximone and milrinone, which have been associated with increased cardiovascular mortality. Although the mechanism of this adverse effect on mortality is not yet fully elucidated, it appears likely to involve an increase in sudden death, presumably related to increased cAMP levels. That this effect is most prominent in NYHA class IV patients and associated with digoxin administration may reflect the increased sensitivity of such patients to arrhythmias. It appears that if phosphodiesterase inhibitors are to be used in the future, they must be used at lower doses and with great caution in patients who are particularly susceptible to adverse effects.

A promising approach may be the combination of two or more positive inotropic mechanisms, such as phosphodiesterase inhibition, calcium sensitization, or ion channel effects. By combining mechanisms of action, it may be possible to benefit from the hemodynamic effects of each mechanism while minimizing their potential adverse effects. The results of controlled trials with oral administration of pimobendan and OPC-8212 are encouraging in this regard, but will require confirmation and establishment of long-term safety.

REFERENCES

1. Colucci WS, Wright RF, Braunwald E. New positive inotropic agents in the treatment of congestive heart failure. Mechanisms of action and recent clinical developments. N Engl J Med 1986; 314:290–299.
2. Katz AM. A new inotropic drug: its promise and a caution. N Engl J Med 1978; 299:1409–1410.
3. Packer M. Protagonist's viewpoint. J Am Coll Cardiol 1988; 12:559–569.
4. Fedida D, Shimoni Y, Giles WR. A novel effect of norepinephrine on cardiac cells is mediated by α_1-adrenoceptors. Am J Physiol 1989; 256:H1500–H1504.
5. Iijima T, Taira N. Membrane current changes responsible for the positive inotropic effect of OPC-8212, a new positive inotropic agent, in single ventricular cells of guinea pig heart. J Pharmacol Exp Ther 1987; 240:657–662.
6. Scholtysik G. Cardiac Na^+ channel activation as a positive inotropic principle. J Cardiovasc Pharmacol 1989; 14:S24–S29.
7. Lathrop DA, Schwartz A. Evidence for possible increase in sodium channel open time and involvement of Na/Ca exchange by a new positive inotropic drug: OPC-8212. Eur J Pharmacol 1985; 117F:391–392.

8. Blinks JR, Endoh M. Modification of myofibrillar responsiveness to Ca^{++} as an inotropic mechanism. Circulation 1986; 73:III-85–III-97.
9. Ruegg JC. Effects of new inotropic agents on Ca^{++} sensitivity of contractile proteins. Circulation 1986; 73:III-78–III-83.
10. Ruegg JC, Morano I. Calcium-sensitivity modulation of cardiac myofibrillar proteins. J. Cardiovasc Pharmacol 1989; 14:S20–S23.
11. Schmitz W, von der Leyen H, Meyer W, Neumann J, Scholz H. Phosphodiesterase inhibition and positive inotropic effects. J Cardiovasc Pharmacol 1989; 14:S11–S14.
12. Jaski BE, Fifer MA, Wright RF, Braunwald E, Colucci WS. Positive inotropic and vasodilator actions of milrinone in patients with severe congestive heart failure. Dose-response relationships and comparison to nitroprusside. J Clin Invest 1985; 75:643–649.
13. Alousi AA, Farah AE, Lesher GY, Opalka CJ Jr. Cardiotonic activity of amrinone-WIN 40680 [5-amino-3′,4′-bipyridine-6(1H)-one]. Circ Res 1979; 45:666–677.
14. Feldman MD, Copelas L, Gwathmey JK, Phillips P, Warren SE, Schoen FJ, Grossman W, Morgan JP. Deficient production of cyclic AMP: pharmacologic evidence of an important cause of contractile dysfunction in patients with end-stage heart failure. Circulation 1987; 75:331–339.
15. Bristow MR, Hershberger RE, Port JD, Gilbert EM, Sandoval A, Rasmussen R, Cates AE, Feldman AM. β-Adrenergic pathways in nonfailing and failing human ventricular myocardium. Circulation 1990; 82:I-12–I-25.
16. Colucci WS, Denniss AR, Leatherman GF, Quigg RJ, Ludmer PL, Marsh JD, Gauthier DF. Intracoronary infusion of dobutamine to patients with and without severe congestive heart failure. Dose-response relationships, correlation with circulating catecholamines, and effect of phosphodiesterase inhibition. J Clin Invest 1988; 81:1103–1110.
17. Gage J, Rutman H, Lucido D, LeJemtel TH. Additive effects of dobutamine and amrinone on myocardial contractility and ventricular performance in patients with severe heart failure. Circulation 1986; 74:367–373.
18. Colucci WS. Do the bipyridines exert a positive inotropic action in patients with congestive heart failure? In: Braunwald E, Julian D, eds. The Acute Therapy of Heart Failure. Intravenous Milrinone—A New Therapeutic Option. Royal Society of Medicine Services Intl. Cong. Symp. Series No. 172. Royal Society of Medicine Services Limited, 1991:11–17.
19. Wilmshurst PT, Thompson DS, Jenkins BS, Coltart DJ, Webb-Peploe MM. Haemodynamic effects of intravenous amrinone in patients with impaired left ventricular function. Br Heart J 1983; 49:77–82.
20. Ludmer PL, Wright RF, Arnold MO, Ganz P, Braunwald E, Colucci WS. Separation of the direct myocardial and vasodilator actions of milrinone administered by an intracoronary infusion technique. Circulation 1986; 73:130–137.

21. Benotti JR, Grossman W, Braunwald E, Davolos DD, Alousi AA. Hemodynamic assessment of amrinone. A new inotropic agent. N Engl J Med 1978; 299:1373–1377.
22. LeJemtel TH, Keung E, Sonnenblick EH, Ribner HS, Matsumoto M, Davis R, Schwartz W, Alousi AA, Davolos D. Amrinone: a new non-glycosidic, non-adrenergic cardiotonic agent effective in the treatment of intractable myocardial failure in man. Circulation 1979; 59:1098–1104.
23. Massie B, Bourassa M, DiBianco R, et al. Long-term oral adminsitration of amrinone for congestive heart failure: lack of efficacy in a multicenter controlled trial. Circulation 1985; 71:963–971.
24. Alousi AA, Stankus GP, Stuart JC, Walton LH. Characterization of the cardiotonic effects of milrinone, a new and potent cardiac bipyridine, on isolated tissues from several animal species. J. Cardiovasc Pharmacol 1983; 5:804–811.
25. Maskin CS, Sinoway L, Chadwick B, Sonnenblick EH, LeJemtel TH. Sustained hemodynamic and clinical effects of a new cardiotonic agent, WIN 47203, in patients with severe congestive heart failure. Circulation 1983; 67:1065–1070.
26. Baim DS, McDowelkl AV, Cherniles J, Monrad ES, Parker JA, Edelson J, Braunwald E, Grossman W. Evaluation of a new bipyridine inotropic agent—milrinone—in patients with severe congestive heart failure. N Engl J Med 1983; 309:748–756.
27. DiBianco R, Shabetai R, Kostuk W, Moran J, Schlant RC, Wright R, for the Milrinone Multicenter Trial Group. A comparison of oral milrinone, digoxin, and their combination in the treatment of patients with chronic heart failure. N Engl J Med 1989; 320:677–683.
28. Packer M, Carver JR, Rodeheffer RJ, Ivanhoe RJ, DiBianco R, Zeldis SM, Hendrix GH, Bommer WJ, Elkayam U, Kukin ML, Mallis GI, Sollano JA, Shannon J, Tandon PK, DeMets DL, on behalf of the PROMISE Study Research Group. Effect of oral milrinone on mortality in severe chronic heart failure. N Engl J Med 1991; 325:1468–1475.
29. Packer M, Francis GS, Abrams J, Cobb FR, Eichhorn EJ, Giles TD, Kahl FR, Tandon PK, and the PROMISE Investigators. Oral milrinone increases the risk of sudden death in severe chronic heart failure: the PROMISE trial (abstr). Circulation 1991; 84(suppl II):II-310.
30. Mancini DM, Benotti JR, Elkayam U, Francis GS, Hess ML, Massie BM, Rodeheffer RJ, Tandon PK, Packer M, and the PROMISE Investigators. Antiarrhythmic drug use and high serum levels of digoxin are independent adverse prognostic factors in patients with chronic heart failure (abstr). Circulation 1991; 84(suppl II):II-243.
31. Uretsky BF, Generalovich T, Reddy PS, Spangenberg RB, Follansbee WP. The acute hemodynamic effects of a new agent, MDL 17,043, in the treatment of congestive heart failure. Circulation 1983; 67:823–828.

32. Crawford MH, Richards KL, Sodums MT, Kennedy GT. Positive inotropic and vasodilator effects of MDL 17,043 in patients with reduced left ventricular performance. Am J Cardiol 1984; 53:1051–1053.
33. Uretsky BF, Generalovich T, Verbalis JG, Valdes AM, Reddy PS. MDL 17,043 therapy in severe congestive heart failure: Characterization of the early and late hemodynamic, pharmacokinetic, hormonal and clinical response. J Am Coll Cardiol 1985; 5:1414–1421.
34. Choraria SK, Taylor D, Pilcher J. Double-blind crossover comparison of enoximone and placebo in patients with congestive heart failure. Circulation 1987; 76:1307–1311.
35. Uretsky BF, Jessup M, Konstam MA, Dec W, Leier CV, Benotti J, Murali S, Herrmann HC, Sandberg JA, for the Enoximone Multicenter Trial Group. Multicenter trial of oral enoximone in patients with moderate to moderately severe congestive heart failure. Lack of benefit compared with placebo. Circulation 1990; 82:774–780.
36. Schleman MM, for the Enoximone Study Group, Marion Merrell Dow Inc. Double-blind, placebo-controlled (P) 12 week trial of low dose enoximone (E) in patients with mild to moderate congestive heart failure (CHF) (abstr). Circulation 1991; 84(suppl II):II-243.
37. Ruegg JC, Pfitzer G, Eubler D, Zeugner C. Effect on contractility of skinned fibres from mammalian heart and smooth muscle by a new benzimidazole derivative, 4,5-dihydro-6-[2](4-methoxyphenyl)-1H-benzimidazol-5-y]-5-methyl-3(2H)-pyridazinone. Arzneim-Forsch Drug Res 1984; 34:1736–1738.
38. Fujino K, Sperelakis N, Solaro RJ. Sensitization of dog and guinea pig heart myofilaments to Ca^{2+} activation and the inotropic effect of pimobendan: comparison with milrinone. Circ Res 1988; 63:911–922.
39. Berger C, Meyer W, Scholz H, Starbatty K. Effects of the benzimidazole derivatives pimobendan and 2-(4-hydroxy-phenyl)-5-(5-methyl-3-oxo-4,5-di-hydro-2H-6-pyridazinyl)benzimidazole-HCL on phosphodiesterase activity and force of contraction in guinea pig hearts. Arzneim-Forsch Drug Res 1985; 35(II):1668–1673.
40. Hasenfuss G, Holubarsch C, Heiss HW, Rattert B, Just HJ. Influence of the calcium-sensitizer UDCG-115 on hemodynamics and myocardial energetics in patients with idiopathic dilated cardiomyopathy. Comparison with nitroprusside. In: Just HJ, Holubarsch CH, Scholz H, eds. Inotropic Stimulation and Myocardial Energetics. New York: Springer-Verlag, 1989:225–233.
41. Katz SD, Kubo SH, Jessup M, Brozena S, Troha JM, Wahl J, Cohn JN, Sonnenblick EH, LeJemtel TH. A multicenter, randomized, double-blind, placebo-controlled trial of pimobendan, a new cardiotonic and vasodilator agent, in patients with severe congestive heart failure. Am Heart J 1992; 123:95–103.
42. Kubo SH, Gollub S, Bourge R, Rahko P, Cobb F, Jessup M, Brozena S, Brodsky M, Kirlin P, Shanes J, et al. Beneficial effects of pimobendan on exercise tolerance and quality of life in patients with heart failure: results of a multicenter trial. Circulation 1992; 85:942–949.

43. Romey G, Quast U, Pauron D, Frelin C, Renaud JF, Lazdunski M. Na^+ channels as sites of action of the cardioactive agent DPI 201-106 with agonist and antagonist enatiomers. Proc Natl Acad Sci USA 1987; 84:896–900.
44. Hajjar RJ, Gwathmey JK, Briggs GM, Morgan JP. Differential effect of DPI 201-106 on the sensitivity of the myofilaments to Ca^{2+} in intact and skinned trabeculae from control and myopathic human hearts. J Clin Invest 1988; 82:1578–1584.
45. Gwathmey JK, Slawsky MT, Briggs GM, Morgan JP. Role of intracellular sodium in the regulation of intracellular calcium and contractility. Effects of DPI 201-106 on excitation-contraction coupling in human ventricular myocardium. J Clin Invest 1988; 82:1592–1605.
46. Kihara Y, Gwathmey JK, Grossman W, Morgan JP. Mechanisms of positive inotropic effects and delayed relaxation produced by DPI 201-106 in mammalian working myocardium: effects on intracellular calcium handling. Br J Pharmacol 1989; 96:927–939.
47. Kostis JB, Lacy CR, Raia JJ, Dworkin JH, Warner RG, Casazza LA. DPI 201-106 for severe congestive heart failure. Am J Cardiol 1987; 60:1334–1339.
48. Thormann J, Kramer W, Kindler M, Kremer FP, Schlepper M. Comparative efficacy of the new cardiotonic agent DPI 201-106 versus dobutamine in dilated cardiomyopathy: Analysis by serial pressure/volume relations and "on-line" MVO_2 assessment. J Cardiovasc Pharmacol 1986; 8:749–757.
49. Yatani A, Imoto Y, Schwartz A, Brown AM. New positive inotropic agent OPC-8212 modulates Ca^{2+} channels in ventricular myocytes of guinea pig. J Cardiovasc Pharmacol 1989; 13:812–819.
50. Lathrop DA, Varro A, Schwartz A. Rate-dependent electrophysiological effects of OPC-8212: comparison to sotalol. Eur J Pharmacol 1989; 164:487–496.
51. Sasayama S, Inoue M, Asanoi H, Kodama K. Hori M, Sakurai T, Kawai C. Acute hemodynamic effects of a new inotropic agent, OPC-8212, on severe congestive heart failure. Heart Vessels 1986; 2:23–28.
52. OPC-8212 Multicenter Research Group. A placebo-controlled, randomized, double-blind study of OPC-8212 in patients with mild chronic heart failure. Cardiovasc Drugs Ther 1990; 4:419–426.
53. Feldman AM, Baughman KL, Lee WK, Gottlieb SH, Weiss JL, Becker LC, Strobeck JE. Usefulness of OPC-8212, a quinolinone derivative, for chronic congestive heart failure in patients with ischemic heart disease or idiopathic dilated cardiomyopathy. Am J Cardiol 1991; 68:1203–1210.

16

Heart Transplantation

Spencer H. Kubo
*University of Minnesota Medical School,
Minneapolis, Minnesota*

INTRODUCTION

Although heart transplantation has been performed for 25 years, it has changed dramatically over the last decade. In the first 15 years, it was considered an experimental procedure, and the 1-year survival rate of transplant recipients was only 20% to 25%. Since the introduction of cyclosporine in 1983, there has been an explosive increase in the number of transplants performed annually as well as a dramatic increase in the 1-year survival rate to 80% to 90%. Heart transplantation is now a well-established treatment for patients with end-stage heart failure, and every physician caring for patients with this clinical syndrome must have some understanding of the indications for heart transplantation as well as its potential success and limitations. This chapter will review the current status of heart transplantation, the selection criteria for potential recipients used at the University of Minnesota, and finally, some of the more common complications of transplantation.

OVERVIEW OF CURRENT STATUS

Registry data on more than 13,000 heart transplants performed worldwide are maintained by the International Society for Heart Transplantation (ISHT)

(1). The rapid growth of transplant centers and the number of transplants performed annually are summarized in Figures 1 and 2. In 1980, only 17 centers were performing heart transplantation. This number has grown steadily, so that in 1989 there were 148 transplant centers in the United States and another 88 centers outside of the United States. The number of orthotopic transplants performed annually also increased rapidly in the 1980s. Indeed, more than 85% of all heart transplants have been performed since 1985. However, this exponential increase has clearly plateaued, and in fact, there were only 2437 transplants in 1989 compared with 2654 in 1988. This plateau is most likely due to the limited donor supply. Thus, while the number of potential recipients is increasing, it is expected that, unless there are changes in the potential donor pool, the expansion of transplantation will be limited.

The age distribution of transplant recipients is shown in Figure 3 (1). In contrast to the relatively restricted age range of transplant patients before 1980, there is now a wide age distribution. In 1989, 9% of all transplants were performed in children (aged 0 to 18 years), primarily because of the increase in neonatal transplantation. Transplants at the other end of the age spectrum have also been increasing. In 1984, only 3% of all transplants were performed in patients over the age of 55. In contrast, in 1989, 40% of all transplants were performed in patients over the age of 50 years. The sex distribution of adult patients receiving transplants is

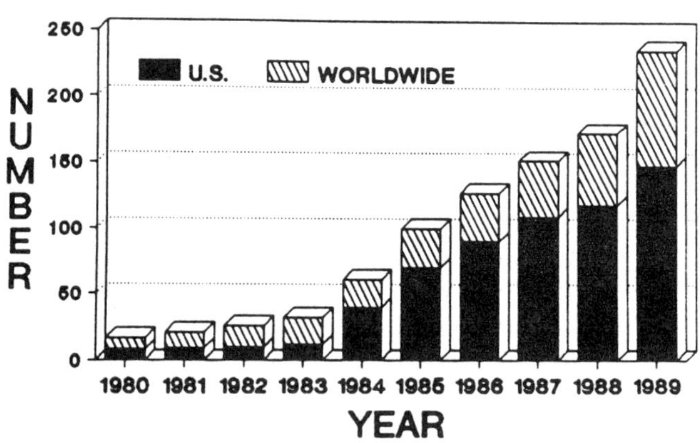

Figure 1 International Society for Heart Transplantation (ISHT) registry data summarizing the continued growth in the number of transplant centers by year in the United States (solid area) and outside of the United States (hatched area). (From Ref. 1.)

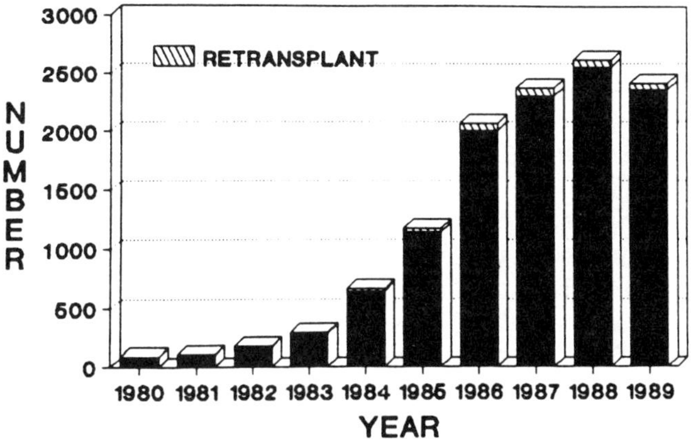

Figure 2 ISHT registry data summarizing the growth in the number of transplants performed each year. After several years of large increases, there is a clear plateau in the number of transplants performed annually. In 1989, there were only 2437 transplants, compared with 2654 in 1988. (From Ref. 1.)

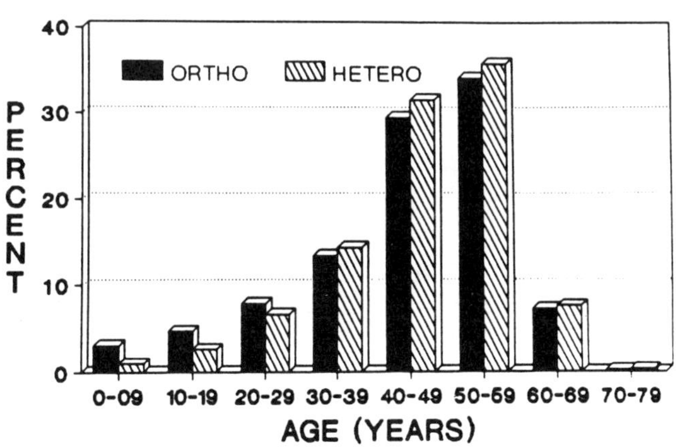

Figure 3 ISHT registry data summarizing the age distribution of transplant recipients in 1989. There is a wide age distribution due to the increase in neonatal transplants as well as in patients over the age of 50. (From Ref. 1.)

predominantly male (83%), and this is probably related to the incidence of atherosclerosis and ischemic cardiomyopathy. However, the sex distribution among children is slightly different, with 62% of recipients being male and 38% female.

Figure 4 summarizes actuarial survival with orthotopic heart transplantation (1). At 5 years, there is a 72% actuarial survival rate. This should be contrasted to the anticipated 10% to 20% 5-year survival rate of patients with end-stage heart failure who are treated medically (2).

Many of these same trends are reflected in the experience of a single center (Fig. 5). At the University of Minnesota, heart transplants have been performed since 1978. Since December 1983, there has been a progressive increase in the number of transplants performed annually, with large increases in 1986 and 1987. However, as the growth in the number of transplant centers exceeds the limited donor supply, the number of transplants annually has been decreasing over the last 3 years. Of the first 28 transplant patients, only 11 (39%) are still alive. Since the early years, the survival of patients has dramatically increased. The actuarial 5-year survival rate of patients on triple-drug immunosuppression at our institution is 78% (3).

PATIENT SELECTION CRITERIA

It is important to review patient selection criteria for heart transplantation carefully, so that the most appropriate patients are considered and the

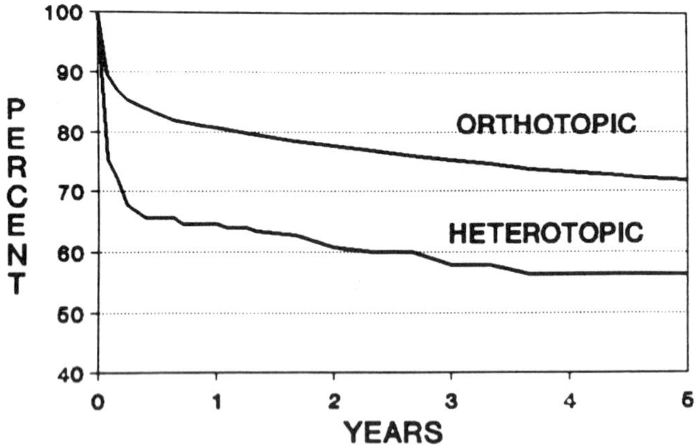

Figure 4 ISHT registry data showing actuarial survival with orthotopic transplantation. At 5 years, there is a 72% actuarial survival rate.

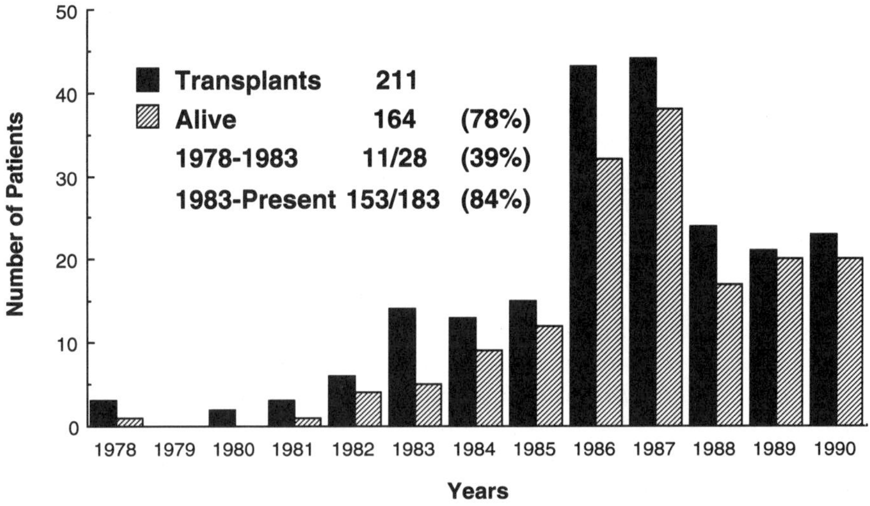

Figure 5 Transplant activity by year at the University of Minnesota. The number of transplants reflect the ISHT trends, with large increases in transplants from 1983 to 1987 and a more recent plateau. Eighty-four percent of patients treated with triple-drug immunosuppression since 1983 are still alive.

limited donor pool can be optimally utilized. These criteria have changed greatly over the past decade (4–7). During the early stages of transplantation, these criteria were empiric and based on the experience and expertise of transplant programs. For example, patients older than 45 years of age or those with insulin-dependent diabetes mellitus were excluded on the basis of anticipated difficulties with the operative procedure and an immunosuppression regimen that utilized high doses of steroids. With the dramatic increase in the survival rate and the introduction of cyclosporine (3,8,9), several modifications of patient selection criteria have been investigated (10,11). At present, patients with uncomplicated diabetes mellitus and those more than 45 years of age are routinely given transplants. In fact, the major factor limiting further expansion of the potential recipient pool is the continued shortage of appropriate donor organs. Lack of donor availability has therefore produced a somewhat paradoxical and ironic situation in which transplant centers have become increasingly judicious and selective about the optimal transplant patient in a period of unparalleled success of transplantation.

At the University of Minnesota, we require that all patients being considered for heart transplantation for end-stage heart failure fulfill five criteria (Table 1). All patients should have evidence of severe left ventricular systolic dysfunction with an ejection fraction less than 35%. This criterion is quite liberal, since most patients with refractory symptoms of heart failure will have an ejection fraction less than 25%. Second, patients should be receiving maximal medical treatment including the combination of digitalis, diuretics, and vasodilators. If they are not able to tolerate these drugs, there should be at least two attempts to initiate therapy. Third, the patient should report refractory or intolerable symptoms that limit the ability to complete the activities of daily life either at work or at home. This criterion is difficult to evaluate, since many patients will change their activity patterns to avoid producing symptoms and may accept increasing limitations as part of the disease and aging process. However, it is important that the patient can *independently* confirm the disability, since a patient with satisfactory activity levels is less likely to perceive benefit and may be less willing to accept the side effects associated with immunosuppressant therapy after transplantation. Fourth, there should be an intensive search for reversible factors, such as ischemia and surgically correctable valvular lesions. Some patients will benefit from high-risk surgery and not require transplantation (12,13). Furthermore, "refractory" heart failure in some patients is related to noncompliance with medication regimens and dietary sodium restriction. Finally, all patients should have an estimated 1-year survival rate of less than 50%. This criterion should focus efforts on the sickest patients who are at highest risk of dying and thus limit premature transplantation. However, this is a difficult parameter to estimate, since previous studies assessing survival in patients with heart failure (2,14,15) describe *group* trends rather than predicting survival for an *individual* patient.

These five criteria identify a very broad population of potential candidates for transplantation. Table 2 lists several additional clinical characteristics that either indicate a poor short-term prognosis or corroborate a poor functional capacity. Although there are few controlled data to test the predictive value of these factors, we have found them to be important supportive criteria confirming the need to strongly consider transplantation for an individual patient.

Table 1 Selection Criteria

1. Left ventricular ejection fraction <35%
2. Maximal medical therapy
3. Refractory symptoms
4. Absence of reversible factors
5. Expected 1-year survival <50%

Table 2 Other Factors Indicating the Need for Transplantation

1. Peak oxygen consumption <12 ml/kg/min
2. Plasma norepinephrine >600 pg/ml
3. Loss of muscle mass
4. Vasodilator intolerance
5. Requirement of intravenous inotropic agents
6. Familial dilated cardiomyopathy
7. Decompensations with trivial events
8. Onset of atrial fibrillation
9. Deterioration in measures of ventricular function or functional capacity

The results of a symptom-limited exercise test with measurement of peak oxygen consumption (peak VO_2) have been particularly useful in assessing the need for transplantation. Patients with a peak VO_2 less than 12 ml/kg/min have severely limited aerobic capacity and a very poor short-term prognosis (16,17). These patients are therefore urgent candidates for transplantation. Furthermore, for patients who are unable to provide reproducible estimates of functional capacity or who may deny limitations, a reduced peak VO_2 may confirm the necessity of transplantation. Conversely, a patient with a relatively preserved aerobic capacity (peak VO_2 > 18 ml/kg/min) may not derive substantial benefit with transplantation, since some studies have suggested that peak VO_2 after transplantation ranges from 18 to 24 ml/kg/min (18,19).

Many factors have been associated with decreased survival among patients with heart failure. However, it has not been possible to create a model utilizing all of the important variables that can predict *short-term* mortality for an individual patient (2). In our experience, an elevated plasma norepinephrine level (> 600 pg/ml) and the presence of cachexia and severe muscle wasting may help identify those patients with the most severe heart failure and the highest short-term mortality risk (20,21).

Patients who are intolerant of vasodilators because of hypotension and/or renal insufficiency also have an increased mortality risk, possibly because of inadequate cardiac reserve and renal perfusion. Conversely, both the VHeFT and the CONSENSUS trials have demonstrated that vasodilator therapy provides an important survival benefit in patients with moderate to severe heart failure (22–24). Thus, patients who are intolerant of vasodilators despite multiple attempts are strongly considered for transplantation. Similarly, we expedite the evaluation of patients who have required intravenous inotropic support or who have clinical decompensations with trivial events. Despite the restoration of clinical stability, we consider these patients to be at high risk for future decompensations.

Although atrial fibrillation is a nonspecific finding in many patients with heart failure (25), Middlekauff et al. (26) recently reported in preliminary form an association with increased mortality, possibly as a result of severe reductions in left ventricular function and left atrial distention. Patients with familial dilated cardiomyopathy may also have a higher mortality risk when compared with patients with similar reductions in left ventricular function due to other causes (27). Finally, when follow-up tests of ventricular function and aerobic capacity indicate a trend for deterioration, these patients are considered to be urgent transplantation candidates.

OTHER INDICATIONS FOR TRANSPLANTATION

Although refractory heart failure is the most common indication for transplantation, there are a number of other conditions that have been successfully treated with transplantation (Table 3). These cases account for only a small percentage of transplants and are considered on an individual basis.

Patients with refractory angina pectoris are considered transplant candidates if their symptoms limit exercise or result in frequent hospitalizations. It is important to document myocardial ischemia either by elevations in cardiac enzymes or by reversible electrocardiographic changes during pain episodes, or with positive thallium scintigraphy or gated blood pool scans during exercise. High-risk coronary bypass surgery is always extensively considered as an alternative, but may not be possible because of previous surgeries, inadequate distal vessels, or concomitant mitral insufficiency. In many patients life-threatening ventricular arrhythmias can be successfully controlled with an implantable defibrillator, and several centers have now reported 5-year survival rates of approximately 90% (28,29). However, it is clear that some patients are still at high risk for early mortality and should be considered for transplantation, particularly patients

Table 3 Other Indications for Transplantation

1. Refractory angina pectoris
2. Life-threatening ventricular arrhythmias
3. Allograft vasculopathy
4. Congenital heart disease
5. Infective endocarditis
6. Cardiac tumors
7. Amyloid (controversial)
8. Hypertrophic cardiomyopathy
9. Restrictive cardiomyopathy

with clinical heart failure or those who experience frequent defibrillations. Patients who develop allograft vasculopathy following cardiac transplantation are at risk for myocardial infarction, arrhythmias, heart failure, and death (9). Since there are no accepted treatments for allograft vasculopathy, patients are considered for retransplantation when coronary angiography detects these changes. Successful transplantation has also been reported in patients with congenital heart disease, infective endocarditis, cardiac tumors, amyloid, hypertrophic cardiomyopathy, and restrictive cardiomyopathy (30–32).

CONTRAINDICATIONS

Table 4 lists the contraindications to transplantation that are used by most transplant centers. These contraindications have been extensively revised over the past decade with increased experience in high-risk groups. Each factor is generally considered to be a relative contraindication, and in most cases a patient will be excluded from transplantation because of a combination of factors, rather than a single absolute contraindication.

Most of these factors are self-explanatory, but several deserve comment. Previous studies have shown that pulmonary hypertension and pulmonary vasoconstriction are associated with increased perioperative mortality, which is probably due to the failure of the donor ventricle to function in the presence of high pressures (33,34). We currently consider patients with a resting pulmonary vascular resistance greater than 6 Wood units and/or a transpulmonary gradient greater than 15 mm Hg to be high-risk candidates. We will accept these patients only if pharmacological interventions are capable of reducing the pulmonary vascular resistance to less than 4 Wood units.

Patients with preexisting renal and hepatic insufficiency are also high-risk candidates because of the known renal and hepatic toxicity of cyclos-

Table 4 Contraindications

1. Age >60–65 yr
2. Pulmonary hypertension
3. Infection
4. Irreversible renal/hepatic dysfunction
5. Complicated diabetes mellitus
6. Severe lung disease
7. Symptomatic cerebral or peripheral vascular disease
8. Malignancy
9. Poor compliance; psychosocial issues

porine and azathioprine (35–37). These patients are at increased risk for more prolonged multiorgan failure after transplantation and may not be able to tolerate full doses of immunosuppression, thus potentially incurring an increased risk of rejection. In selected cases, we have observed improvements in both renal and hepatic function with intravenous dobutamine and vasodilator therapy, which suggests that these abnormalities may reverse with aggressive therapy and should not necessarily exclude patients from transplantation. In general, patients are excluded with a serum creatinine level greater than 2.5 mg/dl, creatinine clearance less than 50 ml/min, bilirubin greater than 2.0 mg%, transaminases more than two to three times normal, or an elevated prothrombin time.

Comorbid diseases are relatively strong contraindications for transplantation because of the possibility that a noncardiac process might independently limit survival. Despite case reports of satisfactory short-term results in patients with malignancies (38), it is still prudent to consider transplantation only if there is demonstration of medical or surgical "cure," or at least a 3- to 5-year disease-free interval before consideration of transplantation. Insulin-dependent diabetes mellitus by itself was formerly a contraindication to transplantation. Currently, diabetics are considered candidates in the absence of target organ complications including retinopathy, neuropathy, nephropathy, and peripheral or cerebral vascular disease.

Finally, psychosocial issues and the ability to comply with a complex medical regimen are very important factors influencing the long-term success of transplantation (4–6). However, it is difficult, before transplantation, to predict compliance and adherence to medical programs. In the absence of well-defined criteria, the optimal candidates will have sufficient motivation and cognitive function to be able to administer medications independently and follow specific instructions. Candidates with psychiatric illnesses such as schizophrenia or who engage in illicit drug use are not candidates for transplantation. Patients who currently smoke or consume alcohol in excess are considered candidates only after a 4- to 6-month period of abstinence.

COMPLICATIONS

There are many complications of transplantation that are carefully considered during routine follow-up (Table 5). Since these complications have been reviewed in detail (9), the remainder of this chapter will discuss rejection, infection, and allograft vasculopathy.

Table 5 Complications

1. Rejection
2. Infection
3. Malignancy
4. Hypertension
5. Allograft vasculopathy
6. Pericardial effusion
7. Renal insufficiency
8. Osteoporosis
9. Problems associated with cyclosporine: hypertension, renal insufficiency, hirsutism, gingival hyperplasia, seizures, hepatotoxicity, malignancy, tremors
10. Problems associated with steroids: diabetes, gout, osteoporosis, bone fractures, hypercholesterolemia, cataracts, skin fragility, myopathy, peptic ulcers

REJECTION

The diagnosis, treatment, and prevention of acute rejection remains one of the most critical determinants of the short- and long-term success of cardiac transplantation. It is clear that refinements in the technique of endomyocardial biopsy (39) and the introduction of cyclosporine to the immunosuppression regimen (3,36) were important contributions to the dramatic success of transplantation in the last 10 years. Before these developments, rejection was more common, was detected relatively late in its course, and was associated with symptoms of heart failure, arrhythmias, and a high mortality rate. However, rejection is now far less common and can be diagnosed with surveillance biopsies before the development of clinical signs and symptoms. Thus, with early detection and early treatment, deaths due to rejection have been markedly reduced.

Despite the ability to obtain endomyocardial biopsy material safely and repeatedly, there is still some confusion about the exact diagnosis of acute cardiac rejection, in part because of the multiplicity of classification schemata. However, a recent working group published a modification of the original Billingham grading scales (40) that it is hoped will encourage standardization of diagnostic criteria (41). In this schema, "mild" rejection is characterized by focal perivascular or interstitial lymphocytic infiltrates (IA) or a diffuse but sparse infiltrate (IB), or by a single focus of aggressive infiltration possibly associated with myocyte damage (II). Grade III ("moderate") rejection is characterized by multifocal aggressive infiltrates and/ or myocyte damage (IIIA) or a diffuse inflammatory process with necrosis

(IIIB). Finally, grade IV rejection shows evidence of a diffuse aggressive polymorphous infiltrate, possibly associated with edema, hemorrhage, vasculitis, and necrosis.

Since acute rejection in patients treated with cyclosporine-based immunosuppression regimens is only rarely associated with clinical signs and symptoms of heart failure, routine surveillance endomyocardial biopsies are performed frequently in the first year. Although the exact schedule differs among centers, the schedule at the University of Minnesota includes biopsies every 2 weeks for the first 3 months, monthly for the next 3 months, and then every 3 months until the second-year anniversary. Data from the Working Group of Transplant Cardiologists (WGTC) for over 700 patients who received transplants in 1989 have demonstrated that 90% of all rejection episodes occur within the first 6 months after transplant (42). After this period, rejection is rare unless there has been a significant change in immunosuppression, possibly due to the development of a malignancy or noncompliance with medication regimens (9). On average, 46% of the patients in the WGTC series had no rejection, 30% had a single rejection, and 24% had more than one rejection during the first year of follow-up.

Although endomyocardial biopsy is the "gold standard" for rejection and can be performed safely, this test is still invasive. Many attempts have been made to define the utility of a noninvasive test as a screening method for cardiac rejection. Techniques such as echocardiography, electrocardiography, nuclear heart scans, magnetic resonance imaging, and immunologic monitoring of peripheral lymphocyte numbers or lymphocyte surface markers have been examined (43–48). However, none of these techniques has sufficient sensitivity or specificity to replace endomyocardial biopsy in the diagnosis of rejection.

Several different immunosuppression regimens have been successfully used to prevent rejection (9). The largest experience has been with "triple-drug immunosuppression" with cyclosporine, azathioprine, and prednisone (3,49). This combination utilizes lower doses to minimize the side effects associated with each component. An alternative strategy uses "induction" therapy with high doses of agents in the early stages of transplant, when the risk of rejection is highest. These protocols utilize either polyclonal agents (e.g., antilymphocyte globulin), or monoclonal preparations developed against the T3 cell surface antigen found in mature T cells (OKT3) (50,51). However, there are few controlled data that have directly compared the efficacy of these strategies in the prevention of rejection. Finally, many new immunosuppressive agents are being developed, including rapamycin (52) and FK-506 (53,54), but their exact role and potential advantages over cyclosporine-based regimens are not known.

INFECTION

One problem that limits the intensity of all immunosuppression regimens is the increased susceptibility to potentially life-threatening infections. It remains important to achieve the delicate balance between the prevention of rejection and an acceptable incidence of opportunistic infections.

There are two peak incidences of infection after transplantation, each associated with a different spectrum of organisms (55–57). In the early stages after transplantation with the highest intensity of immunosuppression to prevent rejection, the rate of bacterial nosocomial infections is high, predominantly as a result of gram-negative and *Staphylococcus* infections. After the first few weeks, other opportunistic viral, fungal, and protozoan infections have increased frequency. Viral infections (e.g., herpes simplex, herpes zoster, or cytomegalovirus) can either occur as a reactivation of infection or be transmitted by the donor. Fungal pathogens such as Aspergillus often require long-term amphotericin-B treatment. Other opportunistic infections such as *Pneumocystis carinii* infection and toxoplasmosis are also seen frequently. It should be emphasized, however, that bacterial infections can still occur in the later phases.

The diagnosis of an opportunistic infection requires the same intensity that is applied to the evaluation of any immunocompromised host. We have aggressively pursued documentation of infection with viral titers and frequently with invasive procedures to obtain a specific culture of the offending organism. Antibacterial treatment is aggressive and frequently requires surgery (e.g., for cholelithiasis and cholecystitis). Many fungal infections will not respond completely to amphotericin-B, since such therapy is frequently complicated by renal toxicity and may require surgery. The treatment of systemic viral infections has been improved recently with the availability of high-dose acyclovir and ganciclovir (58–60).

Several regimens have been successfully employed as prophylaxis against opportunistic infections. Most programs utilize trimethoprim-sulfamethoxazole to prevent infections with *Pneumocystis, Nocardia*, and *Toxoplasma*, and acyclovir for herpes simplex, herpes zoster, and cytomegalovirus (61–62). Ganciclovir is also being used by some centers for cytomegalovirus prophylaxis.

ALLOGRAFT VASCULOPATHY

One of the most serious complications of heart transplantation is allograft vasculopathy, which is the leading cause of death after the first year following transplantation (9,63). This complication is associated with myocardial infarction, heart failure, and arrhythmias and is the most common indication for retransplantation. This accelerated form of coronary artery disease has been previously described as transplant coronary artery disease, chronic vascular rejection, accelerated graft arteriosclerosis, and transplant coronary vasculopathy. Since this entity appears to involve veins as well as arteries, and is pathophysiologically distinct from atherosclerosis in the general population, "allograft vasculopathy" is one of the preferred terms.

It has been difficult to determine the true incidence of allograft vasculopathy. Many patients will not develop symptoms related to coronary insufficiency, and therefore many, but not all, transplant centers perform routine surveillance coronary angiograms on an annual basis. These studies have demonstrated that up to 50% of patients surviving for 3 years will have abnormalities on coronary angiography (64,65). However, it is likely that even this invasive methodology may seriously underestimate the incidence of coronary abnormalities. This is based on the observation of autopsy-proven allograft vasculopathy within months of a "normal" angiographic study (66) and the finding of significant abnormalities with intravascular ultrasound in angiographically normal vascular segments (67). Finally, autopsy studies of patients who have survived at least 1 year after transplant almost uniformly demonstrate pathologic evidence of allograft vasculopathy (68,69).

Given these problems, most centers define allograft vasculopathy as the appearance of any luminal irregularity on coronary angiography. Gao et al. (64) have described three common angiographic patterns including (1) a focal irregular stenosis that gives the appearance of typical atherosclerosis; (2) rapid tapering with diffuse obliteration of distal vessels; and (3) luminal irregularities that diffusely involve the length of the artery. When compared with typical atherosclerosis, the lesions in transplant patients tend to be more distal and are less likely to be associated with collateral vessels. Another important feature of allograft vasculopathy is that it can progress very rapidly, to total occlusion within months. Furthermore, using quantitative angiography, Gao et al. have demonstrated progressive luminal narrowing at rates that were significantly faster than with typical atherosclerosis (70).

There are several distinct pathological features of allograft vasculopathy (63,71,72). In contrast to focal atherosclerotic plaque, this process involves the entire length of the coronary artery. The typical findings are a proliferation of smooth muscle cells and macrophages, an accumulation of collagen and ground substance within the endothelium, and characteristic foam cells in the intima. Deposition of cholesterol is also seen, but the atherosclerotic plaques in allograft vasculopathy are more cellular and less calcified than in typical atherosclerosis. Although the pathogenesis of allograft vasculopathy is not known, it appears to result from an immunologic injury to the endothelium (73–75), mediated by a T-lymphocyte infiltration of intimal cells.

Other investigators have identified factors that appear to predispose transplant recipients to allograft vasculopathy, including hypercholesterolemia (73,76), obesity (77), donor ischemic time (78), the appearance of circulating cytotoxic antibodies against donor class I and class II antigens (79,80), and the number of cellular rejection episodes (81). However, not all studies have confirmed these associations. Recently, we and others (82–84) have demonstrated an association between cytomegalovirus infection and the development of allograft vasculopathy.

To date, there are no effective therapies for allograft vasculopathy. Many patients are treated with aspirin and/or dipyridamole, but there is no evidence that these antiplatelet agents are effective in preventing this complication. Recently, Schroeder et al. (85) demonstrated that the calcium channel blocking agent diltiazem inhibited the progressive narrowing of coronary arteries during follow-up angiograms. Palliative treatments have included percutaneous angioplasty for patients with focal stenoses (86), but this intervention will probably be limited by the small number of appropriate lesions. Retransplantation has also been offered to patients, but the success of second transplants has been limited (87). At Stanford, the 1- and 2-year survival rates are only 55% and 22%, respectively, which is strikingly decreased from the results of primary transplantation. Based on these disappointing results, and in view of the long waiting lists for donor organs, many centers do not offer retransplantation to patients with allograft vasculopathy.

REFERENCES

1. Kriett JM, Kaye MP. The Registry of the International Society for Heart Transplantation. Seventh official report—1990. J Heart Transplantation 1990; 9:323–330.
2. Francis GS, Kubo SH. Prognostic factors affecting diagnosis and treatment of congestive heart failure. Curr Prob Cardiol 1989; 14:631–671.
3. Olivari MT, Kubo SH, Braunlin EA, et al. Five year experience with triple drug immunosuppressive therapy in cardiac transplantation. Circulation 1990; 82(suppl IV):276–280.
4. Jessup M, Brozena SC. Identification and management of potential heart transplant recipients. Cardiology Clinics 1990; 8:11–21.
5. Hastillo A, Hess ML: Selection of patients for cardiac transplantation. In: Thompson ME, ed. Cardiac Transplantation. Philadelphia: FA Davis, 1990:107–120.

6. O'Connell JB, Renlund DG, Bristow MR. Cardiac transplantation: emerging role of the internist/cardiologist. J Intern Med 1989; 225:147–156.
7. Copeland JG, Emery RW, Levinson MM, et al. Selection of patients for cardiac transplantation. Circulation 1987; 75:2–9.
8. Bolman RM, Elick B, Olivari MT, et al. Improved immunosuppression for heart transplantation. J Heart Transplant 1985; 4:315–318.
9. Miller LW. Long-term complications of cardiac transplantation. Prog Cardiovasc Dis 1991; 33:229–282.
10. Rhenman MJ, et al. Diabetes and heart transplantation. J Heart Transplant 1988; 7:356.
11. Olivari MT, Antolick A, Kaye MP, Jamieson DV, Ring WS. Heart transplantation in elderly patients. J Heart Transplant 1988; 7:258–264.
12. Alderman EL, Fisher LD, Litwin P, et al. Results of coronary artery surgery in patients with poor left ventricular function (CASS). Circulation 1983; 68:785–795.
13. Pigott JD, Kouchoukos NJ, Oberman A, Cutter GR. Late results of surgical and medical therapy for patients with coronary artery disease and depressed left ventricular function. J Am Coll Cardiol 1985; 5:1036–1045.
14. Unverferth DV, Magorien DR, Moeschberger ML, et al. Factors influencing the one year mortality of dilated cardiomyopathy. Am J. Cardiol 1984; 54:147–152.
15. Wilson JR, Schwartz JS, St. John Sutton M, et al. Prognosis in severe heart failure: relation to hemodynamic measurements and ventricular ectopic activity. J Am Coll Cardiol 1983; 2:403–410.
16. Mancini DM, Revin A, Mull R, Eisen H, Kussmaul W, Edmunds LH, Wilson JR. Value of peak oxygen consumption to risk stratify cardiac transplant candidates. Circulation 1990; 82:III-713.
17. Szlachcic J, Massie BM, Kramer BL, et al. Correlates and prognostic implication of exercise in chronic congestive heart failure. Am J Cardiol 1985; 1037–1042.
18. Stevenson LW, Sietsma K, Tillish JH, et al. Exercise capacity for survivors of cardiac transplantation or sustained medical therapy for stable heart failure. Circulation 1990; 81:78–85.
19. Johnson TH, Kubo SH, McGinn AL, et al: Physiologic importance of sympathetic reinnervation after cardiac transplantation. J Heart Lung Transplant 1991; 10:178.
20. Cohn JN, Levine TB, Olivari MT, et al: Plasma norepinephrine as a guide to prognosis in patients with chronic congestive heart failure. N Engl J Med 1984; 311:819–823.
21. Mancini DM, et al: Skeletal muscle atrophy contributes to exercise intolerance in heart failure. J Am Coll Cardiol 1991; 17:88A.
22. Stevenson LW, Dracup KA, Tillisch JH. Efficacy of medical therapy tailored for severe congestive heart failure in patients transferred for urgent cardiac transplantation. Am J Cardiol 1989; 63:461–464.

23. Cohn JN, Archibald DG, Ziesche S, et al. Effect of vasodilator therapy on mortality in chronic congestive heart failure: results of a Veterans Administration Cooperative Study. N Engl J Med 1986; 314:1547–1552.
24. The CONSENSUS Trial Study Group. Effects of enalapril on mortality in severe congestive heart failure: results of the Cooperative North Scandinavian Enalapril Survival Study (CONSENSUS). N Engl J Med 1987; 316:1429–1435.
25. Carson P, et al. Atrial fibrillation does not decrease survival in congestive heart failure. J Am Coll Cardiol 1991; 87:90A.
26. Middlekauff HR, Stevenson WG, Stevenson LW, Walden JA. Adverse prognosis of atrial fibrillation in advanced heart failure: A study of 390 patients. J Am Coll Cardiol 1991; 17:87A.
27. Valantine JA, Hunt SA, Fowler MB, Billingham ME, Schroeder JS. Frequency of familial nature of dilated cardiomyopathy and usefulness of cardiac transplantation in this subset. Am J Cardiol 1989; 959–963.
28. Winkle RA, Mead RJ, Ruder MA, et al. Long-term outcome with the automatic implantable cardioverter-defibrillator. J Am Coll Cardiol 1989; 13:1353–1361.
29. Tschou PJ, Kadri N, Anderson J, et al. Automatic implantable cardioverter defibrillators and survival of patients with left ventricular dysfunction and malignant ventricular arrhythmias. Am J Med 1988; 109:529–534.
30. Menkis AH, McKenzie FN, Novick RJ, et al. Special considerations for heart transplantation in congenital heart disease. J Heart Transplant 1990; 9:602–607.
31. Valantine HE, Billingham ME. Recurrence of amyloid in a cardiac allograft four months after transplantation. J Heart Transplant 1989; 8:337–341.
32. Armitage JM, Griffith BP, Kormos RL, et al. Cardiac transplantation in patients with malignancy. J Heart Transplant 1989; 8:89.
33. Kirklin JK, Naftel DC, Kirklin JW, et al. Pulmonary vascular resistance and the risk of heart transplantation. J Heart Transplant 1988; 7:331–336.
34. Addonizio LJ, Gersony WM, Robbins RC, et al. Elevated pulmonary vascular resistance and cardiac transplantation. Circulation 1987; 76(suppl V):V52–V55.
35. Myers BD, Ross J, Newton L, et al. Cyclosporine associated chronic nephropathy. N Engl J Med 1987; 311:699–705.
36. Miller LW, Pennington DL, McBride LR. Long-term effects of cyclosporine in cardiac transplantation. Transplant Proc 1990; 22:15–20.
37. Ireland P, Rashid A, von Lichtenberg F, et al. Liver disease in kidney transplant patients receiving azathioprine. Arch Intern Med 1973; 132:29–37.
38. Edwards BS, Hunt SA, Fowler B, et al. Cardiac transplantation in patients with preexisting neoplastic diseases. Am J Cardiol 1990; 65:501–504.
39. Caves PK, Stinson EB, Billingham ME, et al. Diagnosis of human cardiac allograft rejection by serial cardiac biopsy. J Thorac Cardiovasc Surg 1978; 66:461–466.

40. Billingham ME. Diagnosis of cardiac rejection by endomyocardial biopsy. J Heart Transplant 1981; 1:25–30.
41. Billingham ME, Cary NRB, Hammond ME, et al. A working formulation for the standardization of nomenclature in the diagnosis of heart and lung rejection. Heart Rejection Study Group. J Heart Transplant 1990; 9:587–593.
42. A report of the Working Group of Transplant Cardiologists. J Heart Transplant 1990; 9:61.
43. Valantine HA, Fowler MB, Hunt SA, et al. Changes in Doppler echocardiographic indexes of left ventricular function as potential markers of acute rejection. Circulation 1987; 76(suppl V):V86–V92.
44. Desruennes M, Corcos T, Cabrol C, et al. Doppler echocardiography for the diagnosis of acute cardiac allograft rejection. J Am Coll Cardiol 1988; 12:63–70.
45. Rodman ST, Miller LW, Tsai CC. Role of interleukin-2 receptors in immunologic monitoring following cardiac transplantation. Transplantation 1988; 45:1050–1056.
46. Hanson CA, Bolling SF, Stoolman LM, et al. Cytoimmunologic monitoring and heart transplantation. J Heart Transplant 1988; 7:424–429.
47. Addonizio LJ. Detection of cardiac allograft rejection using radionuclide techniques. Prog Cardiovasc Dis 1990; 33:73–83.
48. Lund G, Morin RT, Olivari MT, Ring WS. Serial myocardial T^2 relaxation time measurements in normal subjects and heart transplant recipients. J Heart Transplant 1988; 7:274–279.
49. Stinson EB, Dong E Jr, Bieber CP, et al. Cardiac transplantation in man. II. Immunosuppressive therapy. J Thorac Cardiovasc Surg 1969; 58:326–343.
50. Hegewald MG, O'Connell JB, Renlund DG, et al. OKT3 monoclonal antibody given for 10 vs. 14 days as immunosuppression prophylaxis in cardiac transplantation. J Heart Transplant 1989; 8:303–309.
51. O'Connell JB, Renlund DG, Lee HR, et al. Newer techniques of immunosuppression in cardiac transplantation. Cardiac Surg 1988; 2:607–615.
52. Sehgal SN, Chang JY. Rapamycin: A new immunosuppressive macrolide. Transplant Immunol Lett 1990; 7:12.
53. Starzl TE: FK-506. A potential breakthrough in immunosuppression. Transplant Proc 1987; 19:103–104.
54. Ochiai T, Nakajima K, Nagata M, et al. Studies of the induction and maintenance of long-term graft acceptance by treatment with FK506 in heterotopic cardiac allotransplantation in rats. Transplantation 1989; 44:734–738.
55. Dummer JS, Hardy A, Poorsattar A, et al. Early infections in kidney, heart and liver transplant recipients on cyclosporine. Transplantation 1983; 36:259–267.
56. Dummer SJ. Infectious complications of transplantation. In: Thompson ME, Brest AN, eds. Cardiac transplantation. Philadelphia: FA Davis, 1990:163–178.

57. Linder J. Infection as a complication of heart transplantation. J Heart Transplant 1988; 7:390–394.
58. Dummer JS, White LT, Ho M, et al. Morbidity of cytomegalovirus infection in recipients of heart or heart-lung transplants who received cyclosporine. J Infect Dis 1985; 152:1182–1191.
59. Icenogle TB, Peterson E, Ray G, et al. DHPG effectively treats CMV infection in heart and heart-lung transplant patients: a preliminary report. J Heart Transplant 1987; 6:199–203.
60. Preiksaitis JK, Rosno S, Grumet C, et al. Infections due to herpes viruses in cardiac transplant recipients: role of the donor heart and immunosuppressive therapy. J Infect Dis 1983; 147:947–981.
61. Hughes WT, Rivera GK, Schell MJ, et al. Successful intermittent chemoprophylaxis for *Pneumocystis carinii* pneumonitis. N Engl J Med 1987; 316:1627–1632.
62. Balfour HH, Chace BA, Stapleton JT, et al. A randomized, placebo-controlled trial of oral acyclovir for the prevention of cytomegalovirus disease in recipients of renal allografts. N Engl J Med 1989; 320:1381–1387.
63. Billingham ME. Cardiac transplant atherosclerosis. Transplant Proc 1987; 19:19–25.
64. Gao SZ, Alderman EL, Schroeder JS, et al. Accelerated coronary vascular disease in the heart transplant patient: Coronary arteriographic findings. J Am Coll Cardiol 1988; 12:334–340.
65. Olivari MT, Homans DC, Wilson RF, Kubo SH, Ring WS. Coronary artery disease in cardiac transplant patients receiving triple drug immunosuppressive therapy. Circulation 1989; 80(suppl III):III-111–III-115.
66. Mason JW, Strefling A. Small vessel disease of the heart resulting in myocardial necrosis and death despite angiographically normal coronary arteries. Am J Cardiol 1979; 44:171–176.
67. St. Goar FG, Pinto FJ, Alderman EL, Valantine HA, Popp RL. Intracoronary ultrasound in cardiac transplant recipients: in vivo evaluation of angiographically silent intimal thickening. J Am Coll Cardiol 1991; 17:102A.
68. Johnson DE, Gao SZ, Schroeder JS, et al. The spectrum of coronary artery pathologic findings in human cardiac allografts. J Heart Transplant 1989; 8:349–359.
69. Pucci AM, Clarke Forbes RD, Billingham ME. Pathologic features in long-term cardiac allografts. J Heart Transplant 1990; 9:339–345.
70. Gao S, Alderman EL, Schroeder JS, Hunt SA, Wiederhold V, Stinson EB. Progressive coronary luminal narrowing after cardiac transplantation. Circulation 1990; 82(suppl IV):IV-269–IV-275.
71. Bieber CP, Stinson EB, Shumway NE, et al. Cardiac transplantation in man. VII. Cardiac allograft pathology. Circulation 1970; 41:753–772.
72. Uys CJ, Rose AG. Pathologic findings in long-term cardiac transplants. Arch Pathol Lab Med 1984; 108:112–116.

73. Alonso DR, Starek PK, Minick CR. Studies on the pathogenesis of atheroarteriosclerosis induced in rabbit cardiac allografts by the synergy of graft rejection and hypercholesterolemia. Am J Pathol 1977; 87:415–442.
74. Lurie KG, Billingham ME, Jamieson SW, et al. Pathogenesis and prevention of graft arteriosclerosis in an experimental heart transplant model. Transplantation 1981; 31:41–47.
75. McManus BM, Winters GL, Radio SJ, et al. Ubiquity and centrifugal intensification of T-cell mediated coronary arteritis in failed human heart allografts. Lab Invest 1988; 58:624.
76. Stinson EB, Payne R, Griepp RB, et al. Correlation of histocompatability matching with graft rejection and survival after cardiac transplantation in man. Lancet 1971; 459–461.
77. Winters GL, Kendall TJ, Radio SJ, et al. Post-transplant obesity and hyperlipidemia: major predictors of severity of coronary arteriopathy in failed human heart allografts. J Heart Transplant 1990; 9:364–371.
78. Kormos RL, Donato W, Hardesty RL, Griffith BP, Kiernan J, Trento A. The influence of donor organ stability and ischemia time on subsequent cardiac recipient survival. Transplant Proc 1988; 20:980–983.
79. Hess ML, Hastillo A, Mohanakumar T, et al. Accelerated atherosclerosis in cardiac transplantation: role of cytotoxic B cell antibodies and hyperlipidemia. Circulation 1983; 68(suppl 2):94–101.
80. Rose EA, Smith CR, Petrossian GA, et al. Humoral immune responses after cardiac transplantation: Correlation with fatal rejection and graft atherosclerosis. Surgery 1989; 106:203–208.
81. Uretsky BF, Murali S, Reddy PS, et al. Development of coronary artery disease in cardiac transplant patients receiving immunosuppressive therapy with cyclosporine and prednisone. Circulation 1987; 76:827–834.
82. McDonald K, Rector TS, Braunlin EA, et al. Association of coronary artery disease in cardiac transplant recipients with cytomegalovirus infection. Am J Cardiol 1989; 64:359–362.
83. Grattan MT, Cabral-Moreno CE, Starnes VA, Oyer PE, Stinson EB, Shumway NE. Cytomegalovirus infection is associated with cardiac allograft rejection and atherosclerosis. JAMA 1989; 261:3561–3566.
84. Loebe M, Schuler S, Zais O, et al. Role of cytomegalovirus infection in the development of coronary artery disease in the transplanted heart. J Heart Transplant 1990; 9:707–711.
85. Schroeder JS, Gao SZ, Alderman EL, et al. Diltiazem inhibits development of early accelerated transplant coronary disease—an interim report (abstr). Circulation 1990; 82:III257.
86. Halle A, Di Sciascio G, Wilson RF, et al. Coronary angioplasty in cardiac transplant patients: Results of a multicenter study. J Am Coll Cardiol 1991; 14:103A.
87. Gao SZ, Schroeder JS, Hunt S, et al. Retransplantation for severe accelerated coronary artery disease in heart transplant recipients. Am J Cardiol 1988; 62:876–881.

17

Sudden Death and Arrhythmias Complicating Heart Failure

Ronald W.F. Campbell
University of Newcastle-Upon-Tyne, Newcastle-Upon-Tyne, United Kingdom

INTRODUCTION

Arrhythmias are a common complication of heart failure, but until recently they have not received the attention that they deserve (1–3). Admittedly, many are trivial and are unlikely to cause symptoms or to have prognostic import, but others are serious and may have a profound or even fatal implication for the patient. It has been suggested that a sizable proportion of the 50% of heart failure sufferers who die suddenly do so as a consequence of an arrhythmia (4). However, the role of arrhythmias in heart failure, with respect to both symptoms and prognosis, involves more complex considerations than those related to potentially fatal ventricular tachyarrhythmias alone. Pathological arrhythmias may cause heart failure, and arrhythmias that might be innocuous in relatively normal persons can have devastating consequences for those in whom ventricular function is seriously compromised. The process of heart failure may in itself encourage arrhythmia development, particularly through the electrophysiological effects of abnormal wall stresses at both the atrial and the ventricular level (5), but arrhythmias may also be a consequence of treatment strategies designed to improve cardiovascular performance. Thus, inotropic agents (6) and diuretics (7) may be incriminated in arrhythmogenesis. At a time when medical therapy has been shown to improve the prognosis of patients with the most serious forms of heart failure (8,9), it is important to establish sound strategies for the management of arrhythmias complicating heart failure, lest treatment do more harm than good (10,11).

MECHANISMS OF DEATH IN HEART FAILURE

It is easy to imagine that death for most heart failure patients must come through an inexorable progression of mechanical dysfunction leading to low cardiac output and organ failure. In this setting, a fatal arrhythmic event would not be unexpected but would not be the primary lethal event. Information about the natural history of the disease, however, suggests that up to 50% of heart failure patients who die do so suddenly, at a time when their disease appears relatively stable (4). At least a portion of this sudden "unexpected" death may be arrhythmic and in these circumstances can hardly be considered agonal.

Equating sudden death with an arrhythmia is unsatisfactory; arrhythmias are just one mechanism by which patients may succumb rapidly or near-instantaneously. Twenty-four hour electrocardiogram recordings in ischemic patients have provided support for the importance of arrhythmias as a mechanism of sudden death (12,13), but similar systematic evidence for heart failure patients is scant (14). Lethal arrhythmias in patients not in heart failure probably are restricted to the major bradyarrhythmias and tachyarrhythmias (asystole, ventricular tachycardia, ventricular fibrillation), but in patients with severe myocardial dysfunction, arrhythmias such as atrial flutter, atrial fibrillation, and junctional tachycardias may be life-threatening.

Descriptors of death can be useful, but mortality categorization is rarely as objective as definitions might suggest. "Instantaneous death" is unambiguous but can never be inferred unwitnessed. "Sudden cardiac death" is a useful concept, but definitions vary, and death during sleep (plus other unwitnessed episodes) confounds secure scientific analysis. Heart failure presents special challenges. Is it possible for a patient in severe heart failure to die suddenly? The importance of this problem has been illustrated by the CONSENSUS study, in which it was suggested that the mortality benefits of enalapril probably were achieved through mechanical rather than antiarrhythmic actions (8). This assertion was based on the fact that sudden cardiac death appeared relatively uninfluenced by enalapril therapy. The reliability of this observation, which depends on the definition of sudden cardiac death in patients with severe heart failure, is questionable.

MECHANISMS OF ARRHYTHMIAS IN HEART FAILURE

Heart failure is a complex process, the clinical manifestations of which owe as much to the primary disease process and compensatory mechanisms (15) as to the features of impaired cardiac performance. Cardiac arrhythmias may be a consequence of one or more of these elements, with the superadded arrhythmogenic contribution that treatment may bring. No arrhythmia is specific to heart failure. Most arrhythmias probably depend on a complex interplay of factors that, on the one hand, diversifies management options but, on the other, involves a level of diagnostic complexity currently beyond available clinical electrophysiological techniques. Thus, much that has been learned of arrhythmia management in heart failure has come from empirical trial and error.

The Primary Disease Process

Every primary disease process that can cause heart failure may in itself generate arrhythmias. Ischemic heart disease, hypertension, hypertrophic cardiomyopathy, valvular heart disease, dilated cardiomyopathies, and acute myocarditides all in their own right have arrhythmic complications. Many of these pathological processes are associated with arrhythmias having a probable reentrant mechanism. Cardiac failure is unlikely to materially alter a fixed anatomic arrhythmia substrate such as supports postinfarction ventricular tachycardia, but failure-related arrhythmias may operate as trigger mechanisms for reentrant arrhythmias. Arrhythmias arising from the primary disease process are likely to be less well tolerated in patients with heart failure, and there is a particular risk that atrial arrhythmias will degenerate to atrial fibrillation and ventricular ones to ventricular fibrillation.

Electrolyte Disturbances

Hypokalemia

Hypokalemia has important arrhythmogenic consequences (16,17). It is one of the few mechanisms by which a completely normal heart may fibrillate. During the acute phase of myocardial infarction, the risk of primary ventricular fibrillation shows a weak correlation with potassium levels (17,18). Hypokalemia is not uncommon in heart failure, but the extent to which this electrolyte upset is responsible for clinically relevant arrhythmias is unknown. Diuretic therapy plays an important role in creating hypokalemia (7,19).

Hyperkalemia

Hyperkalemia is a less common problem in heart failure than hypokalemia but may arise from a combination of antifailure therapy and renal impairment. Although theoretically a cause of arrhythmias, it is unlikely to be of great clinical relevance.

Hypomagnesemia

The importance of hypomagnesemia in arrhythmia generation is only now receiving attention (20). Magnesium administration in early-stage myocardial infarction has been reported to prevent ventricular fibrillation and reduce mortality (21,22), but in another study (23) prophylactic magnesium appeared to achieve benefit by vasodilatory rather than electrophysiological actions. Anecdotal reports have hinted at a role for magnesium therapy in managing drug-induced torsade de pointes (24), although success has not been uniform (25). The arrhythmogenic role of magnesium imbalance is unknown, but it may be relevant in heart failure patients, particularly those on diuretic therapy.

Mechanico-Electrical Feedback

Heart failure is characterized by abnormal wall stress—this is probably one of the signal mechanisms for hypertrophy. It has been known for some time that mechanical loading conditions in myocardial tissue modify electrophysiology (5,26). Stretch of normal muscle shortens action potential duration (27,28) and may eventually give rise to spontaneous electrical activity. In animal models ventricular dilatation produces dispersion of refractoriness (29). It has been suggested that the mechanism for these changes lies in alterations in transmembrane calcium flux (30), either through an electrogenic Na/Ca exchange (31) or by a calcium-activated inward current (32). Mechanico-electrical (contraction/excitation) feedback may well be an important mechanism for generating atrial and ventricular ectopic beats but is unlikely to be the basis for sustained stable tachyarrhythmias. The generated ectopic beats, however, may trigger reentrant arrhythmias with stable characteristics.

Catecholamines

Catecholamine levels correlate with the prognosis and severity of heart failure (33). Elevation of circulating catecholamines and activation of the sympathetic nervous system are part of the neurohumoral response to heart failure and, at least in their early stages, are beneficial. Current evidence suggests that in many individuals, these responses eventually become detrimental. High levels of circulating catecholamines and activation of the sympathetic nervous system are potent factors for arrhythmogenesis. They can create substrate capable of supporting reentry; they may provide trigger beats or disturbances of heart rate to initiate reentrant arrhythmias; and they may accelerate an established arrhythmia or encourage its degeneration to fibrillation.

Arrhythmogenicity of Drugs Used to Treat Heart Failure

Treatment strategies for heart failure may provoke or aggravate arrhythmias. However, separating the arrhythmogenic contribution of diuretics, digoxin, and sympathomimetic amines from the primary disease and the electrophysiology of heart failure is all but impossible.

Diuretics

The arrhythmogenic effects of diuretics are much discussed, but remarkably little scientific evidence of the phenomenon is available. A weak relationship of ventricular fibrillation to hypokalemia and of hypokalemia to the use of non-potassium-sparing diuretics in acute myocardial infarction patients has been established (17,18). Induced hypokalemia has been suggested as an explanation for the failure of diuretic therapy to reduce cardiovascular mortality in hypertensive patients. Diuretic therapy has long been a traditional component of heart failure management. Hypokalemia, if not hypomagnesemia, is common, and the role of diuretics in heart failure needs reappraisal, given that their chronic use is not associated with increased cardiac performance and that the potential risks of hypokalemic arrhythmogenesis may be high (7,19).

Digoxin

The role of digoxin in heart failure management is controversial (34–36). Its utility for the treatment of the heart failure patient in atrial fibrillation is uncontested, but its value for the patient in sinus rhythm is debated. One study suggested that digoxin was at best of benefit in only 25% of heart failure patients in sinus rhythm (37). Whether in the other 75% it was without effect or detrimental is unknown.

Digoxin is a potent antiarrhythmic agent with profound effects on atrioventricular (AV) nodal function. It commonly produces first-degree heart block, or at least a longer than expected PR interval for rate, and, with high doses or in susceptible individuals, second- or third-degree heart block. The latter probably would be poorly tolerated by heart failure patients.

Digoxin also reduces the refractory period of atrial and ventricular tissue. Homogeneous changes of refractory periods are not arrhythmogenic, but with myocardial disease and heart failure, patchy changes may occur and encourage the development of atrial or even ventricular fibrillation. Surveys of postinfarction and postcoronary artery bypass graft patients treated with or without digoxin have suggested that the prognosis in those receiving digoxin is worse than that of the nondigoxin comparison group (38–40). This, however, does not prove that digoxin is responsible; patients requiring digoxin therapy were probably different.

Digoxin can provoke ectopic beats, both atrial and ventricular, through its effect on oscillatory membrane potentials. This is the most likely mechanism of paroxysmal atrial tachycardia with block, the arrhythmia characteristics of digoxin toxicity.

Sympathomimetic Amines

Sympathomimetic amines usually are reserved for management of patients in advanced heart failure. The therapy is controversial, particularly as such patients often have high levels of endogenous sympathetic drive and may have relatively few β-adrenoreceptor sites available for stimulation (41). Studies suggest that sympathomimetic amines offer modest benefit to selected patients (42). Arrhythmogenesis, principally the precipitation of ventricular tachyarrhythmias, has been noted in many studies (6,43).

MECHANISMS OF ANTIARRHYTHMIC ACTIONS IN HEART FAILURE

"Classical" Antiarrhythmic Drugs

The actions of the classical antiarrhythmic drugs are not significantly modified by heart failure except insofar as electrolyte disturbances may be present.

Modification of Mechanical Electrical Feedback

Vasodilators and digoxin theoretically can modify atrial and ventricular wall tension and may thereby have an antiarrhythmic action. At present, there is limited evidence that this effect may occur with digoxin (44), nitrates (45,46), hydralazine, and the angiotensin converting enzyme (ACE) inhibitors (47,48). The antiarrhythmic effects of magnesium (21–23) may in part be related to its vasodilator action. Much remains to be learned in this area. The prospect of arrhythmia control by modifying the mechanical elements responsible for the arrhythmias has great attraction, particularly at a time when the risks of antiarrhythmic therapy have been forcibly brought to attention by the Cardiac Arrhythmia Suppression Trial (CAST) results (49).

Modification of Hypertrophy

Vasodilator therapy may also usefully arrest or regress the hypertrophy and remodeling that is an integral part of the body's response to heart failure. Myocardial hypertrophy brings some initially useful mechanical benefits, but, particularly when it occurs as a response to disease, inhomogeneous electrophysiology may result and be arrhythmogenic.

INOTROPISM AND ANTIARRHYTHMIC DRUGS

Drug management of arrhythmias in the context of heart failure is fraught with problems. Most antiarrhythmic drugs depress left ventricular contractility (50) and so may aggravate cardiac decompensation. It is difficult to establish the relative negative inotropic effect of these agents; few direct comparative studies have been performed, and none has addressed antiarrhythmic efficacy *and* left ventricular depression. The Vaughan Williams class Ic drugs, the most potent of the sodium channel blockers, are considered the most depressant (51–53), but they are among the most effective agents for ventricular tachycardia (54) and have an increasingly important role in the management of atrial fibrillation (55,56). They may achieve arrhythmia control at such low doses that they can be given to patients in heart failure. The Vaughan Williams class Ib drugs have least negative inotropic potential but are useful only for ventricular arrhythmias (57), for which their efficacy is generally lower than that of the Ic compounds. Disopyramide is a Vaughan Williams class Ia agent with powerful antiarrhythmic actions but has gained a reputation as being poorly tolerated by heart failure patients (58). The effect of beta-blockers on left ventricular function is complex. Their slowing of heart rate can improve left ventricular filling time, although their sympathetic blockade may reduce sympathetically driven inotropism. Beta-blockers have even been advocated as treatment for heart failure (59–61), but patient selection must be meticulous and dose titration cautious. Beta-blockers have powerful antiarrhythmic effects (62,63); their contribution in managing heart failure arrhythmias has not yet been studied in detail. The partial β_1-agonist xamoterol was designed to manage heart failure and was expected to stop detrimentally high levels of sympathetic drive while underpinning heart rate and contractility by its intrinsic sympathomimetic activity (64,65). In patients with severe heart failure, an excess mortality was noted when the drug was used, and xamoterol is now reserved for the management only of those with mild and moderate heart failure. Xamoterol may have antiarrhythmic potential, particularly for patients with heart failure.

Class III antiarrhythmic drugs act by prolonging the plateau phase of the action potential through their effect on the potassium channel. Amiodarone, the most important agent of this class, probably has a minimal negative inotropic effect, but this is offset by its peripheral vasodilator action (66). Not only is amiodarone the most "powerful" antiarrhythmic drug currently available, but it is also well tolerated even by patients in severe heart failure (67). Unfortunately, the noncardiac toxicity of amiodarone (68) and the likely need for chronic suppressive antiarrhythmic therapy in heart failure dictate that amiodarone be reserved for situations in which other therapy is ineffective, not tolerated, or contraindicated.

The electrophysiologically active calcium channel blockers (verapamil, diltiazem) are also vasodilators. This action is insufficient to mask their negative inotropic effects. They are very well tolerated for the management of narrow-QRS tachyarrhythmias in patients with normal or near-normal ventricular function but should be used with caution, if at all, in heart failure.

Digoxin is a positive inotropic drug. Its useful electrophysiological actions are relatively restricted to its AV nodal effect, which slows the ventricular rate in atrial fibrillation. There is a suggestion that it may offer a useful antiarrhythmic effect against ventricular arrhythmias through its potential to modify wall stress (44).

HEART FAILURE AND ANTIARRHYTHMIC DRUG KINETICS

The state of heart failure may dramatically alter the pharmacokinetics of drugs (69). Absorption from the gastrointestinal tract may be slow and incomplete (reduced bioavailability). Alterations in hepatic blood flow may reduce first-pass hepatic metabolism (increased bioavailability), and reduced hepatic function may extend the biological half-life of drugs or alternatively may reduce the formation of active metabolites. Impaired renal function will reduce the excretion of drugs normally eliminated by this route.

Safe use of antiarrhythmic drugs in heart failure patients mandates an awareness of the effects heart failure has on drug kinetics. All doses and routes of administration should be selected carefully and reviewed regularly, particularly in the face of changing cardiovascular status. In arrhythmia management, there is often a choice of potentially effective agent, permitting selection of the one most appropriate for the patient's need and least likely to suffer pharmacokinetic disturbance. Mexiletine and disopyramide are *not* identical antiarrhythmic drugs, but in some circumstances (e.g., suppression of troublesome symptomatic ventricular ectopic beats in a heart failure patient with only minimal left ventricular decompensation but marked renal impairment), the hepatic degradation of mexiletine is an advantage when compared with the renal excretion of disopyramide.

As in other situations of arrhythmia management, the lowest effective dose of the "safest" therapy should be selected.

EXPRESSION OF ARRHYTHMIAS

All types of arrhythmias can occur in heart failure patients. As previously discussed, some may reflect primary disease, others treatment strategies, and others yet again are related to specific features of the heart failure process itself.

Supraventricular Ectopic Beats

Supraventricular ectopic beats are common in normal healthy individuals, who usually are unaware of their presence and for whom they have no prognostic significance. Supraventricular ectopic beats are very frequent in heart failure patients, but here too they rarely cause symptoms despite their possibly more profound hemodynamic impact. Frequent supraventricular ectopic beats may herald and initiate atrial fibrillation, although proof of this relationship is weak.

Management

Supraventricular ectopic beats usually require no treatment. There is no evidence that suppression of supraventricular beats is useful in the prophylaxis of atrial fibrillation.

Atrial Fibrillation

Atrial fibrillation is the most common important arrhythmia to complicate heart failure. A primary atrial myocardial pathology favors but is not essential, for its occurrence. Abnormal wall tension in the atria appears sufficient in itself to destabilize atrial electrophysiology and allow fibrillation to occur.

Atrial fibrillation is a serious arrhythmia in heart failure patients. Loss of atrial transport, loss of regular ventricular contraction, and excessively rapid ventricular response rates have serious implications for patients whose ventricular function is already compromised. Atrial fibrillation usually produces marked symptoms (lassitude, breathlessness, dizziness) and may precipitate further cardiac decompensation.

Management

Restoration of sinus rhythm is the best option but is difficult to achieve. Unless the primary disease process can be arrested or suppressed, success rates for electrical cardioversion to sinus rhythm are poor. Medical cardioversion is similarly unrewarding and may involve the use of antiarrhythmic drugs with potentially negative inotropic effects (quinidine, disopyramide, propafenone, flecainide, etc.). In most patients, initial management comprises rate control, amelioration of heart failure status, and then consideration of cardioversion.

Rate control is best offered by digoxin. Digoxin may also offer a useful positive inotropic effect in some but certainly not all patients. An initial rapid digitalizing dose is needed. Although heart failure alters digoxin kinetics (through renal function alterations), the standard digitalizing dose of 1 mg is unchanged and should be given parenterally. Subsequent maintenance doses will be dictated by renal function, by drug effect, and by clinical status. If rate control is not achieved with digoxin alone, an adjunctive therapy can be considered. Neither of the two classical options—a beta-blocker and verapamil—is immediately appealing to give to a compromised patient in heart failure. Both may depress cardiac performance. The better of these alternatives has not been established by scientific research, but given the high levels of sympathetic response in heart failure, cautious administration of a beta-blocker would seem most appropriate. Small, frequent doses of a cardioselective beta-blocker, e.g., metoprolol, are appropriate. There is theoretic merit in considering a partial β_1-agonist such as xamoterol for the purpose—it might provide beta-sympathetic blocker yet, through its intrinsic sympathomimetic activity, prevent a devastating loss of all sympathetic drive. Early studies have suggested benefit (65), but these agents should not be used routinely in heart failure for this purpose until their place has been more securely established.

All patients in atrial fibrillation should be considered at risk of thromboembolism. Those in heart failure are especially at risk, and some form of protection should be given unless otherwise contraindicated. Standard warfarin regimens have been shown to benefit. Low-dose warfarin (70) and aspirin (71) may be useful, but at present the evidence is controversial.

Atrial Flutter

Atrial flutter is an organized atrial arrhythmia probably based on a macroreentrant circuit involving the low right atrium (72). Its consequences when complicating heart failure are similar to those of atrial fibrillation. Atrial flutter, however, rarely is chronic. The abnormal hemodynamic state in heart failure encourages an early degeneration to atrial fibrillation.

Management

The management of sustained atrial flutter is similar to that of atrial fibrillation, although there is a greater prospect for restoration of sinus rhythm by DC cardioversion. Vaughan Williams class I antiarrhythmic drug therapy carries a risk that by slowing the atrial flutter rate without influencing AV nodal conduction, it will change the AV conduction ratio, with an acceleration of ventricular response (73). In heart failure patients with atrial flutter it is most unlikely that negative inotropic drugs such as disopyramide would be used without digoxin.

Ventricular Ectopic Beats

Ventricular ectopic beats occur in normal individuals but are increased in frequency and complexity in almost every cardiac disease. Regardless of their pathological setting, most ventricular ectopic beats cause no symptoms. Each is a single self-contained event. Susceptible patients who are aware of ventricular ectopic beats may notice the succeeding augmented normal beat rather than the premature abnormal beat. Ventricular ectopic beats that complicate the late phase of infarction (74) and aortic stenosis (75) have been associated with an adverse prognosis.

Ventricular ectopic beats are very frequent in patients with heart failure. Depending on frequency they have prognostic implications (76).

Management

Ventricular ectopic beats in themselves rarely merit treatment. Very occasionally they cause sufficient palpitatory distress to warrant considering their suppression. This is a delicate area of therapeutic endeavor. The risk-benefit ratio of ventricular ectopic beat suppression in heart failure is not advantageous (77). Most effective ventricular ectopic beat suppressants have adverse effects on myocardial contractility. The first step should be to identify and correct potentially remediable precipitating causes such as hypokalemia. As with normal individuals, occasionally coffee, tea, or alcohol (to be deprecated in any heart failure patient) may be relevant to ventricular arrhythmogenesis. The patient should be reassured that the ventricular ectopic beats in themselves are harmless. Only rarely will more definitive action be necessary. The best choice of antiarrhythmic agent is mexiletine, a Vaughan Williams class lb antiarrhythmic drug with a highly selective effect on ventricular arrhythmias and with the most minimal negative inotropic effect (57). Its use is limited by unwanted gastrointestinal and central nervous system effects, but with judicious dosing these can usually be contained. Other class I antiarrhythmic drugs may be useful, but none offers such an attractive risk-benefit profile in this context. In patients free of heart failure, a beta-blocker would be the drug of first choice when ventricular ectopic beats need to be suppressed. In heart failure patients, similarly, a beta-blocker may be useful, but dosing must be cautious and the minimum consistent with the desired end result of symptom control. This may be achieved without necessarily completely suppressing the arrhythmia.

The prognostic implication of ventricular ectopic beats in heart failure has prompted investigation of whether the outlook for heart failure might be ameliorated by their suppression. This strategy was recently proven to be contraindicated in survivors of myocardial infarction, in whom flecainide, encainide, and moricizine were associated with an increased mortality in comparison with placebo-treated counterparts (49). Many of the patients enrolled in these studies had significant impairment of left ventricular function, although none were in overt heart failure. The disastrous results of these trials have been echoed by similar findings in studies using mexiletine (78,79), tocainide (80,81), and phenytoin (82,83).

The prospect that antiarrhythmic drugs will ameliorate the prognosis of heart failure patients is not good. Although no large-scale studies have been performed, numerous small studies have failed to show benefit of conventional antiarrhythmic drugs (84–86). None were of sufficient size or of adequate duration to detect a prognostic change. In the absence of hard evidence, there is little to commend ventricular ectopic beat modification in the expectation that prognosis can be improved in heart failure. Rather, the detection of prognostically important ventricular ectopic beats should prompt improved management of the failure itself.

Therapy with ACE inhibitors can reduce the frequency of ventricular ectopic beats in heart failure patients (47,48). The effect is relatively modest and is an order of magnitude less than the suppression that might be obtained from conventional antiarrhythmic therapy. Nonetheless, this modulating effect on ventricular ectopic beats was sufficient to encourage optimism that ACE inhibitors might reduce sudden death in heart failure patients. In the CONSENSUS study (8), patients in severe heart failure (New York Heart Association [NYHA] class III, IV) were randomized to receive either enalapril or a placebo. Mortality was significantly reduced in those receiving the active ACE inhibitor. It appeared to be mechanical death rather than sudden, presumptively arrhythmic death that was reduced. The problems of categorizing mode of death in heart failure have already been alluded to, and it remains possible that ACE inhibitors can offer prognostic improvement through an antiarrhythmic effect. Indeed, in the VHeFT II study, sudden death was reduced (87). The effect was most obvious in patients with less severe heart failure (NYHA class II), raising the possibility that any stretch- and tension-related antiarrhythmic benefits of ACE inhibitor therapy can be gained only at a time when there is an adequate mass of drug-sensitive cells, i.e., before major fibrosis occurs.

Ventricular Tachycardia

Ventricular tachycardia covers a wide range of arrhythmias ranging from those that are little more than a brief salvo of ventricular ectopic beats to a rapid sustained arrhythmia that may directly threaten life. Sustained monomorphic ventricular tachycardia is a special form of ventricular tachycardia that is almost always based on a fixed structural anatomic abnormality and a reentrant electrophysiological mechanism. This form of ventricular tachycardia is very rare as a complication of heart failure. If it does occur, it is likely to reflect the primary pathology—e.g., postinfarction left ventricular aneurysm. The ventricular tachycardia that complicates heart failure characteristically is of relatively brief duration (less than 10 consecutive beats) and is polymorphic and irregular. Reentry is unlikely to be the mechanism, as judged by these features and by the anecdotal evidence that the arrhythmia is unlikely to be provokable by programmed electrical stimulation. The symptoms and immediate implications of such episodes of ventricular tachycardia are difficult to predict. Surprisingly, many patients are unaware of their occurrence despite their considerable but brief effects on cardiac output. As in this and many other situations of cardiovascular disease, the presence of ventricular tachycardia has serious prognostic implications (76, 84).

Management

Not all ventricular tachycardia must be treated, although at present, all ventricular tachycardia in heart failure must be considered to signify a bad prognosis. As with ventricular ectopic beats, a search for remediable causes should be a first priority. When an antiarrhythmic drug is necessary, the smallest dose of the least toxic drug should be tried first. In anecdotal experience, mexiletine, propafenone, flecainide, and quinidine have proved useful, but in most cases the potential for left ventricular depression is high, and this may preclude use of an effective antiarrhythmic dose. Amiodarone has an important place in management. It is well tolerated by patients even when left ventricular function is dramatically impaired. Its remarkable efficacy overshadows its unwanted-effect profile, particularly in the context of the heart failure patient with ventricular tachycardia.

Ventricular tachycardia as a complication of heart failure carries a higher level of prognostic risk than is reflected by ventricular ectopic beats alone. The arrhythmia thus identifies a high-risk subgroup of the heart failure population who can be identified electrocardiographically. That prognosis might be improved if ventricular tachycardia were suppressed seems logical, but as has been seen with the CAST results, the hypothesis may not be valid (88). As for ventricular ectopic beats, no definitive study has been reported in heart failure. Anecdotes suggest that little or no prognostic benefit is obtainable using antiarrhythmic therapy, but no study has yet had an adequate sample size, involved a reasonable duration of follow-up, and carefully defined the clinical characteristics of recruited patients.

Ventricular Fibrillation

Ventricular fibrillation may be an "agonal" rhythm in heart failure patients. The term implies that the arrhythmia is merely the final electrophysiological disturbance in a heart that is irreversibly diseased and metabolically abnormal. In the context of acute myocardial infarction such ventricular fibrillation may be labeled "secondary" (secondary to heart failure or shock) (89), with the implication that there is a poor immediate prognosis (i.e., for successful conversion to sinus rhythm by DC shock) and late prognosis (90). Evidence from victims of secondary ventricular fibrillation confirms that the success rate for restoration of sinus rhythm is low but suggests that survivors have a reasonable long-term prognosis (91). Thus, in acute myocardial infarction there is a possibility of hemodynamic and metabolic improvement. In most situations of heart failure, such improvements are unlikely. Moreover, unlike infarction, heart failure often is not heralded by an easily recognizable new clinical event; rather, it is a chronic process. Thus, few heart failure patients are hospitalized, and even fewer will be electrocardiographically monitored. As a consequence, very little is known about the antecedents and pattern of ventricular fibrillation in heart failure unassociated with infarction.

Management

Ventricular fibrillation in heart failure is managed as in other situations: with immediate basic resuscitation and DC shock. Success rates for restoration of sinus rhythm are low. Multiple shocks and adjunctive measures are likely to be tried (adrenaline, lignocaine, etc.), but nothing has been shown scientifically to improve the success rate of DC energy alone. Electrolyte abnormalities are likely to be present in heart failure ventricular fibrillation. Correction would seem appropriate, but little or nothing is known of its value or safety.

If sinus rhythm can be restored, the metabolic and electrophysiological milieu that was responsible for ventricular fibrillation will probably still persist. Recurrence of ventricular fibrillation is common. Standard practice is to administer intravenous lignocaine as a prophylactic strategy. Lignocaine, a Vaughan Williams class lb drug, has rapid onset and offset effects on the sodium channel, and although it is not entirely devoid of left ventricular depressant properties, given cautiously it is well tolerated by heart failure patients. The standard regime comprises 100 mg intravenously over 3 min followed by an infusion of 4 mg per min for 1 h, reduced thereafter to 2 or 3 mg/h for 24 h. In patients with compromised circulation and poor hepatic blood flow, lignocaine may accumulate, with plasma concentrations rising to toxic levels. Clinical examination for tremor—an important and useful but often overlooked clinical sign—can help predict and prevent the problem. Otherwise, empiric dose reduction or estimation of plasma lignocaine concentrations may be appropriate. Despite the widespread use of lignocaine after resuscitation from ventricular fibrillation, there are no data to indicate that this is a useful therapy (92). In infarction patients, the incidence of ventricular fibrillation has been high despite "adequate" lignocaine therapy. No alternative treatment possibilities have been investigated. This situation is far from satisfactory and should be resolved by controlled studies.

Heart failure patients resuscitated from ventricular fibrillation should be reviewed urgently. Common sense would indicate that electrolytes be checked and normalized, that antifailure therapy be reviewed lest it be arrhythmogenic, and finally that the hemodynamic status of the patient be improved if at all possible.

Asystole

Asystole—cessation of electrical activity in the ventricles (often also in the atria)—potentially is a lethal arrhythmia. It reflects profound and extreme electrophysiological disturbances within the myocardium, as manifested by the complete failure of support ectopic pacemakers to emerge. It may be heralded by short asystolic periods (with or without symptoms), but these are not infrequent on 24-h monitoring of heart failure patients, and at present no reliable electrocardiographic predictors of asystole have been identified.

Management

Asystole is treated first by basic cardiopulmonary resuscitation, which should maintain life until either ventricular pacing is established (the ideal intervention) or an isoprenaline infusion is started. The latter is difficult to control: there is a risk of producing a ventricular tachyarrhythmia and creating a situation in which the patient's rhythm alternates uncontrollably from ventricular fibrillation to asystole and vice-versa. Very few heart failure patients survive asystole. Pacing often fails to excite the ventricle, or if it does there is electromechanical dissociation. If resuscitation from asystole is successful, recurrences are likely. Prophylactic short-term pacing facilitates clinical management but may not materially influence the prognosis. Implantation of a permanent pacemaker is rarely if ever warranted.

Heart Block

Disturbances of AV nodal conduction are common in heart failure patients and may reflect the primary disease process, the effect of antifailure therapy, or electrolyte disturbances. These arrhythmias are not specific to heart failure. Neither first-degree nor second-degree AV block needs treatment, but review of the patient's cardiovascular state and adjustment of therapy are appropriate. Complete heart block is serious and is unlikely to be tolerated by the heart failure patient.

Management

Complete heart block needs active intervention. Circulatory support is the first activity. This may require pacing (ideal) or an isoprenaline infusion. Correction of precipitating factors is logical, but careful assessment will be necessary to establish whether complete heart block is reliably reversible (e.g., when it is a consequence of hypokalemic and digoxin therapy). Long-term treatment, if necessary, will involve permanent pacemaking with a system that optimizes cardiac output (e.g., DDD and VVIR).

PROGNOSIS IN HEART FAILURE

The prognosis for heart failure is poor. The 1-year survival rate for those in severe heart failure (NYHA class IV) is no better than 30% to 50%. At least some of the mortality is arrhythmic, but whether primary or merely as a final agonal event is difficult to establish. The mortality improvements reported by the CONSENSUS study (8) were initially thought to have been mediated by amelioration of cardiac mechanical performance, but the possibility of an antiarrhythmic effect has not been excluded. This will be important to establish, particularly as ACE inhibitor therapy is now being used in milder degrees of heart failure and in some circumstances as a prophylactic measure to prevent postinfarction cardiac dilatation and subsequent failure (93). The SAVE study (93) showed a significant mortality reduction by captopril in postmyocardial infarction patients with left ventricular damage but without heart failure. In the SOLVD study (94), a trend for mortality improvement was reported, and hospitalization for heart failure was significantly reduced. The failure of the CONSENSUS II study (95) questions the wisdom of very early postinfarction ACE inhibitor treatment. First-dose hypotension appeared to be the problem; there was no evidence to suggest that ACE inhibitor therapy caused arrhythmias.

Prophylactic use of antiarrhythmic drugs to improve prognosis has had some successes in situations other than heart failure; amiodarone in high-risk patients with hypertrophic cardiomyopathy (96) (although inefficacy has also been claimed) (97); beta-blockers in the congenital long-QT syndromes (62); and possibly beta-blockers (98) and amiodarone (99) after infarction. Prophylactic antiarrhythmic drug failures have attracted more attention; for example, encainide, flecainide, and moricizine after infarction (49). Several relatively small studies of antiarrhythmic drug use in heart failure patients have been reported (84–86). None showed benefit, and although all were limited by the small sample size, there is little promise for this intervention. Of course, antiarrhythmic drug use is limited in heart failure—most agents have important negative inotropic effects and are an unattractive intervention for patients whose left ventricular performance is already suboptimal. For this reason, amiodarone has attracted attention. Amiodarone is remarkably well tolerated even by patients in severe heart failure. It has almost no negative inotropic effects and is a modest vasodilator. It is active against a wide range of arrhythmias and has antifibrillatory effects. Moreover, in the management of such a serious condition as heart failure, its toxicity profile may be acceptable. Disappointingly, in one reported study, neither total mortality nor sudden (presumptively arrhythmic) death was reduced (100). The study was small; its result could conceal a mortality benefit of up to 10%, but to establish that would require a very large investigation. Although this could be undertaken, there would be major difficulties as ACE inhibitor therapy becomes more aggressively used. The study would need to examine the interaction of amiodarone and ACE inhibitors.

THE IMPLANTABLE CARDIOVERTER DEFIBRILLATOR IN HEART FAILURE

The implantable cardioverter defibrillator (ICD) is an important antiarrhythmic development. It reduces mortality in patients whose lives are threatened by primary ventricular tachycardia or fibrillation (101,102). It will not help those in whom ventricular tachycardia or ventricular fibrillation reflects irreversible myocardial damage or biochemical catastrophe. It is inappropriate for patients with very frequent episodes of these arrhythmias (a limitation related to battery life). Some but not all heart failure patients will be excluded by these caveats. Those who have survived one documented cardiac arrest (due to ventricular tachycardia or ventricular fibrillation) would be ideal candidates. The value of the ICD for prophylactic therapy in heart failure is unknown but is under investigation. Implantable cardioverter defibrillators are not without their problems. Many of the difficulties are of a general nature and are independent of heart failure status (infection, device longevity, failure to sense, etc.). For some problems, heart failure has relevance. These include inappropriate shock delivery (especially related to atrial fibrillation with fast ventricular responses—more common in heart failure patients), patch thresholds (increased in heart failure), implantation mortality (increased in heart failure patients to around 3%), and postimplantation cardiac decompensation (possibly related to restriction from epicardial patches).

Heart failure patients may benefit from the ICD, but recipients need to be selected carefully. More liberal implantation policies should depend on the results of well-designed clinical studies.

NONPHARMACOLOGICAL ARRHYTHMIA MANAGEMENT RELEVANT TO HEART FAILURE

Nonpharmacological management of arrhythmias offers the attraction of arrhythmia cure rather than palliation. Arrhythmic surgery, DC or radio frequency ablation, and transplantation are the commonly available procedures.

Arrhythmia Surgery

There are surgical approaches for atrial fibrillation (103,104), the reciprocating tachycardias utilizing bypass pathways (105), intra- and para-AV nodal reentry tachycardia (106,107), true atrial tachycardia (108), and ventricular tachycardia (109). Some are more successful and better developed than others. These arrhythmias, if sustained, may *cause* heart failure, in which case they may merit surgical treatment. Atrial fibrillation and ventricular tachycardia are the two most important rhythms to complicate heart failure; their surgical management is possible but may not be desirable.

Surgery for Atrial Fibrillation

Atrial fibrillation is common in heart failure. Its medical treatment is less than satisfactory, but neither of the two current surgical strategies has great appeal. In the corridor procedure (103), the free walls of the right and left atria are disarticulated from the central and septal atrium, which becomes a corridor connecting the sinus and AV nodes. Sinus rhythm and control of the ventricle is achieved, but the free atria may continue to fibrillate, with an attendant loss of atrial transport and the risk of emboli. In the maze procedure (104), the critical mass of the atria is reduced by establishing a tortuous conduction pathway. The atria are dissected in a complex pattern and repaired. Sinus rhythm is achieved in a high proportion of patients, but overall experience is still small, and the procedure is a major one. Both operations carry a considerable operative risk for patients in heart failure.

Surgery for Ventricular Tachycardia

Surgical management of ventricular tachycardia is principally confined to postinfarction patients whose ventricular tachycardia is sustained and monomorphic and is unresponsive to medical therapy (109). Many of these patients have underlying left ventricular aneurysm, and the vast majority have seriously impaired left ventricular function. A proportion present in frank heart failure. Surgery is usually map-guided and involves endocardial resection. Concomitant aneurysmectomy has been traditional, but overenthusiastic resection of myocardium may be detrimental. Nonetheless, surgery for ventricular tachycardia offers an opportunity to improve left ventricular performance, reduce heart failure, and control the arrhythmia. Were it not for the surgical mortality, this option would be very attractive. Mortality rates vary from 7% to 30%, but the variation reflects the initial selection of patients more than surgical expertise (110). Excellent surgical results can be established by restricting the procedure to patients with "slow" ventricular tachycardia and "good" left ventricular function. The real problem, however, is the patient in heart failure with a low ejection fraction, with "fast" ventricular tachycardia that is recurring frequently and does not respond to antiarrhythmic therapy. Surgery for such a patient carries a high risk. In many centers patients such as this are refused surgery. Aneurysmectomy or infarctectomy alone carries a high operative mortality. An added antiarrhythmic procedure adds more risk, but the rewards of success are substantial. Investigation of optimal myocardial remodeling by resection might revitalize surgery as a therapeutic option, particularly when poor left ventricular performance is no longer seen as a bar to revascularization procedures. Surgery has little or no role to play in the management of brief paroxysms of polymorphic ventricular tachycardia, which are common in heart failure patients. The major importance of these episodes of ventricular tachycardia relates to long-term prognosis rather than to their immediate hemodynamic impact.

Ablation

True atrial tachycardia and reciprocating tachycardias using bypass pathways can be successfully ablated by radio frequency or DC energy. The results of ablation of ventricular tachycardia are poor regardless of left ventricular function. Atrioventricular node ablation is of limited applicability to heart failure patients in whom drugs have failed to stop excessive and uncontrollable ventricular rate responses to atrial fibrillation. Since ablation damages the heart, it should be used as a last resort. There is evidence that DC shocks may cause extensive "blast" damage, which is apparent as both acute and chronic heart failure. In the heart failure patient, radio frequency ablation may be safer. It is believed not to carry a risk of early and late heart failure, but follow-up studies of this procedure are still relatively few and most are short-term.

Transplantation

Cardiac transplantation is an important management option for patients with severe heart failure. It has many attractions in respect to arrhythmia management in such patients, and many large cardiac transplant series contain some patients operated on for the combination of heart failure and drug-refractory arrhythmias.

ARRHYTHMIAS THAT CAUSE HEART FAILURE

Any sustained tachyarrhythmia may cause heart failure. Fortunately, sustained incessant ventricular tachycardia is very uncommon. When it occurs, the electrocardiogram usually is easily diagnosed and the primary role of the arrhythmia is apparent.

Incessant narrow-QRS tachycardias pose a greater challenge. They can easily be mistaken for sinus tachycardia, which might not be unexpected in a patient with heart failure due to another cause. Moreover, echocardiography and angiocardiography will show a nonspecific dilated ventricle, adding momentum to the misdiagnosis that the primary problem is in the ventricular myocardium, with secondary sinus tachycardia. In heart failure, sinus tachycardia rarely exceeds 120 beats/min at rest. Narrow-QRS tachycardia at rates in excess of 120 beats/min should arouse suspicion that the arrhythmia is not of sinus origin. The electrocardiogram should be scrutinized for the P-to-QRS relationship, P wave morphology, and the response to vagal maneuvers.

True atrial tachycardia (automatic) and the reciprocating tachycardias using accessory pathways (particularly a unidirectional ventriculoatrial conduction pathway) are the two arrhythmias most likely to be incessant and to be sufficiently rapid to decompensate an initially normal ventricle. Reciprocating tachycardia is an important cause of heart failure in infancy. On stopping the arrhythmia, hemodynamic restitution may take a long time. Impaired left ventricular contractility and left ventricular dilatation may persist for months after arrhythmia control, raising doubts about initial myocardial normality. Whether any dilated cardiomyopathy presenting late may have initially been due to a sustained arrhythmia is unknown but is probably unlikely.

SPECIAL CAUSES OF HEART FAILURE WITH ARRHYTHMIA IMPLICATIONS

Although any primary myocardial process may cause either heart failure or arrhythmias, three deserve special mention: alcohol, viruses, and Chagas' disease.

Alcohol

Alcohol is increasingly recognized as a cause of heart failure through its direct myocardial effect. Arrhythmias are also a feature of excessive alcohol intake. Alcohol has been particularly incriminated in both paroxysmal and sustained forms of atrial fibrillation. There is anecdotal evidence that with abstinence, atrial fibrillation may stop and myocardial function can improve. The extent and reliability of such reversibility is unknown.

Viruses

Viral myocarditis may present as an acute condition with severe cardiac decompensation. Ventricular arrhythmias are a common accompaniment but rarely are sustained. Arrhythmia treatment should be given only if absolutely necessary, as, for instance, when ventricular fibrillation is occurring (111). At least some patients who survive severe acute myocarditis may be left with a chronic arrhythmia necessitating long-term therapy.

Chagas' disease

Chagas' disease is common in South America (112) but rare elsewhere. It is frequently complicated by ventricular arrhythmias, which may be very resistant to medical therapy. Anecdotal reports suggest that amiodarone may have a particular role to play in the management of this condition.

THE FUTURE

Heart failure management is a major clinical challenge. Its scientific basis is not well established, but heart failure is such a common condition that improved treatment protocols must be a priority. Despite the many years over which heart failure has been recognized as a clinical entity, surprisingly little is known of whether arrhythmias are merely epiphenomena or whether they directly contribute to the process of deterioration and subsequent death. Current opinion is that arrhythmias may be an important mechanism of *premature* mortality in heart failure patients. If this can be established, therapy directed at preserving the electrical integrity of the myocardium will become important. Success may demand antiarrhythmic strategies quite unlike those currently in use. The ACE inhibitors have shown that antiarrhythmic effects can be achieved through mechanisms other than direct actions on transmembrane ionic gates. On a more traditional note, although few of the currently available antiarrhythmic agents offer attractive properties for use in patients with compromised ventricular function, amiodarone and new class III antiarrhythmic drugs that are under development may yet prove to have a role to play in improving the outlook for heart failure sufferers.

REFERENCES

1. Anderson JL. Should complex ventricular arrhythmias in patients with congestive heart failure be treated? A protagonist's viewpoint. Am J Cardiol 1990; 66:447–450.
2. Kjekshus J. Arrhythmias and mortality in congestive heart failure. Am J Cardiol 1990; 65:421–481.
3. Rehnquist N. Arrhythmias and their treatment in patients with heart failure. Am J Cardiol 1989; 64:61J–64J.
4. Packer M. Sudden unexpected death in patients with congestive heart failure: a second frontier. Circulation 1985; 72:681–685.
5. Dean JW, Lab MJ. Arrhythmia in heart failure: role of mechanically induced changes in electrophysiology. Lancet 1989; i:1309–1312.
6. Ferrick KJ, Fein SA, Ferrick AM, Doyle JT. Effect of milrinone on ventricular arrhythmias in congestive heart failure. Am J Cardiol 1990; 66:431–434.
7. Myers MG, Diuretic therapy and ventricular arrhythmias in persons 65 years of age and older. Am J Cardiol 1990; 65:599–603.
8. The CONSENSUS Trial Study Group. Effects of enalapril on mortality in severe congestive heart failure. Results of the Cooperative North Scandinavian Summit Study. N Engl J Med 1987; 316:1429–1435.
9. Cohn JN, Archibald DG, Ziesche S, Franciosa JA, Harston WE, Tristani FE, Dunkman WB, Jacobs W, Francis GS, et al. Effect of vasodilator therapy on mortality in chronic congestive heart failure. Results of a Veterans Administration Cooperative study. N Engl J Med 1986; 314:1547–1552.
10. Anderson JL. Should complex ventricular arrhythmias in patients with congestive heart failure be treated? A protagonist's veiw. Am J Cardiol 1990; 66:447–450.
11. Podrid PJ, Wilson JS. Should asymptomatic ventricular arrhythmia in patients with congestive heart failure be treated? An antagonist's viewpoint. Am J Cardiol 1990; 66:451–457.
12. Roelandt J, Klootwijk J, Lumsen J, Janse MJ. Sudden death during longterm ambulatory monitoring. Eur Heart J 1984; 5:7–20.
13. Milner PG, Platia EV, Reid PR, Griffith LSC. Ambulatory electrocardiographic recordings at the time of fatal cardiac arrest. Am J Cardiol 1985; 55:146–151.

14. Luu M, Stevenson WG. Diverse mechanisms of unexpected cardiac arrest in advanced heart failure. Circulation 1989; 80:1675–1680.
15. Francis GS. Neuro-humoral mechanisms involved in congestive heart failure. Am J Cardiol 1985; 55:15A–21A.
16. Podrid PJ. Potassium and ventricular arrhythmias. Am J Cardiol 1990; 65:33E–44E.
17. Campbell RWF, Higham D, Adams PC, Murray A. Potassium: its relevance for arrhythmias complicating acute myocardial infarction. J Cardiovasc Pharmacol 1987; 10:S25–S30.
18. Nordrehaug JE, VanderLippe G. Hypokalemia and ventricular fibrillation in acute myocardial infarction. Br Heart J 1983; 50;525–529.
19. Stewart DE, Ikram H, Espiner EA, Nicholls MG. Arrhythmogenic potential of diuretic induced hypokalemia in patients with mild hypertension and ischaemic disease. Br Heart J 1985; 54:290–297.
20. Keller PK, Aronson RS. The role of magnesium in cardiac arrhythmias. Prog Cardiovasc Dis 1990; 32:433–448.
21. Shechter M, Hod H, Marks N. Beneficial effect of magnesium sulfate in acute myocardial infarction. Am J Cardiol 1990; 66:271–274.
22. Rasmussen HS, McNair P, Norregard P, Backer V, Lindeneg O, Balslev S. Intravenous magnesium in acute myocardial infarction. Lancet 1986; i:234–236.
23. Woods KL, Fletcher S, Roffe C, Haider Y. Intravenous magnesium sulphate in suspected acute myocardial infarction: Results of the second Leicester Intravenous Magnesium Intervention Trial (LIMIT-2). Lancet 1992; 339:1553–1558.
24. Tzivoni D, Keren A, Cohen AM, Loebel H, Zahavi I, Chenzbraun A, Stern S. Magnesium therapy for torsade de pointes. Am J Cardiol 1984; 53:528–530.
25. Toivonen LK, Leinonen H. Limited effect of magnesium sulphate on torsades de pointes ventricular tachycardia. Int J Cardiol 1986; 12:260–262.
26. Dudel J, Trautwein W. Das aktionspotential und mechanogram des herzmuskels unter dem einflus der dehnung. Cardiologie 1954; 25:344–362.
27. Taggart P, Sutton PMI, Treasure T, et al. Monophasic action potentials at discontinuation of cardiopulmonary bypass: evidence for contraction-excitation feedback in man. Circulation 1988; 77:1266–1275.
28. Levine JH, Guarnieri T, Kadish AH, White RI, Calkins H, Kan JS. Changes in myocardial repolarization in patients undergoing balloon valvuloplasty for congenital pulmonary stenosis: evidence for contraction-excitation feedback in humans. Circulation 1988; 77:70–77.
29. Reiter MJ, Synhorst DP, Mann DE. Electrophysiological effects of acute ventricular dilatation in the isolated rabbit heart. Circulation Res 1988; 62:554–562.
30. Lab MJ, Allen D, Orchard C. The effects of shortening on myoplasmic calcium concentration and on the action potential in mammalian ventricular muscle. Circulation Res 1984; 55:825–829.

31. Mullins LJ. The generation of electric currents in cardiac fibres by Na/Ca exchange. Am J Physiol 1979; 263:C103–C110.
32. Colquhoun D, Neher E, Reuter H, Stevens H. Inward current channels activated by intracellular Ca^{2+} in cultured cardiac cells. Nature 1981; 294:752–754.
33. Cohn JN, Levine TB, Olivari MT, Garberg V, Lura D, Francis GS, Simon AB, Rector T. Plasma norepinephrine as a guide to prognosis in patients with chronic congestive heart failure. N Engl J Med 1984; 311:819–823.
34. Fleg JL, Gottlieb SH, Lakatta EG. Is digoxin really important in the treatment of compensated heart failure? A placebo-controlled crossover study in patients in normal sinus rhythm. Am J Med 1982; 73:244–250.
35. Guyatt GH, Sullivan MJJ, Fallen EL, Tihal H, Rideout E, Halcrow S, Nogradi S, Townsend M, Taylor DW. A controlled trial of digoxin in congestive heart failure. Am J Cardiol 1988; 61:371–375.
36. Arnold SB, Byrd RC, Meister W, Melmon K, Cheitlin MD, Brestow JD, Parmley WW, Chatterjee K. Long-term digitalis therapy improves left ventricular function in heart failure. New Engl J Med 1980; 303:1443–1448.
37. Pugh SE, White NJ, Aronson JK, Grahame-Smith DG, Bloomfield JG. Clinical, haemodynamic, and pharmocological effects of withdrawal and reintroduction of digoxin in patients with heart failure in sinus rhythm after long term treatment. Br Heart J 1989; 61:529–539.
38. Madsen EB, Gilpin E, Henning H, Ahnve S, LeWinter M, Mazur J, Shabetai R, Collins D, Ross JJN. Prognostic importance of digitalis after acute myocardial infarction. J Am Coll Cardiol 1984; 3:681–689.
39. Bigger JT, Fleiss JL, Rolnitzky LM, Merab JP, Ferrick KJ. Effect of digitalis treatment on survival after myocardial infarction. Am J Cardiol 1985; 55:623–630.
40. Ryan TJ, Bailey KR, McCabe CH, Luk S, Fisher LD, Mock MB, Killip T. The effects of digitalis on survival in high risk patients with coronary artery disease. The Coronary Artery Surgery Study (CASS). Circulation 1983; 67:735–742.
41. Bristow MR, Ginsberg R, Minobe W, Cubiccioti RS, Sageman WS, Lurie K, Billingham ME, Harrison DC, Stinson EB. Decreased catecholamine sensitivity and beta-adrenergic-receptor density in failing human hearts. N Engl J Med 1982; 307:205–211.
42. Baim DS, McDowell AV, Cherniles J, Monrad ES, Parker JA, Edelson J, Braunwald E, Grossman W. Evaluation of a new bipyridine inotropic agent—milrinone—in patients with severe congestive heart failure. N Engl J Med 1983; 309:748–756.
43. DiBianco R, Shabetai R, Kostuk W, Moran J, Schlant R, Wright R. A comparison of oral milrinone, digoxin, and their combination in the treatment of patients with chronic heart failure. N Engl J Med 1989; 320:677–683.

44. Gradman AH, Cunningham M, Harbison MA, Berger HJ, Zaret BL. Effects of oral digoxin on ventricular ectopy and its relation to left ventricular function. Am J Cardiol 1983; 51:765–769.
45. Bussman WD, Neuman K, Kaltenbach M. Effect of intravenous nitroglycerine on ventricular ectopic beats in acute myocardial infarction. Am Heart J 1984; 107:940–944.
46. Gnecchi M, DeMarzio P, Morelli S, Aguglia F. Suppression of complex ventricular arrhythmias by isosorbide dinitrate in a case of congestive heart failure. Cardiologia 1985; 30:401–404.
47. McKenna WJ, Hayward GA. The role of ACE inhibitors in the treatment of arrhythmias. J Clin Cardiol 1990; 13(suppl VII):49–52.
48. Webster MWI, Fitzpatrick MA, Nicholls MG, Ikram H, Wells JE. Effect of enalapril on ventricular arrhythmias in congestive heart failure. Am J Cardiol 1985; 56:566–569.
49. The Cardiac Arrhythmia Suppression Trial (CAST) Investigators. Preliminary report: effect of encainide and flecainide on mortality in a randomized trial of arrhythmia suppression after myocardial infarction. N Engl J Med 1989; 321:406–412.
50. Bourke JP, Cowan JC, Tansuphaswadikul S, Campbell RWF. Antiarrhythmic drug effects on left ventricular performance. Eur Heart J 1987; 8:105–111.
51. Hoffmeister HM, Hepp A, Seipel L. Negative inotropic effect of class-1 antarrhythmic drugs: comparison of flecainide with disopyramide and quinidine. Eur Heart J 1987; 8:1126–1132.
52. Gottlieb SS, Kukin ML, Medina N, Yushak M, Packer M. Comparative hemodynamic effects of procanamide, tocainide, and encainide in severe chronic heart failure. Circulation 1990; 81:860–864.
53. Brodsky MA, Allen BJ, Abate D, Henry WL. Propafenone therapy for ventricular tachycardia in the setting of congestive heart failure. Am Heart J 1985; 110:794–799.
54. Lal R, Chapman PD, Naccarrelli GV, Troup PJ, Rinkenberger RL, Dougherty AH, Ruffy R. Short and long-term experience with flecainide acetate in the management of refractory life-threatening ventricular arrhythmias. J Am Coll Cardiol 1985; 6:772–779.
55. Porterfield JG, Porterfield LM. Therapeutic efficacy and safety of oral propafenone for atrial fibrillation. Am J Cardiol 1989; 63:114–116.
56. Borgeat A, Goy JJ, Maendly R, Kaufmann, U, Grbic M, Sigwart U. Flecainide versus quinidine for conversion of atrial fibrillation to sinus rhythm. Am J Cardiol 1986; 58:496–498.
57. Campbell RWF. Mexiletine. N Engl J Med 1987; 316:29–34.
58. Podrid PJ, Schoeneberger A, Lown B. Congestive heart failure caused by oral disopyramide. N Engl J Med 1980; 302:614–617.
59. Swedberg K, Hjalmarson A, Waagstein F, Wallentin I. Beneficial effects of long-term beta-blockade in congestive cardiomyopathy. Br Heart J 1980; 44:117–133.

60. Waagstein F, Hjalmarson A, Varnauskas E, Wallentin I. Effect of chronic beta-adrenergic receptor blockade in congestive cardiomyopathy. Br Heart J 1975; 37:1022–1036.
61. Gilbert EM, Anderson JL, Deitchman D, Yanowitz FG, O'Connell JB, Renlund DG, Bartholomew M, Mealey P, Bristow MR. Long-term beta-blocker vasodilator therapy improves cardiac function in idiopathic dilated cardiomyopathy; a double-blind randomized study of bucindolol versus placebo. Am J Med 1990; 88:223–229.
62. Schwartz PJ. The idiopathic long QT syndrome. The need for a prospective registry. Eur Heart J 1983; 4:529–531.
63. Singh S, Cohen A, Chen Y, Wish M, Thoben-O'Grady L, Peralba J, Gottdiener J, Fletcher R. Sotalol for refractory sustained ventricular tachycardia and nonfatal cardiac arrest. Am J Cardiol 1988; 62:399–402.
64. Campbell RWF. The management of heart failure and the scope for new therapies: what role for xamoterol. Br J Clin Pharmacol 1989; 28:59S–64S.
65. The German and Austrian Xamoterol Study Group. Double-blind placebo-controlled comparison of digoxin and xamoterol in chronic heart failure. Lancet 1988; i:489–493.
66. Cote P, Bourassa MG, Delaye J, Janin A, Froment R, David P. Effects of amiodarone on cardiac and coronary hemodynamics and myocardial metabolism in patients with coronary artery disease. Circulation 1979; 59:1165–1172.
67. Cleland JGF, Dargie HJ, Findlay IN, Wilson JT. Clinical, haemodynamic, and antiarrhythmic effects of long term treatment with amiodarone of patients in heart failure. Br Heart J 1987; 57:436–445.
68. Adams PC, Gibson GJ, Morley AR, Wright AJ, Corris PA, Reid DS, Campbell RWF. Amiodarone pulmonary toxicity: clinical and subclinical features. Quarterly J Med 1986; 59:449–471.
69. Dunselman PHJM, Edgar B, Scaf AHJ, Kuntze CEE, Wesseling H. Pharmacology of felodipine after intravenous and chronic oral administration in patients with congestive heart failure. Br J Clin Pharmacol 1989; 28:45–52.
70. Boston Area Anticoagulation Trial for Atrial Fibrillation Investigators. Effect of low-dose warfarin on the risk of stroke in patients with nonrheumatic atrial fibrillation. N Engl J Med 1990; 323:1505–1511.
71. Preliminary report of the stroke prevention in atrial fibrillation study. N Engl J Med 1990; 322:863–868.
72. Waldo AL, Maclean WAH, Karp RB, Kouchoukos NT, James TN. Entrainment and interruption of atrial flutter with atrial pacing: studies in man following open heart surgery. Circulation 1978; 56:737–745.
73. Robertson CE, Miller HC. Extreme tachycardia complicating the use of disopyramide in atrial flutter. Br Heart J 1980; 44:602–603.
74. Kostis JB, Byington R, Friedman LM, Goldstein S, Furberg C. Prognostic significance of ventricular ectopic activity in survivors of acute myocardial infarction. J Am Coll Cardiol 1987; 10:231–242.

75. Chizner MA, Pearle DL, de Leon AC. The natural history of aortic stenosis in adults. Am Heart J 1980; 99:419–424.
76. Cleland JGF, Dargie HJ, Ford I. Mortality in heart failure: clinical variables of prognostic value. Br Heart J 1987; 58:572–582.
77. Campbell RWF. Assessment of the risk-benefit ratio for antiarrhythmic drug use. Drugs 1988; 36:616–632.
78. Chamberlain DA, Jewitt DE, Julian DG, Campbell RWF, Boyle DMcC, Shanks RG. Oral mexiletine in high-risk patients after myocardial infarction. Lancet 1980; ii:1324–1327.
79. Impact Research Group. International mexiletine and placebo antiarrhythmic coronary trial: I. Report on arrhythmia and other findings. J Am Coll Cardiol 1984; 4:1148–1163.
80. Ryden L, Arnman K, Conradson T-B, Hofvendahl S, Mortensen O, Smedgard P. Prophylaxis of ventricular tachyarrhythmias with intravenous and oral tocainide in patients with and recovering from acute myocardial infarction. Am Heart J 1980; 100:1006–1012.
81. Bastian BC, Macfarlane PW, McLauchlan JH, Ballantyne D, Clark R, Hillis WS, Rae AP, Hutton I. A prospective randomized trial of tocainide in patients following myocardial infarction. Am Heart J 1980; 100:1017–1022.
82. Peter T, Ross D, Duffield A, Luxton M, Harper R, Hunt D, Sloman G. Effect on survival after myocardial infarction of long-term treatment with phenytoin. Br Heart J 1978; 40:1356–1360.
83. Collaborative Group. Phenytoin after recovery from myocardial infarction. Controlled trial in 568 patients. Lancet 1971; ii:1055–1057.
84. Chakko S, Gheorghiade M. Ventricular arrhythmias in severe heart failure: incidence, significance and effectiveness of therapy. Am Heart J 1985; 109:497–504.
85. Unverferth DV, Magorien RD, Moeschberger ML, Baker PB, Fetters JK, Leier CV. Factors influencing one-year mortality of dilated cardiomyopathy. Am J Cardiol 1984; 57:147–152.
86. Parmley WW, Chatterjee K. Congestive heart failure and arrhythmia: an overview. Am J Cardiol 1986; 57(Suppl 3):34B–37B.
87. Cohen JN, Johnson G, Ziesche S, VA Cooperative Study Group: V-HeFT II. A comparison of enalapril with hydralazine-isosorbide dinitrate in the treatment of chronic congestive heart failure. N Engl J Med 1991; 325:303–310.
88. Akhtar M, Breithardt G, Camm AJ, Coumel P, Janse MJ, Lazzara R, Myerburg RJ, Schwartz PJ, Waldo AL, et al. CAST and Beyond: Implications of the cardiac arrhythmia suppression trial. Circulation 1990; 81:1123–1127.
89. Oliver MF, Julian DG, Donald KW. Problems in evaluating coronary care units. Their responsibility and their relation to the community. Am J Cardiol 1967: 20:465–474.

90. Goldberg R, Szklo M, Kennedy H, Tonascia J. Short and long-term prognosis of myocardial infarction complicated by ventricular fibrillation or cardiac arrest (abstr). Circulation 1978; 4(suppl 2):89.
91. Dougeni-Christacou V, Dougenis D, Tai YT, McComb J, Campbell RWF. Hospital mortality of ventricular tachycardia and fibrillation (abstr). Br Heart J 1989; 61:125.
92. Kertes P, Hunt D. Prophylaxis of primary ventricular fibrillation in acute myocardial infarction. The case against lignocaine. Br Heart J 1984; 52:241–247.
93. Pfeffer, et al. Results of the SAVE Trial. Effect of captopril on mortality and morbidity in patients with left ventricular dysfunction after myocardial infarction. N Engl J Med 1992; 327:669–677.
94. Yusuf et al. The SOLVD Investigators. Effect of enalapril on mortality and the development of heart failure in asymptomatic patients with reduced left ventricular ejection fractions. N Engl J Med 1992; 327:685–691.
95. Swedberg et al. The CONSENSUS II Study Group. Effects of the early administration of enalapril on mortality in patients with acute myocardial infarction. N Engl J Med 1992; 327:678–684.
96. McKenna WJ, Harris L, Perez G, Krikler DM, Oakley C, Goodwin JF. Arrhythmias in hypertropic cardiomyopathy. II Comparison of amiodarone and verapamil in treatment. Br Heart J 1981; 46:173–178.
97. Fananapazir L, Leon MB, Bonow RO, Tracy CM, Cannon RO, Epstein SE. Sudden death during empiric amiodarone therapy in symptomatic hypertrophic cardiomyopathy. Am J Cardiol 1991; 67:169–174.
98. Hjalmarson A, Herlitz J, Holmberg S. The Goteborg Metoprolol Trial: Effects on mortality and morbidity in acute myocardial infarction. Circulation 1983; 67(suppl I):26–32.
99. Burkart FF, Pfisterer M, Kiowski W, Follath F, Burckhardt D, Jordi H. Effect of antiarrhythmic therapy on mortality in survivors of myocardial infarction with asymptomatic complex ventricular arrhythmias: Basel Antiarrhythmic Study of Infarct Survival (BASIS). J Am Coll Cardiol 1990; 16:1711–1718.
100. Stewart RA, McKenna WJ, Poloniecki JD, Michelson JK, Das SK, Morady F, Schork MA, Pitt B, Nicklas JM. Prospective randomised double blind placebo controlled trial of low dose amiodarone in patients with severe heart failure and frequent ventricular extrasystoles. Br Heart J 1989; 61:459–460.
101. Kay GN, Plumb VJ, Dailey SM, Epstein AE. Current role of the automatic implantable cardioverter-defibrillator in the treatment of life-threatening ventricular arrhythmias. Am J Med 1990; 88:25N–34N.
102. Tchou PJ, Kadri N, Anderson J, Caceres JA, Jazayeri M, Akhtar M. Automatic implantable cardioverter defibrillators and survival of patients with left ventricular arrhythmias. Ann Intern Med 1988; 109:529–534.
103. Guiraudon GM, Pineda EA, Klein GJ, Sharma Ad, Yee R. Early clinical results of corridor surgery for treatment of chronic atrial fibrillation. J Am Coll Cardiol 1988; 11:111 (Abstr).

104. Cox JL, Boineau JP, Schuessler RB, Ferguson TB Jr, Cain ME, Lindsay BD, Corr PB, Kater KM, Lappas DG. Successful surgical treatment of atrial fibrillation. JAMA 1991; 266:1976–1980.
105. Sealy WC, Anderson RW, Gallagher JJ. Surgical treatment of supraventricular tachyarrhythmias. J Thorac Cardiovasc Surg 1977; 73:511–522.
106. Guiraudon M, Klein GJ, Van Hemel N, Guiraudon CM, Yee R, Vermeulen FEE. Anatomically guided surgery to the AV node. AV nodal skeletonization: experience in 46 patients with AV nodal reentrant tachycardia. Eur J Cardiothorac Surg 1990; 4:461–465.
107. Ross DL, Johnson DC, Denniss AR, Cooper MJ, Richards DA Uther JB. Curative surgery for atrioventricular junctional (AV nodal reentrant tachycardia). J Am Coll Cardiol 1985; 6:1383–1392.
108. Furniss SS, Bourke JP, Campbell RWF. Surgery for atrial arrhythmias. In: Attuel P, Coumel P, Janse MJ, eds. Atrium in Health and Disease. New York: Futura, 1989:239–248.
109. Bourke JP, Hilton CJ, McComb JM, Cowan JC, Tansuphaswadikul S, Kertes PJ, Campbell RWF. Surgery for control of recurrent life-threatening ventricular tachyarrhythmias within 2 months of myocardial infarction. J Am Coll Cardiol 1990; 16:42–48.
110. Borgreffe M, Podczek A, Ostermeyer J, Breithardt G, and and the Surgical Ablation Registry. Long-term results of electrophysiologically guided antitachycardia surgery in ventricular tachyarrhythmias: a collaborative report on 665 patients. In: Breithardt G, Borgreffe M, Zipes DP, eds. Nonpharmacological Therapy of Tachyarrhythmias. New York: New Futura, 1987:109–132.
111. Fiddler GI, Campbell RWF, Pottage A, Godman MJ. Varicella myocarditis presenting with unusual ventricular arrhythmias. Br Heart J 1977; 39:1150–1153.
112. Rosenbaum MB. Chagasic myocardiopathy. Prog Cardiovasc Dis 1964; 7:199–225.

Index

About the Editors

DAVID B. BARNETT is Professor of Clinical Pharmacology and Therapeutics and Honorary Cardiovascular Physician, University of Leicester and the Leicester Royal Infirmary, England. The author or coauthor of over 150 journal articles, book chapters, and abstracts, he is a fellow of the Royal College of Physicians and a member of the British Pharmacological Society, the British Cardiac Society, and the Association of Physicians of Great Britain and Ireland. Dr. Barnett received the M.B. degree (1967) and the M.D. degree (1979) from the University of Sheffield, England.

HUBERT POULEUR is Professor, Department of Physiology and Pharmacology and Division of Cardiology, School of Medicine, the University of Louvain, Brussels, Belgium. The author or coauthor of over 300 journal articles, book chapters, and abstracts, he is a Fellow of the Council on Circulation of the American Heart Association and of the American College of Cardiology. Dr. Pouleur received the M.D. (1973) and the Ph.D. (1980) degrees from the University of Louvain, Brussels, Belgium.

GARY S. FRANCIS is Professor of Medicine, Cardiovascular Division, the University of Minnesota Medical School, Minneapolis, and Director of Acute Cardiac Care at the University Hospital, Minneapolis, Minnesota.

The author or coauthor of nearly 300 journal articles and book chapters, Dr. Francis serves on several journal editorial boards, including *Circulation*, the *Journal of the American College of Cardiology*, the *American Journal of Cardiology*, and the *American Heart Journal*. He is a Fellow of the American College of Physicians, the Council on Circulation and the Council on Basic Science of the American Heart Association, and the American College of Cardiology. Dr. Francis received the M.D. degree (1969) from Creighton University School of Medicine.